T0263289

Precision Oncology and Cancer Surgery

Editor

JASON K. SICKLICK

SURGICAL ONCOLOGY CLINICS OF NORTH AMERICA

www.surgonc.theclinics.com

Consulting Editor
TIMOTHY M. PAWLIK

April 2024 • Volume 33 • Number 2

ELSEVIER

1600 John F. Kennedy Boulevard • Suite 1800 • Philadelphia, Pennsylvania, 19103-2899

http://www.theclinics.com

SURGICAL ONCOLOGY CLINICS OF NORTH AMERICA Volume 33, Number 2
April 2024 ISSN 1055-3207, ISBN-13: 978-0-443-13025-0

Editor: John Vassallo (j.vassallo@elsevier.com)
Developmental Editor: Malvika Shah

© **2024 Elsevier Inc. All rights are reserved, including those for text and data mining, AI training, and similar technologies.**

This periodical and the individual contributions contained in it are protected under copyright by Elsevier, and the following terms and conditions apply to their use:

Photocopying
Single photocopies of single articles may be made for personal use as allowed by national copyright laws. Permission of the Publisher and payment of a fee is required for all other photocopying, including multiple or systematic copying, copying for advertising or promotional purposes, resale, and all forms of document delivery. Special rates are available for educational institutions that wish to make photocopies for non-profit educational classroom use. For information on how to seek permission visit www.elsevier.com/permissions or call: (+44) 1865 843830 (UK)/(+1) 215 239 3804 (USA).

Derivative Works
Subscribers may reproduce tables of contents or prepare lists of articles including abstracts for internal circulation within their institutions. Permission of the Publisher is required for resale or distribution outside the institution. Permission of the Publisher is required for all other derivative works, including compilations and translations (please consult www.elsevier.com/permissions).

Electronic Storage or Usage
Permission of the Publisher is required to store or use electronically any material contained in this periodical, including any article or part of an article (please consult www.elsevier.com/permissions). Except as outlined above, no part of this publication may be reproduced, stored in a retrieval system or transmitted in any form or by any means, electronic, mechanical, photocopying, recording or otherwise, without prior written permission of the Publisher.

Notice
No responsibility is assumed by the Publisher for any injury and/or damage to persons or property as a matter of products liability, negligence or otherwise, or from any use or operation of any methods, products, instructions or ideas contained in the material herein. Because of rapid advances in the medical sciences, in particular, independent verification of diagnoses and drug dosages should be made.

Although all advertising material is expected to conform to ethical (medical) standards, inclusion in this publication does not constitute a guarantee or endorsement of the quality or value of such product or of the claims made of it by its manufacturer.

Surgical Oncology Clinics of North America (ISSN 1055-3207) is published quarterly by Elsevier Inc., 360 Park Avenue South, New York, NY 10010-1710. Months of publication are January, April, July, and October. Business and Editorial Offices: 1600 John F. Kennedy Blvd., Ste. 1800, Philadelphia, PA 19103-2899. Customer Service Office: 3251 Riverport Lane, Maryland Heights, MO 63043. Periodicals postage paid at New York, NY and additional mailing offices. Subscription prices are $345.00 per year (US individuals), $100.00 (US student/resident), $385.00 (Canadian individuals), $100.00 (Canadian student/resident), $499.00 (foreign individuals), and $205.00 (foreign student/resident). For institutional access pricing please contact Customer Service via the contact information below. Foreign air speed delivery is included in all *Clinics* subscription prices. All prices are subject to change without notice. **POSTMASTER**: Send address changes to *Surgical Oncology Clinics of North America*, Elsevier Health Science Division, Subscription Customer Service, 3251 Riverport Lane, Maryland Heights, MO 63043. **Customer Service: 1-800-654-2452 (US and Canada). 314-447-8871 (outside US and Canada). Fax: 314-447-8029. E-mail: journalscustomerservice-usa@elsevier.com (for print support); journalsonlinesupport-usa@elsevier.com (for online support)**.

Reprints. For copies of 100 or more, of articles in this publication, please contact the Commercial Reprints Department, Elsevier Inc., 360 Park Avenue South, New York, New York 10010-1710. Tel. 212-633-3874; Fax: 212-633-3820; E-mail: reprints@elsevier.com.

Surgical Oncology Clinics of North America is covered in *MEDLINE/PubMed (Index Medicus) and EMBASE/ Excerpta Medica, Current Contents/Clinical Medicine, and ISI/BIOMED.*

Contributors

CONSULTING EDITOR

TIMOTHY M. PAWLIK, MD, MPH, PhD, FACS, FRACS (Hon)
Professor and Chair, Department of Surgery, The Urban Meyer III and Shelley Meyer Chair for Cancer Research, Professor of Surgery, Oncology, and Health Services Management and Policy, Surgeon in Chief, The Ohio State University, Wexner Medical Center, Columbus, Ohio, USA

EDITOR

JASON K. SICKLICK, MD, FACS
Executive Vice Chair of Research, Professor, Division of Surgical Oncology, Department of Surgery, Adjunct Professor, Department of Pharmacology, Co-Leader, Structural and Functional Genomics Program, Moores Cancer Center, University of California, San Diego, La Jolla, California, USA

AUTHORS

ALI BENJAMIN ABBASI, MD
Resident, Department of Surgery, San Francisco Breast Care Center, University of California, San Francisco, California, USA

SUDEEP BANERJEE, MD, MAS
Colorectal Surgeon, Division of Colorectal Surgery, Department of General Surgery, Kaiser Permanente San Jose Medical Center, Kaiser Permanente Northern California, San Jose, California, USA

HANNAH BANK, MD, PhD
Resident, Department of Surgery, Massachusetts General Hospital, Boston, Massachusetts, USA

JEAN-YVES BLAY, MD, PhD
Professor, Department of Medical Oncology, Centre Leon Berard and the University of Lyon, Lyon, France

GENEVIEVE BOLAND, MD, PhD
Vice Chair of Research, Department of Surgery, Massachusetts General Hospital, Massachusetts General Hospital Cancer Center, Associate Professor, Harvard Medical School (HMS), Boston, Massachusetts, USA

PATRICK BOU-SAMRA, MD
General Surgery Resident, Division of Thoracic Surgery, The University of Pennsylvania Perelman School of Medicine, Philadelphia, Pennsylvania, USA

JULIA A. ELVIN, MD, PhD
Senior Vice President, Pathology and Diagnostic Medicine, Foundation Medicine, Inc, Cambridge, Massachusetts, USA

RAMEZ N. ESKANDER, MD
Professor, Division of Gynecologic Oncology, Department of Obstetrics, Gynecology and Reproductive Sciences, Center for Personalized Cancer Therapy, Moores Cancer Center, University of California San Diego, La Jolla, California, USA

LAURA J. ESSERMAN, MD, MBA
Professor, Department of Surgery, San Francisco Breast Care Center, University of California, San Francisco, California, USA

ADAM M. FONTEBASSO, MD, PhD
Fellow, Division of Surgical Oncology, Department of Surgery, University of Toronto, Mount Sinai Hospital, Sinai Health Systems, Princess Margaret Cancer Centre, University Health Network, Toronto, Ontario, Canada

YU FUJIWARA, MD
Fellow, Department of Medicine, Roswell Park Comprehensive Cancer Center, Buffalo, New York, USA

REBECCA A. GLADDY, MD, PhD
Associate Professor, Division of Surgical Oncology, Department of Surgery, University of Toronto, Mount Sinai Hospital, Sinai Health Systems, Princess Margaret Cancer Centre, University Health Network, Toronto, Ontario, Canada

MOHAMED A. GOUDA, MD, MSc
Clinical Fellow, Department of Investigational Cancer Therapeutics, The University of Texas MD Anderson Cancer Center, Houston, Texas, USA

SHUMEI KATO, MD
Clinical Associate Professor, Division of Hematology and Oncology, Department of Medicine, Center for Personalized Cancer Therapy, Moores Cancer Center, University of California San Diego La Jolla, California, USA

DANIEL M. KEREKES, MD, MHS
Resident, Department of General Surgery, Division of Surgical Oncology, Yale University, New Haven, Connecticut, USA

SAJID A. KHAN, MD, FACS, FSSO
Associate Professor and Chief of Hepatopancreatobiliary and Mixed Tumors, Department of Surgery, Yale University, New Haven, Connecticut, USA

EUGENE S. KIM, MD
Professor of Surgery and Pediatrics, Director, Division of Pediatric Surgery, Vice Chair, Department of Surgery, Cedars-Sinai Medical Center, Los Angeles, California, USA

JOSEPH KIM, MD, FACS, FSSO
Professor and Chief, Department of General Surgery, Division of Surgical Oncology, The University of Kentucky, Lexington, Kentucky, USA

RAZELLE KURZROCK, MD
Professor, Genomic Sciences and Precision Medicine Center, Medical College of Wisconsin, Froedtert and Medical College of Wisconsin Cancer Center and Linda T. and John A. Mellowes Center for Genomic Sciences and Precision Medicine, Milwaukee, Wisconsin; WIN Consortium, Paris, France; University of Nebraska, Lincoln, Nebraska, USA

JULIE E. LANG, MD, FACS
Associate Professor, Department of Surgery, Chief of Breast Surgery, Hillcrest Hospital, Cleveland Clinic Breast Services, Cleveland, Ohio, USA

WILLIAM G. LEE, MD
Resident, Department of Surgery, Cedars-Sinai Medical Center, Los Angeles, California, USA

SHOSHANA LEVI, MD
Resident, Department of Surgery, Massachusetts General Hospital, Boston, Massachusetts, USA

HANNAH G. McDONALD, MD
Research Fellow, Department of General Surgery, Division of Surgical Oncology, The University of Kentucky, Lexington, Kentucky, USA

FUNDA MERIC-BERNSTAM, MD
Chair, Department of Investigational Cancer Therapeutics, Division of Cancer Medicine, The University of Texas MD Anderson Cancer Center, Houston, Texas, USA

JOHN MULLINAX, MD
Surgical Oncologist, Sarcoma Department, Moffitt Cancer Center, Tampa, Florida, USA

TIMOTHY E. NEWHOOK, MD
Assistant Professor, Department of Surgical Oncology, Division of Surgery, The University of Texas MD Anderson Cancer Center, Houston, Texas, USA

DAISUKE NISHIZAKI, MD
Postdoctoral Researcher, Division of Hematology and Oncology, Department of Medicine, Center for Personalized Cancer Therapy, Moores Cancer Center, University of California San Diego, La Jolla, California, USA

SANDIP PRAVIN PATEL, MD
Professor, Division of Hematology/Oncology, Department of Medicine, University of California, San Diego, La Jolla, California, USA

WILLIAM B. PEARSE, MD
Assistant Professor of Medicine, Division of Hematology/Oncology, University of California, San Diego Moores Cancer Center, La Jolla, California, USA

ERIN G. REID, MD, MS
Professor of Medicine (Hematology/Oncology), Division of Hematology/Oncology, Moores Cancer Center, University of California, San Diego, La Jolla, California, USA

CHRISTINA L. ROLAND, MD, MS
Associate Professor, Department of Surgical Oncology, The University of Texas MD Anderson Cancer Center, Houston, Texas, USA

JEFFREY D. RYTLEWSKI, MD
Fellow, Department of Internal Medicine University of Colorado School of Medicine, Aurora, Colorado, USA

SHIRUYEH SCHOKRPUR, MD, PhD
Assistant Physician, Division of Hematology/Oncology, Department of Medicine, University of California, San Diego, La Jolla, California, USA

SUNIL SINGHAL, MD
Professor, Division of Thoracic Surgery, The University of Pennsylvania Perelman School of Medicine, Philadelphia, Pennsylvania, USA

VIVEK SUBBIAH, MD
Chief, Early-Phase Drug Development, Sarah Cannon Research Institute, Nashville, Tennessee, USA

SUSAN TSAI, MD, MHS
Chief, Division of Surgical Oncology, Department of Surgery, Ohio State University Comprehensive Cancer Center, Columbus, Ohio, USA

MICHAEL G. WHITE, MD, MSc
Assistant Professor, Department of Colon and Rectal Surgery, The University of Texas MD Anderson Cancer Center, Houston, Texas, USA

BREELYN A. WILKY, MD
Associate Professor, Department of Medicine-Medical Oncology University of Colorado School of Medicine, Aurora, Colorado, USA

VINCENT WU, MD
General Surgery Specialist, Department of Surgery, Cleveland Clinic Breast Services, Cleveland, Ohio, USA

Contents

With multiple molecular targeted therapies available for patients with cancer that correspond to a specific genetic alteration, the selection of the best treatment is essential to ensure therapeutic efficacy. Molecular tumor boards (MTBs) play a key role in this process to deliver personalized medicine to patients with cancer in a multidisciplinary manner. Historically, personalized medicine has been offered to patients with advanced cancer, but the incorporation of molecular targeted therapies and immunotherapy into the perioperative setting requires clinicians to understand the role of the MTB. Evidence is accumulating to support feasibility and survival benefit in patients treated with matched therapy.

Over the past three decades, the landscape of clinically available molecular tests has evolved due to advancements in basic science cancer research and the subsequent utilization of this knowledge to develop DNA, RNA, and protein-based molecular assays for oncology that can be employed for routine clinical use in diagnostics laboratories. Molecular testing of tumors is revealing gaps in previous histopathologic classification systems and opportunities for new, personalized treatment paradigms. Awareness of validated molecular assay options and their general advantages and limitations is crucial for oncology care providers to ensure the optimal test(s) are selected for each patient's circumstances.

Cost-effectiveness analysis of precision oncology can help guide value-driven care. Next-generation sequencing is increasingly cost-efficient over single gene testing because diagnostic algorithms require multiple individual gene tests to determine biomarker status. Matched targeted therapy is often not cost-effective due to the high cost associated with drug treatment. However, genomic profiling can promote cost-effective care by identifying patients who are unlikely to benefit from therapy. Additional applications of genomic profiling such as universal testing for hereditary

important to recognize that breast cancer is a heterogeneous disease that requires treatment based on molecular characteristics. Early endpoints such as pathologic complete response correlate with event-free survival, allowing the opportunity to consider de-escalation of certain cancer treatments to avoid overtreatment. This article discusses clinical trials of tailoring treatment (eg, I-SPY2) and screening (eg, WISDOM) to individual patients based on their unique risk features.

mutations with therapeutic potential and (2) the mechanistic understanding of a tumor-specific immune response. With breakthrough findings in such a relatively short period of time, the treatment of patients with metastatic melanoma has become intensely personalized.

Adam M. Fontebasso, Jeffrey D. Rytlewski, Jean-Yves Blay, Rebecca A. Gladdy, and Breelyn A. Wilky

Soft tissue sarcomas (STSs), including gastrointestinal stromal tumors (GISTs), are mesenchymal neoplasms with heterogeneous clinical behavior and represent broad categories comprising multiple distinct biologic entities. Multidisciplinary management of these rare tumors is critical. To date, multiple studies have outlined the importance of biological characterization of mesenchymal tumors and have identified key molecular alterations which drive tumor biology. GIST has represented a flagship for targeted therapy in solid tumors with the advent of imatinib which has revolutionized the way we treat this malignancy. Herein, the authors discuss the importance of biological and molecular diagnostics in managing STS and GIST patients.

William G. Lee and Eugene S. Kim

Pediatric precision oncology has provided a greater understanding of the wide range of molecular alterations in difficult-to-treat or rare tumors with the aims of increasing survival as well as decreasing toxicity and morbidity from current cytotoxic therapies. In this article, the authors discuss the current state of pediatric precision oncology which has increased access to novel targeted therapies while also providing a framework for clinical implementation in this unique population. The authors evaluate the targetable mutations currently under investigation—with a focus on pediatric solid tumors—and discuss the key surgical implications associated with novel targeted therapies.

William B. Pearse and Erin G. Reid

Although there are more than 100 clinically distinct lymphoid neoplasms with varied prognoses and treatment approaches, they generally share high sensitivity to glucocorticoids, cytotoxic chemotherapy, and radiation. The disease control rates for lymphoid malignancies are higher than many solid tumors, and many are curable even when presenting with extensive involvement. Novel targeted therapies have improved disease control and cure rates for nearly all subtypes of lymphoid neoplasms. Surgical oncologists will primarily be involved in obtaining biopsies of sufficient quality to allow accurate diagnosis. However, there are scenarios in which surgical intervention may be necessary to address an oncologic emergency.

SURGICAL ONCOLOGY CLINICS OF NORTH AMERICA

SERIES OF RELATED INTEREST

Advances in Surgery
https://www.advancessurgery.com
Surgical Clinics of North America
https://www.surgical.theclinics.com
Thoracic Surgery Clinics
https://www.thoracic.theclinics.com

THE CLINICS ARE AVAILABLE ONLINE!
Access your subscription at:
www.theclinics.com

Foreword

Precision Oncology and Cancer Surgery

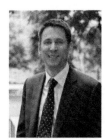

Timothy M. Pawlik, MD, MPH, PhD, FACS, FRACS (Hon)
Consulting Editor

This issue of the *Surgical Oncology Clinics of North America* focuses on Precision Oncology and Cancer Surgery.

Traditionally, treatment approaches for patients with a malignant diagnosis have been designed for the "average patient" using a one-size-fits-all approach based largely on histologic cancer subtype. This approach may be successful for some patients, but often fails in others.

Precision medicine, and the corollary "precision oncology," is an exciting and innovative approach that seeks to tailor treatment considering the differences in individual patient's genes and environments. To that end, precision oncology seeks to bring together innovations in fields such as genomics, metabolomics, biomedical data sciences, and environmental sciences. Recognizing the importance of the field, in a 2015 State of the Union address, President Obama announced a Precision Medicine Initiative to revolutionize how we improve health and research and treat disease. The initiative defined precision medicine as "an emerging approach for disease treatment and prevention that takes into account individual variability in genes, environment, and lifestyle for each person." Since that time, advances in precision medicine have led to important new discoveries and FDA-approved treatments for patients with cancer allowing for a more tailored oncologic therapeutic approach. Currently, it is routine that patients with a variety of cancers undergo molecular testing as part of their care, enabling physicians to select treatments that improve chances of survival and possibly reducing exposure to adverse effects. Given the burgeoning role of precision medicine in the field of cancer, the current issue of *Surgical Oncology Clinics of North America* is an important contribution to our readership. We are especially fortunate to have Jason K. Sicklick as our Guest Editor. Dr Sicklick is an internationally recognized surgical oncologist who specializes in treating gastrointestinal stromal tumors (GIST), abdominal/retroperitoneal

Surg Oncol Clin N Am 33 (2024) xiii–xiv
https://doi.org/10.1016/j.soc.2023.12.019
1055-3207/24/© 2023 Published by Elsevier Inc.
surgonc.theclinics.com

sarcomas, and liver tumors (primary and metastatic). A professor of surgery and pharmacology at UC San Diego School of Medicine, Dr Sicklick conducts clinical research to improve our understanding of complex cancers such as GIST and retroperitoneal sarcomas, as well as enhance precision medicine approaches for treating metastatic cancers. His laboratory focuses on the diversity in the genomic landscape of advanced and metastatic tumors with a focus on combination therapies based on tumor genomic signatures. He is co-leader of the Sarcoma Disease Team at UC San Diego Health and a member of the National Comprehensive Cancer Network Soft-Tissue Sarcoma Committee and GIST Subcommittee, which develops best practices for treating rare and often challenging-to-treat cancers.

The current issue covers multiple important topics that highlight the evolution of precision oncology, personalize medicine, and molecular tumor boards. The issue provides a variety of important perspectives on the landscape of molecular testing, as well as the role of immune-oncology and targeted therapies. In addition to providing insights into foundational precision medicine topics, the authors provide an in-depth look into the role of precision oncology related to breast, lung, gastrointestinal, hepatopancreaticobiliary, soft tissue, and pediatric malignant diseases. In doing this, the various articles provide a comprehensive overview of how precision medicine applies to the care of patients across a wide range of diseases.

I want to thank Dr Sicklick for recruiting a fantastic group of coauthors to contribute to this issue of *Surgical Oncology Clinics of North America*. The authors have done an outstanding job in providing our readership with a key resource to inform their practices on how precision medicine impacts the care of patients with cancer. This issue of *Surgical Oncology Clinics of North America* should be extremely helpful in informing how precision oncology can be utilized to care for our patients to improve their outcomes. Again, thank you to Dr Sicklick, as well as all the contributing authors.

Timothy M. Pawlik, MD, MPH, PhD, FACS, FRACS (Hon)
Professor and Chair, Department of Surgery
The Urban Meyer III and Shelley Meyer Chair for Cancer Research
The Ohio State University
Wexner Medical Center
395 West 12th Avenue, Suite 670
Columbus, OH 43210, USA

E-mail address:
tim.pawlik@osumc.edu

Preface

Precision Oncology and Cancer Surgery

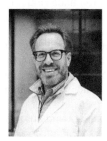

Jason K. Sicklick, MD, FACS
Editor

Historically, research has advanced treatment and understanding of cancer biology by reducing complexity and standardizing treatment for groups of diverse individuals. But we are undergoing a fundamental shift in this philosophy and also in the practice of cancer research and clinical care. We are now leveraging the analysis of high-dimensional, linked clinical and molecular data in novel and powerful ways to obtain a more precise and deeper understanding of cancer biology at the individual patient level. The treatment paradigm is shifting from a drug-centric, one-size-fits-all treatment approach depending upon tumor histology to more *precise*, molecularly driven, and patient-centric (ie, *personalized, or individualized*) approaches guided by deeper analysis of linked molecular and clinical data.

Taking a step back, these precision and personalization concepts are not new to surgical oncologists. Early in our training, we are taught to treat the individual patient, recognizing that everyone's anatomy, tumor biology, and the approach to tumor resection is unique to them. We go into operations with general game plans of how we plan to resect a tumor, knowing that what we see on cross-sectional imaging may be somewhat different from what we discover at the time of surgery. We are trained to be flexible and comfortable with completely changing our approach in real time. We personalize, individualize, and customize each operation; we thus cannot religiously adhere to a prescripted recipe. This goal-oriented but open-minded approach provides us with a unique perspective to embrace changing paradigms to care for patients with cancer, while providing us with new opportunities to expand surgical indications, convert unresectable to resectable tumors, or utilize neoadjuvant and adjuvant therapy to increase cure rates.

With clinical testing provided by both commercial third-party vendors and academic institutional laboratory services, next-generation sequencing–based genomic tests for

Surg Oncol Clin N Am 33 (2024) xv–xvi
https://doi.org/10.1016/j.soc.2023.12.005
1055-3207/24/© 2023 Published by Elsevier Inc.
surgonc.theclinics.com

individual patients continues to expand in oncology. To date, the adoption and expansion of this testing have been slow because many clinicians, including surgeons, are unfamiliar with the rapidly evolving technologies, how to apply these test results to the care of their patients, concerns about toxicities, and the breakneck pace at which new cancer drugs are being developed. Simultaneously, often disconnected from the clinic, exponential development of new platforms for acquiring types of high-density clinical, population, and tumor-specific data (ie, DNA, RNA, proteins, metabolites, epigenetic, and much more), and computational approaches for analyzing them occurs. On the research side, we are even studying these molecular data at the single-cell level to better understand spatial intertumoral (ie, between tumors) and intratumoral (ie, within the same tumor) heterogeneity, as well as temporal evolution with treatment. This revolution in technology and data science has the potential to drive better clinical care through translational investigations that employ large data sets (including population, clinical, genetic, transcriptomic, epigenetic, metabolomic, proteomic, radiomic, and other -omics platforms).

But it may be possible to accelerate this transition in surgical patients and surgically treated cancers if scientists and surgical oncologists spoke the same language, and also, if there were improved understanding and consensus views on how best to clinically translate these rapidly evolving discoveries. Now more than ever, we need to focus on collaboration between surgical, medical, and radiation oncologists, as well as basic, translational, and computational cancer researchers to train the next generation of cancer surgeons as "surgical cancer biologists." This new approach should fully leverage the immense potential of new drug targets and therapies to better focus on the detection, stratification, and treatment of our patients with cancer with the broader goals of improving outcomes in the localized, locally advanced, and metastatic disease settings.

We confront an inflection point in surgical oncology: more effective therapies may play an important role in expanding future surgical indications, while giving rise to previously unappreciated side effects. It is for this reason that this issue was carefully designed to cover the multifaceted aspects of precision oncology care, with a particularly sharp focus on surgical diseases and those cancers where surgeons are frequently called upon to collaborate in the care of these patients. Finally, it should be recognized that a majority of these articles are written by surgical oncologists, because we as a community can and should shape the future of precision oncology that is personalized to our patients.

DISCLOSURE

J.K. Sicklick receives consultant fees from Deciphera, Aadi, and Grand Rounds; serves as a consultant for CureMatch; received speaker's fees from Deciphera, La-Hoffman Roche, Foundation Medicine, Merck, QED, and Daiichi Sankyo; and owns stock in Personalis and CureMatch.

Jason K. Sicklick, MD, FACS
Moores Cancer Center
University of California San Diego School of Medicine
3855 Health Sciences Drive Box# 0987
La Jolla, CA 92093, USA

E-mail address:
jsicklick@health.ucsd.edu

Evolution of Precision Oncology, Personalized Medicine, and Molecular Tumor Boards

Yu Fujiwara, MD[a],*, Shumei Kato, MD[b,c], Razelle Kurzrock, MD[d,e,f]

KEYWORDS

- Histology-agnostic • Personalized medicine • Personalized oncology
- Precision medicine • Tumor-agnostic

KEY POINTS

- Clinicians caring for patients with cancer need to understand the process of precision medicine.
- Precision oncology allows for treatment selection based on molecular profiles of each patient's cancer.
- Precision medicine has been incorporated into definitive and palliative treatments for patients with advanced malignancies regardless of histologic subtype.
- Molecular tumor boards (MTBs) play an important role in the interpretation of genomic profiling tests and recommendations of molecularly matched treatment regimens.
- Many subspecialists take a vital role in the MTB in order to discuss the best personalized treatment for each patient with cancer.

INTRODUCTION

Precision oncology is the concept of providing treatment based on individual patient's tumor mutation profiles. In recent years, new therapeutic options have been approved for specific cancer patient populations based on corresponding gene alterations and

[a] Department of Medicine, Roswell Park Comprehensive Cancer Center, Elm and Carlton Streets, Buffalo, NY 14263, USA; [b] Center for Personalized Cancer Therapy, University of California San Diego Moores Cancer Center, 3855 Health Sciences Drive, La Jolla, CA 92093, USA; [c] Division of Hematology and Oncology, Department of Medicine, University of California San Diego Moores Cancer Center, La Jolla, CA, USA; [d] Genomic Sciences and Precision Medicine Center, Medical College of Wisconsin, Froedtert and Medical College of Wisconsin Cancer Center and Linda T. and John A. Mellowes Center for Genomic Sciences and Precision Medicine, 9200 West Wisconsin Avenue, Milwaukee, WI 53226, USA; [e] WIN Consortium, Paris, France; [f] University of Nebraska, Lincoln, NE, USA
* Corresponding author.
E-mail address: Yu.Fujiwara@RoswellPark.org

Surg Oncol Clin N Am 33 (2024) 197–216
https://doi.org/10.1016/j.soc.2023.12.004
1055-3207/24/© 2023 Elsevier Inc. All rights reserved.

biomarkers.[1] Although biomarker-driven approaches have been developed mainly for patients with advanced cancer, the rapid development of these therapeutics also allows the incorporation of personalized medicine into the adjuvant/neoadjuvant settings along with curative intent surgery and/or radiotherapy. This integration suggests the importance of early molecular profiling testing to determine the best therapy through multidisciplinary discussions for patients with early and advanced-stage cancers.[2]

Therapeutic options for patients with advanced cancer were historically limited to cytotoxic chemotherapy until the discovery of targetable mutations, which revolutionized the cancer treatment landscape. Early examples of these molecular targeted therapies included imatinib for *BCR-ABL* chronic myeloid leukemia and erlotinib for epidermal growth factor receptor (*EGFR*)-mutant lung adenocarcinoma.[3-5] Since the development of these agents, the advent of next-generation sequencing (NGS) has allowed clinicians to rapidly identify targetable molecular alterations with novel drugs that may provide better clinical outcomes than classic cytotoxic chemotherapy.[6,7] These alterations can be observed across cancer types, and molecular targeted therapies may have clinical activity across tumor types.[8,9] Furthermore, recent developments in immunotherapy, including immune checkpoint inhibitors (ICIs), have dramatically changed the paradigm of cancer treatment by providing durable responses in some cancer patients.[10] Several factors such as high programmed death-ligand 1 (PD-L1) expression and high tumor mutational burden (TMB) have been associated with prolonged survival and could potentially be used as biomarkers to select patients before initiating ICIs.[11,12] It is through increased understanding of tumor biology that treatment is evolving.

This article summarizes the development of precision oncology, the role of MTBs, and future directions of personalized medicine for patients with cancer including those who are candidates for surgical intervention.

DISCUSSION
History

The evolution of precision oncology dates back to the late 1990s, when imatinib was found to be effective in chronic myeloid leukemia (CML) harboring *BCR-ABL* rearrangement, leading to approval by the US Food and Drug Administration (FDA) in 2001.[3] Along with the development of techniques such as fluorescence in situ hybridization (FISH) and polymerase chain reaction (PCR), which allowed rapid detection of targetable alterations, several molecular targeted therapies were subsequently developed. One of the first examples of precision medicine for solid tumors was use of a tyrosine kinase inhibitor (TKI), such as erlotinib and gefitinib, for patients with non-small cell lung carcinoma (NSCLC) harboring an *EGFR* mutation. Gefitinib was initially shown to be effective for NSCLC patients, but subgroup analysis suggested that its efficacy was driven by *EGFR*-mutant population, which was subsequently confirmed in a clinical trial limited to patients with an *EGFR* mutation.[5,13,14] Erlotinib was also developed and initially approved specifically for patients with EGFR-mutant NSCLC in 2013.[15] This small molecule inhibitor became the focus of attention, as it inhibits a specific alteration, rendering more efficacy with potentially less toxicity than traditional cytotoxic chemotherapy. Thus, its application was incorporated into the standard of care in patients with malignancy.[6,7]

The initial development of molecular-targeted agents was achieved by dividing a specific cancer type into subtypes according to genomic mutation patterns such as EGFR, anaplastic lymphoma kinase (ALK), and c-ros oncogene 1 (ROS1) inhibitors for NSCLC.[16,17] However, as different types of cancer can share the same genomic alteration, the tumor-agnostic approach has been explored to broaden the application of targeted therapies. In 2019, entrectinib, an neurotrophic tyrosine receptor kinase (NTRK) inhibitor, was approved by the FDA for solid tumors with *NTRK* fusion regardless of cancer type after demonstrating its efficacy (durable overall response rate of 57%).[18] Similarly, pembrolizumab, a programmed cell death protein 1 (PD-1) inhibitor, was approved by the FDA in patients with DNA mismatch repair-deficiency (dMMR) or microsatellite instability-high (MSI-H) tumors in 2017, and in patients high TMB tumors in 2020, respectively.[19,20] These strategies have highlighted the importance of performing NGS to expand treatment options without losing the chance of a potentially long-lasting therapeutic opportunity. As personalized medicine evolves, the treatment landscape becomes more complicated, because each cancer possesses a different genetic profile. Currently, multiple agents are approved for specific alterations in 1 tumor type and for the same alteration across cancer types. For example, there are 5 FDA-approved ALK inhibitors for NSCLC, 3 tumor-agnostic indications for the use of pembrolizumab in solid tumors, and 2 NTRK inhibitors for solid tumors harboring *NTRK* fusions.[18–22] Therefore, discussions in a multidisciplinary fashion at an MTB play a more important role in determining the best treatment for each patient by considering their performance status and comorbidities, the adverse effect profile of the matched agents, and access to clinical trials.[23]

Precision Oncology in Clinic

Historically, precision oncology has been delivered primarily to patients with advanced malignancies after progression on multiple lines of chemotherapy. To explore further therapeutic opportunities such as molecular targeted therapy that are not approved for a specific cancer type and enrollment in clinical trials, genomic profile tests can be performed through NGS. Clinicians need to explain the concept of testing to obtain a genomic profile from tumor tissue or liquid samples, including the benefits and risks of testing to the patients (**Table 1**). In particular, physicians need to explain the potential risk of detecting a germline mutation, as this would affect the medical care for a patient's relatives, such as an increased risk of developing cancer in siblings and children.[23] In this case, consultation for genetic counseling may be necessary. Additionally, the detection rate of effective treatments for a cancer can be relatively low (approximately 5% to 20%) at present, and patients need to understand what the next process looks like if no therapeutic options are available after performing the genomic profiling test.[2] Insufficient amount of tissues and remote tissue samples also make it difficult to perform NGS, and in this case, additional biopsy might be needed. Liquid biopsy is another option that may provide up-to-date genomic information in a noninvasive way.[24,25]

Molecular Tumor Board

Once genomic profiling is obtained from tissues and/or liquid samples, the result and potential treatment options need to be discussed in a multidisciplinary manner to provide the best and most personalized care with the potential for maximum treatment benefit, taking into account factors such as comorbidities and access to care. The MTB plays an integral role in clinical decision making by facilitating discussions with expertise in medical oncology, surgical oncology, bioinformatics, clinical genomics, genetic counseling, and radiation oncology (**Fig. 1**).[23] Genomic data can provide potential treatment options for targetable alterations and biomarkers to predict the efficacy of available therapies. Through multidisciplinary discussions by obtaining perspectives from each specialist, the MTB may suggest consideration of experimental drugs,

Table 1
Risk and benefit upon performing genetic profiling testing for precision medicine

	Benefits	Risks
Therapeutic options	Finding a treatment option available on the market Example: *EGFR* mutation for EGFR TKI	Treatment corresponding to a detected alteration is not available on the market Example: *KRAS G12 V* mutation (only KRAS G12 C inhibitors are available).
Predictive marker	Detecting a predictive biomarker for a specific therapy Example: high TMB for immune checkpoint inhibitors	Can potentially find a factor that negatively predicts the therapeutic efficacy Example: low tumor mutational burden that could potentially decrease the efficacy of immune checkpoint inhibitors
Clinical trials	Finding actionable alterations for which many clinical trials are available	Mutations whose molecular structures make them undruggable. Limited options of clinical trials.
Genetic information	Detection of somatic mutations only Counseling of relatives can be omitted in this case	Possibility of detecting germline mutations that predispose to the risk of developing cancer in relatives Genetic counseling may be necessary

Abbreviations: EGFR, epidermal growth factor receptor; KRAS, Kirsten rat sarcoma viral oncogene homolog; TKI, tyrosine kinase inhibitor.

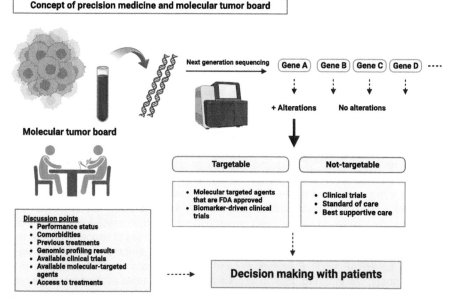

Fig. 1. Concept of precision medicine and role of molecular tumor board. The flowchart to perform precision medicine from specimen sampling, analysis, discussion at molecular tumor board, to treatment suggestions. TMB, Tumor mutational burden. (Created with BioRender. com.)

enrollment in clinical trials, and use of approved agents, based on the available evidence. On top of the genomic profile, information on clinical status such as performance status, active medical issues, and access to health care such as whether patients need to be referred to another institution for clinical trials will be discussed.

The role of MTBs is critical to improve survival outcomes for patients with advanced cancers. Patients with genomic alterations for which targeted therapies are available are more likely to benefit from matched treatments more than those with physician's choice treatment mostly because of the unavailability of agents for their alterations. For example, if patients are matched with agents recommended by the MTB, clinical outcomes such as objective response rate (ORR), disease control rate (DCR), progression-free survival (PFS), and overall survival (OS) may be improved more than those treated with physician's choice treatment.[26] These approaches have been implemented for patients with advanced malignancies, particularly those with limited treatment options after disease progression on several lines of treatment. However, precision medicine approaches are now rapidly being incorporated into earlier lines of therapy for patients with advanced disease, and the curative setting for patients treated with neoadjuvant or adjuvant therapy. Dating back to the 1970s, the hormonal therapy tamoxifen was shown to delay recurrence in early breast cancer. Tamoxifen and aromatase inhibitors have been used for hormone receptor-positive breast cancer.[27] Also in breast cancer, HER2 inhibitors such as trastuzumab and pertuzumab showed survival benefits when used as neoadjuvant and/or adjuvant therapy in those with *ERBB2* amplified tumors.[28–30] Immunotherapy such as ICIs has also been shown to be effective when used perioperatively by improving relapse-free survival and OS in patients with certain cancers.[31–36] Therefore, MTBs are becoming increasingly valuable for input and discussion not only from experts providing systemic therapy, but also from experts providing curative treatment such as surgery and radiotherapy.

Clinical Outcomes by Implementing Precision Medicine and Molecular Tumor Board

Traditionally, clinical trials evaluated patients with a specific cancer, and most did not select patients based on biomarkers that could potentially predict the efficacy of corresponding agents. The era of precision medicine has required novel clinical trial designs that make personalized therapy evaluable and feasible (**Table 2**). Several clinical trial designs have been developed to evaluate the feasibility and efficacy of MTBs and to assess agents selected based on genomic profile information as summarized in a previous review article.[37] Compared with these traditional clinical trials, precision medicine requires the evaluation of genomic profiles and the administration of agents matched with genomic alterations. Trials with master protocols allow assessment of more than 1 drug or 1 tumor within a single clinical trial.[38] Basket and umbrella trials are the first generation of clinical trials implementing precision medicine. Basket trials evaluate agents against a specific genetic alteration regardless of cancer type, leading to the successful development of pembrolizumab, NTRK inhibitors, BRAF and MEK inhibitors for *BRAF* V600 E mutations, and RET inhibitors for *RET* mutation in a tumor-agnostic manner (**Fig. 2**).[39–41] In contrast, umbrella trials evaluate multiple molecular alterations within a single cancer type to address heterogeneity within patients with a specific tumor type.[37] Umbrella trials are advantageous when evaluating common cancers with multiple alterations such as lung cancer and breast cancer.[37] When master protocols evaluate multiple hypotheses in 1 protocol, they are referred to as platform trials. The IMPACT1 trial, a platform trial, demonstrated the feasibility of the efficacy of precision medicine by showing better survival in patients with matched agents than those without matched therapies.[42,43] Several platform trials are ongoing such as IMPACT2 and NCI-MATCH across tumor types to evaluate agents matched to unique genomic alterations.[37,44] In particular, the NCI-MATCH trial comprises 40 treatment arms to evaluate agents matched to alterations of each patient, and demonstrated its feasibility of patient enrollment and performing NGS. Clinical benefit varied across targeted agents; however, approximately 38% of enrolled patients were found to have potential molecular targets, and 18% of patients received matched agents.[45,46]

The next generation of clinical trials implementing precision medicine includes N-of-1 trials.[47] In contrast to conventional clinical trials, N-of-1 trials focus on individualized therapy for patients with cancer. This design aims to evaluate the efficacy and safety at the level of an individual patient. Information gathered from N-of-1 trials may provide a tailored therapeutic strategy for individuals by addressing the interpatient heterogeneity of cancer.[2,47] The Investigation of Profile-Related Evidence Determining Individualized Cancer Therapy (I-PREDICT) trial was the first prospective trial to use the N-of-1 trial design to evaluate personalized treatment suggested by the MTB for patients with advanced cancer. Therapy was suggested based on evaluated biomarkers from tissue NGS, circulating tumor DNA (ctDNA), and immune markers including MSI status, TMB, and PD-L1 expression. Treatment efficacy was assessed by calculating a matching score representing the degree of matched therapies. For example, if a patient had 4 alterations and was given therapy that targets 1 alteration, the matching score was 1/4 (=25% [low]). In contrast, if a patient had 4 alterations and was given therapy that targets 3 alterations, a matching score was calculated as 3/4 (=75% [high]). In this study, higher matching score (>50%) was associated with a statistically better DCR (defined as partial response or stable disease $\geq$ 6 months) and

Table 2
Clinical trial and research design evaluating precision medicine that includes a molecular tumor board

Design	Design Detail	Pros	Cons	Study References
Master protocol				
Basket trial	Tissue-agnostic, assessing agents targeting a common pan-cancer gene alteration	Can broaden the indication of 1 agent to multiple tumor types	Not all driver alterations are successfully targeted because of heterogeneity across tumor types	TAPUR[a] [82-84]
Umbrella trial	Tumor histology-specific, assessing several agents in different genomic subsets	Can address interpatient heterogeneity of a specific tumor type	Difficult to implement clinical trials for rare tumors Hard to determine treatment arms when a patient has multiple actionable alterations	TAPUR[a] [82-84]
Platform trial	Trial allowing assessment of several hypothesis in 1 protocol	Can expand or delete treatment arms even when clinical trials are running Can assess multiple biomarkers and targetable alterations in 1 clinical trial Cost-effective	Complicated clinical trial design High burden on trial administration Complexity of statistical analysis	IMPACT1[42,43] IMPACT2[85] TAPUR[a] [82-84]
Newer generation				
N-of-1 trial	Patient-centered trial evaluating individualized combination treatments The degree of matching to therapy suggested by the molecular tumor board is assessed Outcomes are compared among patients treated with low vs high degree of molecular matching	Can offer individualized combination treatment approaches for each enrolled patient by considering their molecular features	Complexity of calculating the degree of matching Difficult to generalize the trial outcomes to different populations Patients are treated with customized combination therapies that are unique to each patient	I-PREDICT[48,49]

(continued on next page)

Table 2
(continued)

Design	Design Detail	Pros	Cons	Study References
Others				
Real-world data	Analyzing data obtained in electronic medical records and industrial patient data to address unmet needs in real world	Can address unmet needs and clinical questions that arise in daily practice Cost-effective	Patient and treatment selection possess a risk of bias, as real-world data analysis is not a prospective clinical trial	USCD-PREDICT (NCT02478931)[26]

Details of each trial listed and other trials not listed here are summarized in previous review articles.[37,86]

[a] Combination of basket and umbrella trial.

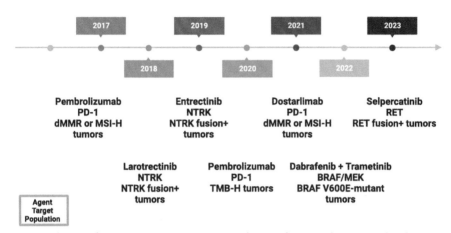

Tumor-agnostic approvals for advanced disease

2017	**2019**	**2021**	**2023**
	2018	**2020**	**2022**

Pembrolizumab
PD-1
dMMR or MSI-H
tumors

Entrectinib
NTRK
NTRK fusion+
tumors

Dostarlimab
PD-1
dMMR or MSI-H
tumors

Selpercatinib
RET
RET fusion+ tumors

Larotrectinib
NTRK
NTRK fusion+
tumors

Pembrolizumab
PD-1
TMB-H tumors

Dabrafenib + Trametinib
BRAF/MEK
BRAF V600E-mutant
tumors

Agent
Target
Population

Fig. 2. Evolution of tumor-agnostic precision oncology in the United States. Each column includes: (1) agent name, (2) targeted alterations, and (3) targeted population. BRAF, V-Raf murine sarcoma viral oncogene homolog B; dMMR, DNA mismatch repair-deficiency; MEK, mitogen-activated protein kinase; MSI-H, microsatellite instability-high; NTRK, neurotrophic tyrosine receptor kinase; PD-1, programmed cell death protein 1; RET, rearranged during transfection. (Created with BioRender.com.)

improved PFS and OS across tumor types when compared to patients who received therapies with a low matching score.[26,48–50] Overall, the I-PREDICT trial showed the feasibility and safety of N-of-1 trials, customizing personalized treatment approaches provided by the MTB.

The number of studies utilizing MTBs for delivering precision medicine is growing. A recent study by the University of California, San Diego, investigating the utility of MTB showed that a higher matching score in patients with colorectal cancer was associated with longer PFS (hazard ratio [HR], 0.41; 95% confidence interval [CI], 0.21–0.81; $P=.01$) with higher clinical benefit rates (41% vs 18%, $P=.058$) than those treated with unmatched therapy. The authors concluded that MTB plays a vital role in treatment decision making and survival improvement in a specific cancer type.[51] Because it is difficult for traditional clinical trials to ensure the feasibility of precision medicine, the authors anticipate that more clinical trials will implement trial designs such as N-of-1 trials. Clinicians involved in the care of patients with cancer need to understand the newer concept of these trials to develop new evidence for patient care through personalized medicine.

PERIOPERATIVE PRECISION ONCOLOGY
Somatic Alterations

Precision oncology through biomarker-based patient selection is now growing in the perioperative setting as neoadjuvant/adjuvant therapy (**Table 3**). Breast cancer was one of the first cancers to consider patient selection based on biologic characteristics. Endocrine therapy such as tamoxifen and aromatase inhibitors are standard adjuvant therapy in hormone receptor-positive patients, and HER2-targeting agents such as

Table 3
Examples of precision oncology in the perioperative setting

Cancer	Example	Population	Agents	References
Breast cancer	Adjuvant hormonal therapy	Hormone-receptor positive	Tamoxifen Aromatase inhibitors	27,87
	Neoadjuvant/adjuvant HER2 inhibitors	ERBB2 amplification	Trastuzumab Pertuzumab Trastuzumab-emtansine (for residual disease)	29,30,88
	Adjuvant PARP inhibitors	*BRCA1/2* mutations HRD	Olaparib	59
	Adjuvant CDK4/6 inhibitors	High-risk hormone-receptor positive	Abemaciclib	52
Colorectal cancer	Neoadjuvant immunotherapy	Mismatch repair-deficient rectal cancer	Dostarlimab[a]	89
Lung cancer	Adjuvant EGFR TKI	*EGFR* mutation	Osimertinib	53
Malignant melanoma	Adjuvant BRAF and MEK inhibitors	*BRAF V600 E* or *V600 K* mutations	Dabrafenib plus trametinib	90
Ovarian cancer	PARP inhibitors	*BRCA1/2* mutations	Olaparib	91

Abbreviations: BRAF, V-Raf murine sarcoma viral oncogene homolog B; BRCA, BReast CAncer gene; CDK, cyclin-dependent kinase; EGFR, epidermal growth factor receptor; ERBB2, erythroblastic oncogene B 2; HER2, human epidermal growth factor receptor 2; HRD, homologous recombination deficiency; MEK, mitogen-activated protein kinase; NSCLC, non-small cell lung cancer; PARP, Poly-ADP ribose polymerase; TKI, tyrosine kinase inhibitor.
[a] Not FDA-approved.

trastuzumab and pertuzumab are now used as a neoadjuvant and adjuvant therapy in locally advanced disease with *ERBB2* amplification.[29,30] Additionally, a CDK4/6 inhibitor, abemaciclib, has been shown to prolong relapse-free survival in hormone receptor-positive breast cancer with high-risk features in the MonerchE trial, expanding further options in patients with breast cancer as a perioperative strategy.[52] In lung cancer, the ADAURA trial showed survival improvement with osimertinib, an EGFR TKI, after definitive surgery with or without adjuvant chemotherapy, expanding further personalized options in other cancer types.[53]

Other than targeted therapy, ICIs are now being incorporated into the standard of care as either neoadjuvant or adjuvant therapy by showing improvement in relapse-free survival and OS in multiple cancer types.[31–33,35,36] In this setting, an appropriate biomarker for patient selection has not yet been established, but PD-L1 expression may be a positive predictor for relapse-free survival based on subgroup analyses in these trials.[32,33,36]

Germline Alterations

In addition to a strategy targeting somatic mutation, patients with germline mutation also benefit from precision medicine. For example, poly-ADP ribose polymerase (PARP) inhibitors such as olaparib improve survival in patients with breast cancer harboring *BRCA1/2* mutations.[54] Subsequently, the maintenance use of PARP inhibitors showed benefit by prolonging relapse-free survival in *BRCA*-mutant ovarian cancer.[55] Their use has also been expanded to other tumor types such as advanced pancreatic cancer and metastatic castration-resistant prostate cancer harboring *BRCA* mutations.[56–58] PARP inhibitors are also being used in the perioperative setting. Adjuvant use of olaparib for HER2-negative early breast cancer harboring *BRCA1* or *BRCA2* germline mutations with high-risk clinical features showed prolonged invasive disease-free survival (HR, 0.58, 99.5% CI, 0.46–0.74, $P < .0001$) and OS (HR, 0.68, 99.5% CI, 0.50–0.91, $P < .0091$) compared with placebo after neoadjuvant or adjuvant chemotherapy, leading to its FDA approval in 2022.[59,60] Thus, the authors anticipate an increase in the number of early stage cancer cases requiring genomic profiling tests before or after surgery to guide appropriate perioperative therapy, including the use of PARP inhibitors. As they are now utilized in upfront therapy, all providers need to understand the long-term risks of PARP inhibitors such as a potential increase in the risk of treatment-related myeloid dysplastic syndrome (MDS) or acute myeloid leukemia (AML), as well as the incidental detection of germline mutations in patients' relatives, resulting in an increase in risk of several cancer types.[23]

The I-SPY 2 trial, implementing perioperative tailored approach, has a framework of an adaptive phase 2 clinical trial design evaluating neoadjuvant therapy for patients with high-risk breast cancer. The trial categories breast cancer into 10 subtypes according to hormone receptor and HER2 status, and 70-gene assay (MammaPrint) score. For randomization, Bayesian methods are used to achieve a higher probability of efficacy in the use of experimental drugs in addition to standard neoadjuvant chemotherapy.[61,62] This platform trial is ongoing to identify new agents combined with standard neoadjuvant chemotherapy and ideal strategies for each patients with early stage high-risk breast cancer.

Precision oncology is now rapidly becoming the standard of care even in the early stage setting as part of neoadjuvant/adjuvant therapy (**Fig. 3**). Performing NGS and molecular profiling tests at the time of cancer diagnosis must be strongly considered to gain maximum therapeutic benefit. Details of treatment for each type of cancer are summarized and discussed in other articles.

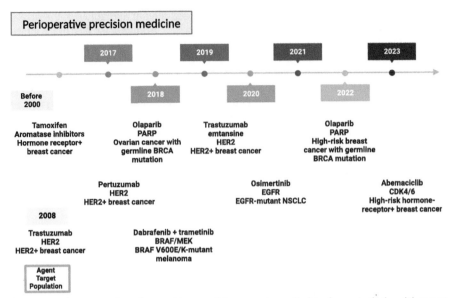

Fig. 3. Development of peri-operative precision oncology. Each column includes: (1) agent name, (2) targeted alterations, and (3) targeted population. BRAF, V-Raf murine sarcoma viral oncogene homolog B; BRCA, BReast CAncer gene; CDK, cyclin-dependent kinase; EGFR, epidermal growth factor receptor; HER2, human epidermal growth factor receptor 2; MEK, mitogen-activated protein kinase; NSCLC, non-small cell lung cancer; PARP, poly-ADP ribose polymerase. (Created with BioRender.com.)

CHALLENGES OF PRECISION MEDICINE AND MOLECULAR TUMOR BOARD
Expertise

Multidisciplinary discussion facilitates treatment consideration and selection at the MTB. However, availability of experts to conduct the MTB can be challenging, particularly in small institutions, rural areas, and developing countries.[23,63] Additionally, time constraints may be another issue, as experts may not be available at the same time. In institutions with limited access to individual subspecialists, creating a tumor board team that works remotely both internally and externally can address this issue.[64] Further, education and lectures created by experienced institutions may also help each clinician improve his or her understanding of the interpretation of genomic test results, resulting in improved feasibility of MTBs in any institution with limited access to experts. Precision oncology using NGS and clinical trials developed primarily in Western countries. Experts in these fields could facilitate the process of holding the MTB in other regions by working remotely, and the feasibility of a virtual MTB has been shown in several studies from Western countries.[63,65] Clinical trials assessing precision medicine are also being performed in Asian countries, and expansion to other regions is expected in the near future.[66–68] Broadening the application of precision oncology in these areas would improve survival outcomes in patients with cancer worldwide by addressing racial and ethnic molecular differences.[69,70] Further global collaborations are needed to address these MTB feasibility issues.

Access to Clinical Trials

However, access to treatment can also be problematic even in larger clinical cancer centers. The MTB suggests tailored therapeutic options for each patient. Oftentimes, clinical trials are the only option that can be suggested as an experimental therapeutic option, which may not be available at the treating physician's institution. Transferring from the original institution could be a burden for patients, and thus, smooth referral to the new clinical site where clinical trials are available is necessary for seamless care. There is a growing demand for collaboration through a clinical trial network to reduce patient burden and ensure access to clinical trials across the country.[23]

Unanticipated Germline Findings

The challenging aspect of genetic testing for is the possibility of detecting germline genomic alterations. A pathogenic germline variant can be detected in approximately 4% to 12% of patients using genomic profiling.[71–74] These findings can lead to prescribing treatments such as PARP inhibitors for *BRCA1/2*-mutant cancers and those with homologous recombination deficiency (HRD), but could also result in family members of these patients being at increased risk of developing cancer in the future because of specific germline mutations. Institutional support such as a genetic counselor must be established at centers where genetic profiling tests are performed. Clinicians should be aware of the psychological burden of detecting germline mutations in patients and their family members. The risk-benefit discussion by providing data such as the detection rate of treatable alterations and germline mutations needs to be carefully conducted with each patient undergoing genomic profiling.

Tumor Heterogeneity and Evolution

Traditional genomic profiling tests have static characteristics, in which tissue or liquid biopsies are collected and analyzed for clinically meaningful expression or actionable genetic alterations at a single time. Although some patients can gain useful information from genomic profiling for treatment decisions, it would be difficult for static analyses to account for tumor heterogeneity and evolution within each patient over time. Recently, the concept of functional precision medicine has been proposed, which is an approach based on exposing patient samples to existing or experimental drugs.[75] In the future, integrating the functional precision medicine approach would allow one to determine which drugs are more potent and effective for each patient. Challenges to functional precision medicine include techniques for handling patient tissues, unclear clinical associations between in vivo analysis and actual patient outcome, and the time from tissue collection, creation of specific models such as cell lines, organoids, and xenograft models, to drug testing.[76] There are ongoing clinical trials evaluating the feasibility and utility of functional precision medicine. The integration of traditional genomics-driven, static precision medicine and functional precision medicine would provide better rationale for combination treatments and facilitate better discussion in the MTB.[76]

Perioperative Toxicity

In the perioperative setting, the toxicity of agents suggested by the MTB needs to be carefully considered, because severe adverse events from targeted therapies or immunotherapy can delay surgery and affect quality of life in patients whose cancer is potentially curable (see article by Nishizaki and Eskander). To implement the personalized medicine in the early setting, future clinical trials incorporating MTB and precision oncology must assess the safety and the impact of toxicity on the outcome of definitive therapy to optimize outcomes.

FUTURE DIRECTIONS

Clinical trials evaluating precision oncology have demonstrated its feasibility and survival benefits across tumor types leading to the rapid expansion of tailored medicine for patients with solid tumors. Particularly, molecular targeted therapies and immunotherapy are being actively incorporated into neoadjuvant and adjuvant therapy with surgery, suggesting the need for the MTB in the perioperative setting to deliver the best personalized therapeutic strategy to increase the chances of cancer cure.

Current issues and challenges with molecular targeted therapy and ICIs are that most patients receiving these agents eventually acquire resistance and show disease progression while receiving these treatments. Precision medicine trials showed feasibility of patient enrollment and sequencing, but have also shown that therapies targeting a single alteration do not provide significant benefit.[44] As cancer cells acquire some escape pathways after exposure to these agents, strategies to combine 2 or more agents have been proposed and evaluated to improve treatment outcomes in recent clinical trials.[77,78] The NCI-ComboMATCH was launched to search for ideal combination therapies based on evidence from preclinical studies.[79] Results from this type of clinical trial will provide useful information to guide treatment decisions at the MTB.

The development of antibody-drug conjugates (ADCs), bispecific antibodies, cellular therapy, and radionuclide therapy will also expand precision medicine. The use of ADCs for cancer treatment is growing dramatically. ADCs are composed of a cytotoxic payload, an antibody to target antigens expressed on tumor cells, and a linker to connect the payload and antibody. Examples of ADCs in oncology include enfortumab vedotin (payload: MMAE, target antigen: nectin-4), trastuzumab deruxtecan (payload: DXd, target antigen: HER2), and sacituzumab govitecan (payload: SN-38, target antigen: Trop-2). Because antigen expression patterns differ between tumor types, ADCs have been evaluated for specific tumor types. Recently, trastuzumab deruxtecan demonstrated a promising objective response rate (37.1% in the entire population; 61.3% in patients with IHC 3+ expression) for HER2 overexpressing tumors in the pan-cancer setting (NCT04482309, DESTINY-PanTumor02), suggesting the utility of ADCs as a tumor-agnostic approach.[80] Additionally, bispecific antibodies and cellular therapy targeting specific tumor-associated antigens on cancer cells also implement the concept of personalized medicine. Radionuclide therapy such as Lutetium-177–PSMA-617 has also been shown to improve PFS in patients with PSMA-positive castration-resistant prostate cancer.[81] All of these treatment modalities have demonstrated clinical benefit by targeting specific antigen expression on tumors, suggesting the importance of dissecting molecular features on tumor cells before determining the treatment plan for each patient.

Addressing challenges such as access to genomic profiling testing and the MTB is also important to resolve health care disparities in the United States and globally. Not all institutions have the capacity to conduct MTBs. Interinstitutional collaboration through the establishment of precision medicine networks, the implementation of virtual meetings at the request of physicians, and education and training in MTBs for health care providers in rural areas may lead to a seamless discussion with patients regardless of the areas in which they live.

MTBs are an integral part of delivering precision medicine to patients with early and advanced cancer. Its presence and role are growing, and multiple clinical trials are underway to evaluate the feasibility of MTB for the implementation of personalized medicine in oncology. The challenges mentioned in this article need to be addressed to eliminate disparities and advance precision oncology, but the future of precision medicine is bright, and MTB will continue to play an important role in offering the best personalized therapy for patients with cancer.

SUMMARY

With multiple molecular targeted therapies available for patients with cancer that correspond to a specific genetic alteration, the selection of the best treatment through discussion is essential to ensure therapeutic efficacy. MTBs play a key role in this decision-making process to deliver personalized medicine to patients with cancer in a multidisciplinary manner. Historically, personalized medicine has been offered to patients with advanced cancer, but the incorporation of molecular targeted therapies and immunotherapy into the perioperative setting requires clinicians, including surgeons, to understand the role of the MTB. Evidence is accumulating to support the feasibility and survival benefit in patients treated with the matched therapy proposed by the MTB, and the MTB will continue to play an integral role in incorporating the growing body of evidence of cancer therapy to provide personalized treatment for each patient with cancer.

CLINICS CARE POINTS

- The MTB is an essential venue for discussing molecular profiling test results and offering personalized therapy including molecular targeted therapy, immunotherapy, and available clinical trials for patients with cancer.
- Precision medicine is being incorporated into the perioperative setting, and, therefore, surgical oncologists should be involved in multidisciplinary MTBs.

DISCLOSURE

Y. Fujiwara does not have conflicts of interest. S. Kato serves as a consultant for Foundation Medicine. He receives speaker's fees from Roche and the advisory board for Pfizer. He has research funding from ACT Genomics, Sysmex, Japan, Konica Minolta and OmniSeq. R. Kurzrock has received research funding from Boehringer Ingelheim, Germany, Debiopharm, Foundation Medicine, United States, Genentech, United States, Grifols, Spain, Guardant, Incyte, Konica Minolta, MedImmune, United States, Merck Serono, Omniseq, Pfizer, United States, Sequenom, Takeda, Japan, and TopAlliance and from the NCI, United States, as well as consultant and/or speaker fees and/or advisory board/consultant for Actuate Therapeutics, AstraZeneca, Bicara Therapeutics, Inc., Biological Dynamics, Caris, Datar Cancer Genetics, Daiichi, EISAI, EOM Pharmaceuticals, Iylon, LabCorp, Merck, NeoGenomics, Neomed, Pfizer, Precirix, Prosperdtx, Regeneron, Roche, TD2/Volastra, Turning Point Therapeutics, X-Biotech. R. Kurzrock has an equity interest in CureMatch Inc.; serves on the Board of CureMatch and CureMetrix, and is a co-founder of CureMatch. R. Kurzrock is funded in part by 5U01CA180888 to 08 and 5UG1CA233198 to 05.

REFERENCES

1. Wu Q, Qian W, Sun X, et al. Small-molecule inhibitors, immune checkpoint inhibitors, and more: FDA-approved novel therapeutic drugs for solid tumors from 1991 to 2021. J Hematol Oncol 2022;15(1):143.
2. Tsimberidou AM, Fountzilas E, Nikanjam M, et al. Review of precision cancer medicine: evolution of the treatment paradigm. Cancer Treat Rev 2020;86:102019.

3. Druker BJ, Talpaz M, Resta DJ, et al. Efficacy and safety of a specific inhibitor of the BCR-ABL tyrosine kinase in chronic myeloid leukemia. N Engl J Med 2001; 344(14):1031–7.

4. Lynch TJ, Bell DW, Sordella R, et al. Activating mutations in the epidermal growth factor receptor underlying responsiveness of non-small-cell lung cancer to gefitinib. N Engl J Med 2004;350(21):2129–39.

5. Mok TS, Wu YL, Thongprasert S, et al. Gefitinib or carboplatin-paclitaxel in pulmonary adenocarcinoma. N Engl J Med 2009;361(10):947–57.

6. Schwaederle M, Zhao M, Lee JJ, et al. Impact of precision medicine in diverse cancers: a meta-analysis of phase II clinical trials. J Clin Oncol 2015;33(32):3817–25.

7. Horak P, Fröhling S, Glimm H. Integrating next-generation sequencing into clinical oncology: strategies, promises and pitfalls. ESMO Open 2016;1(5):e000094.

8. Subbiah V, Puzanov I, Blay JY, et al. Pan-cancer efficacy of vemurafenib in BRAF (V600)-mutant non-melanoma cancers. Cancer Discov 2020;10(5):657–63.

9. Gouda MA, Nelson BE, Buschhorn L, et al. Tumor-agnostic precision medicine from the AACR GENIE database: clinical implications. Clin Cancer Res 2023; 29(15):2753–60.

10. Kiyotani K, Toyoshima Y, Nakamura Y. Personalized immunotherapy in cancer precision medicine. Cancer Biol Med 2021;18(4):955–65.

11. Goodman AM, Kato S, Bazhenova L, et al. Tumor mutational burden as an independent predictor of response to immunotherapy in diverse cancers. Mol Cancer Ther 2017;16(11):2598–608.

12. Doroshow DB, Bhalla S, Beasley MB, et al. PD-L1 as a biomarker of response to immune-checkpoint inhibitors. Nat Rev Clin Oncol 2021;18(6):345–62.

13. Fukuoka M, Yano S, Giaccone G, et al. Multi-institutional randomized phase ii trial of gefitinib for previously treated patients with advanced non–small-cell lung cancer. J Clin Oncol 2003;21(12):2237–46.

14. Maemondo M, Inoue A, Kobayashi K, et al. Gefitinib or chemotherapy for non-small-cell lung cancer with mutated EGFR. N Engl J Med 2010;362(25):2380–8.

15. Khozin S, Blumenthal GM, Jiang X, et al. U.S. Food and Drug Administration approval summary: erlotinib for the first-line treatment of metastatic non-small cell lung cancer with epidermal growth factor receptor exon 19 deletions or exon 21 (L858R) substitution mutations. Oncol 2014;19(7):774–9.

16. Kazandjian D, Blumenthal GM, Chen HY, et al. FDA approval summary: crizotinib for the treatment of metastatic non-small cell lung cancer with anaplastic lymphoma kinase rearrangements. Oncol 2014;19(10):e5–11.

17. Pegram MD, Lipton A, Hayes DF, et al. Phase II study of receptor-enhanced chemosensitivity using recombinant humanized anti-p185HER2/neu monoclonal antibody plus cisplatin in patients with HER2/neu-overexpressing metastatic breast cancer refractory to chemotherapy treatment. J Clin Oncol 1998;16(8):2659–71.

18. Marcus L, Donoghue M, Aungst S, et al. FDA approval summary: entrectinib for the treatment of NTRK gene fusion solid tumors. Clin Cancer Res 2021;27(4): 928–32.

19. Marcus L, Lemery SJ, Keegan P, et al. FDA approval summary: pembrolizumab for the treatment of microsatellite instability-high solid tumors. Clin Cancer Res 2019;25(13):3753–8.

20. Marcus L, Fashoyin-Aje LA, Donoghue M, et al. FDA approval summary: pembrolizumab for the treatment of tumor mutational burden-high solid tumors. Clin Cancer Res 2021;27(17):4685–9.

21. Rijavec E, Biello F, Indini A, et al. Current Insights on the treatment of anaplastic lymphoma kinase-positive metastatic non-small cell lung cancer: focus on brigatinib. Clin Pharmacol 2022;14:1–9.

22. Hong DS, DuBois SG, Kummar S, et al. Larotrectinib in patients with TRK fusion-positive solid tumours: a pooled analysis of three phase 1/2 clinical trials. Lancet Oncol 2020;21(4):531–40.

23. Mateo J, Steuten L, Aftimos P, et al. Delivering precision oncology to patients with cancer. Nat Med 2022;28(4):658–65.

24. Parikh AR, Leshchiner I, Elagina L, et al. Liquid versus tissue biopsy for detecting acquired resistance and tumor heterogeneity in gastrointestinal cancers. Nat Med 2019;25(9):1415–21.

25. Kinugasa H, Nouso K, Miyahara K, et al. Detection of K-ras gene mutation by liquid biopsy in patients with pancreatic cancer. Cancer 2015;121(13):2271–80.

26. Kato S, Kim KH, Lim HJ, et al. Real-world data from a molecular tumor board demonstrates improved outcomes with a precision N-of-One strategy. Nat Commun 2020;11(1):4965.

27. Jordan VC. Tamoxifen: a most unlikely pioneering medicine. Nat Rev Drug Discov 2003;2(3):205–13.

28. Baselga J, Perez EA, Pienkowski T, et al. Adjuvant trastuzumab: a milestone in the treatment of HER-2-positive early breast cancer. Oncol 2006;11(Suppl 1):4–12.

29. Piccart-Gebhart MJ, Procter M, Leyland-Jones B, et al. Trastuzumab after adjuvant chemotherapy in HER2-positive breast cancer. N Engl J Med 2005;353(16):1659–72.

30. von Minckwitz G, Procter M, de Azambuja E, et al. Adjuvant pertuzumab and trastuzumab in early her2-positive breast cancer. N Engl J Med 2017;377(2):122–31.

31. Schmid P, Cortes J, Dent R, et al. Event-free survival with pembrolizumab in early triple-negative breast cancer. N Engl J Med 2022;386(6):556–67.

32. Choueiri TK, Tomczak P, Park SH, et al. Adjuvant pembrolizumab after nephrectomy in renal-cell carcinoma. N Engl J Med 2021;385(8):683–94.

33. Bajorin DF, Witjes JA, Gschwend JE, et al. Adjuvant nivolumab versus placebo in muscle-invasive urothelial carcinoma. N Engl J Med 2021;384(22):2102–14.

34. O'Brien M, Paz-Ares L, Marreaud S, et al. Pembrolizumab versus placebo as adjuvant therapy for completely resected stage IB–IIIA non-small-cell lung cancer (PEARLS/KEYNOTE-091): an interim analysis of a randomised, triple-blind, phase 3 trial. Lancet Oncol 2022;23(10):1274–86.

35. Forde PM, Spicer J, Lu S, et al. Neoadjuvant nivolumab plus chemotherapy in resectable lung cancer. N Engl J Med 2022;386(21):1973–85.

36. Felip E, Altorki N, Zhou C, et al. Adjuvant atezolizumab after adjuvant chemotherapy in resected stage IB-IIIA non-small-cell lung cancer (IMpower010): a randomised, multicentre, open-label, phase 3 trial. Lancet 2021;398(10308):1344–57.

37. Fountzilas E, Tsimberidou AM, Vo HH, et al. Clinical trial design in the era of precision medicine. Genome Med 2022;14(1):101.

38. Park JJH, Siden E, Zoratti MJ, et al. Systematic review of basket trials, umbrella trials, and platform trials: a landscape analysis of master protocols. Trials 2019;20(1):572.

39. Subbiah V, Wolf J, Konda B, et al. Tumour-agnostic efficacy and safety of selpercatinib in patients with RET fusion-positive solid tumours other than lung or thyroid tumours (LIBRETTO-001): a phase 1/2, open-label, basket trial. Lancet Oncol 2022;23(10):1261–73.

40. Salama AKS, Li S, Macrae ER, et al. Dabrafenib and trametinib in patients with tumors with BRAFV600E mutations: results of the NCI-MATCH Trial Subprotocol H. J Clin Oncol 2020;38(33):3895–904.

41. Wen PY, Stein A, van den Bent M, et al. Dabrafenib plus trametinib in patients with BRAF[V600E]-mutant low-grade and high-grade glioma (ROAR): a multicentre, open-label, single-arm, phase 2, basket trial. Lancet Oncol 2022;23(1):53–64.

42. Tsimberidou AM, Iskander NG, Hong DS, et al. Personalized medicine in a phase I clinical trials program: the MD Anderson Cancer Center initiative. Clin Cancer Res 2012;18(22):6373–83.

43. Tsimberidou AM, Hong DS, Wheler JJ, et al. Long-term overall survival and prognostic score predicting survival: the IMPACT study in precision medicine. J Hematol Oncol 2019;12(1):145.

44. O'Dwyer PJ, Gray RJ, Flaherty KT, et al. The NCI-MATCH trial: lessons for precision oncology. Nat Med 2023;29(6):1349–57.

45. Flaherty KT, Gray RJ, Chen AP, et al. Molecular landscape and actionable alterations in a genomically guided cancer clinical trial: national cancer institute molecular analysis for therapy choice (NCI-MATCH). J Clin Oncol 2020;38(33):3883–94.

46. NCI-MATCH Sets. Benchmark of actionability. Cancer Discov 2021;11(1):6–7.

47. Gouda MA, Buschhorn L, Schneeweiss A, et al. N-of-1 trials in cancer drug development. Cancer Discov 2023;13(6):1301–9.

48. Sicklick JK, Kato S, Okamura R, et al. Molecular profiling of cancer patients enables personalized combination therapy: the I-PREDICT study. Nat Med 2019;25(5):744–50.

49. Sicklick JK, Kato S, Okamura R, et al. Molecular profiling of advanced malignancies guides first-line N-of-1 treatments in the I-PREDICT treatment-naïve study. Genome Med 2021;13(1):155.

50. Schwaederle M, Parker BA, Schwab RB, et al. Precision oncology: the UC San Diego Moores Cancer Center PREDICT experience. Mol Cancer Ther 2016;15(4):743–52.

51. Louie BH, Kato S, Kim KH, et al. Precision medicine-based therapies in advanced colorectal cancer: The University of California San Diego Molecular Tumor Board experience. Mol Oncol 2022;16(13):2575–84.

52. Johnston SRD, Harbeck N, Hegg R, et al. Abemaciclib combined with endocrine therapy for the adjuvant treatment of hr+, her2-node-positive, high-risk, early breast cancer (monarchE). J Clin Oncol 2020;38(34):3987–98.

53. Tsuboi M, Herbst RS, John T, et al. Overall Survival with osimertinib in resected EGFR-mutated NSCLC. N Engl J Med 2023;389(2):137–47.

54. Robson M, Im S-A, Senkus E, et al. Olaparib for metastatic breast cancer in patients with a germline BRCA mutation. N Engl J Med 2017;377(6):523–33.

55. Arora S, Balasubramaniam S, Zhang H, et al. FDA approval summary: olaparib monotherapy or in combination with bevacizumab for the maintenance treatment of patients with advanced ovarian cancer. Oncol 2021;26(1):e164–72.

56. Golan T, Hammel P, Reni M, et al. Maintenance olaparib for germline BRCA-mutated metastatic pancreatic cancer. N Engl J Med 2019;381(4):317–27.

57. de Bono J, Mateo J, Fizazi K, et al. Olaparib for metastatic castration-resistant prostate cancer. N Engl J Med 2020;382(22):2091–102.

58. Abida W, Patnaik A, Campbell D, et al. Rucaparib in men with metastatic castration-resistant prostate cancer harboring a BRCA1 or BRCA2 gene alteration. J Clin Oncol 2020;38(32):3763–72.

59. Tutt ANJ, Garber JE, Kaufman B, et al. Adjuvant olaparib for patients with BRCA1- or BRCA2-mutated breast cancer. N Engl J Med 2021;384(25):2394–405.
60. Geyer CE Jr, Garber JE, Gelber RD, et al. Overall survival in the OlympiA phase III trial of adjuvant olaparib in patients with germline pathogenic variants in BRCA1/2 and high-risk, early breast cancer. Ann Oncol 2022;33(12):1250–68.
61. Nanda R, Liu MC, Yau C, et al. Effect of pembrolizumab plus neoadjuvant chemotherapy on pathologic complete response in women with early-stage breast cancer: an analysis of the ongoing phase 2 adaptively randomized I-SPY2 Trial. JAMA Oncol 2020;6(5):676–84.
62. Barker A, Sigman C, Kelloff G, et al. I-SPY 2: an adaptive breast cancer trial design in the setting of neoadjuvant chemotherapy. Clinical Pharmacology & Therapeutics 2009;86(1):97–100.
63. Irwin KE, Ko N, Walsh EP, et al. Developing a virtual equity hub: adapting the tumor board model for equity in cancer care. Oncol 2022;27(7):518–24.
64. Pishvaian MJ, Blais EM, Bender RJ, et al. A virtual molecular tumor board to improve efficiency and scalability of delivering precision oncology to physicians and their patients. JAMIA Open 2019;2(4):505–15.
65. Michele B, Alice B, Gaia G, et al. A fully virtual and nationwide molecular tumor board for gynecologic cancer patients: the virtual experience of the MITO cooperative group. Int J Gynecol Cancer 2022;32(9):1205.
66. Park KH, Choi JY, Lim AR, et al. Genomic landscape and clinical utility in Korean advanced pan-cancer patients from prospective clinical sequencing: K-MASTER program. Cancer Discov 2022;12(4):938–48.
67. Heong V, Syn NL, Lee XW, et al. Value of a molecular screening program to support clinical trial enrollment in Asian cancer patients: The Integrated Molecular Analysis of Cancer (IMAC) Study. Int J Cancer 2018;142(9):1890–900.
68. Nakamura Y, Taniguchi H, Ikeda M, et al. Clinical utility of circulating tumor DNA sequencing in advanced gastrointestinal cancer: SCRUM-Japan GI-SCREEN and GOZILA studies. Nat Med 2020;26(12):1859–64.
69. Moyers JT, Subbiah V. Think globally, act locally: globalizing precision oncology. Cancer Discov 2022;12(4):886–8.
70. Drake TM, Knight SR, Harrison EM, et al. Global Inequities in precision medicine and molecular cancer research. Front Oncol 2018;8:346.
71. Meric-Bernstam F, Brusco L, Daniels M, et al. Incidental germline variants in 1000 advanced cancers on a prospective somatic genomic profiling protocol. Ann Oncol 2016;27(5):795–800.
72. Seifert BA, O'Daniel JM, Amin K, et al. Germline analysis from tumor-germline sequencing dyads to identify clinically actionable secondary findings. Clin Cancer Res 2016;22(16):4087–94.
73. Schrader KA, Cheng DT, Joseph V, et al. Germline variants in targeted tumor sequencing using matched normal DNA. JAMA Oncol 2016;2(1):104–11.
74. DeLeonardis K, Hogan L, Cannistra SA, et al. When should tumor genomic profiling prompt consideration of germline testing? Journal of Oncology Practice 2019;15(9):465–73.
75. Letai A. Functional precision cancer medicine-moving beyond pure genomics. Nat Med 2017;23(9):1028–35.
76. Letai A, Bhola P, Welm AL. Functional precision oncology: testing tumors with drugs to identify vulnerabilities and novel combinations. Cancer Cell 2022;40(1): 26–35.
77. Jin H, Wang L, Bernards R. Rational combinations of targeted cancer therapies: background, advances and challenges. Nat Rev Drug Discov 2023;22(3):213–34.

78. Fujiwara Y, Mittra A, Naqash AR, et al. A review of mechanisms of resistance to immune checkpoint inhibitors and potential strategies for therapy. Cancer Drug Resist 2020;3(3):252–75.
79. Meric-Bernstam F, Ford JM, O'Dwyer PJ, et al. National cancer institute combination therapy platform trial with molecular analysis for therapy choice (Combo-MATCH). Clin Cancer Res 2023;29(8):1412–22.
80. Meric-Bernstam F, Makker V, Oaknin A, et al. Efficacy and safety of trastuzumab deruxtecan (T-DXd) in patients (pts) with HER2-expressing solid tumors: DESTINY-PanTumor02 (DP-02) interim results. J Clin Oncol 2023;41(17_suppl): LBA3000.
81. Sartor O, de Bono J, Chi KN, et al. Lutetium-177–PSMA-617 for metastatic castration-resistant prostate cancer. N Engl J Med 2021;385(12):1091–103.
82. Mangat PK, Halabi S, Bruinooge SS, et al. Rationale and design of the targeted agent and profiling utilization registry (TAPUR) study. JCO Precis Oncol 2018; 2018.
83. Alva AS, Mangat PK, Garrett-Mayer E, et al. Pembrolizumab in patients with metastatic breast cancer with high tumor mutational burden: results from the targeted agent and profiling utilization registry (TAPUR) Study. J Clin Oncol 2021;39(22): 2443–51.
84. Ahn ER, Rothe M, Mangat PK, et al. Pertuzumab plus trastuzumab in patients with endometrial cancer with ERBB2/3 amplification, overexpression, or mutation: results from the TAPUR study. JCO Precis Oncol 2023;7:e2200609.
85. Tsimberidou AM, Hong DS, Fu S, et al. Precision medicine: preliminary results from the Initiative for Molecular Profiling and Advanced Cancer Therapy 2 (IMPACT2) study. NPJ Precis Oncol 2021;5(1):21.
86. Adashek JJ, Subbiah V, Kurzrock R. From tissue-agnostic to N-of-one therapies: (R)evolution of the precision paradigm. Trends Cancer 2021;7(1):15–28.
87. Howell A, Cuzick J, Baum M, et al. Results of the ATAC (Arimidex, Tamoxifen, Alone or in Combination) trial after completion of 5 years' adjuvant treatment for breast cancer. Lancet 2005;365(9453):60–2.
88. von Minckwitz G, Huang C-S, Mano MS, et al. Trastuzumab emtansine for residual invasive HER2-positive breast cancer. N Engl J Med 2018;380(7):617–28.
89. Cercek A, Lumish M, Sinopoli J, et al. PD-1 blockade in mismatch repair-deficient, locally advanced rectal cancer. N Engl J Med 2022;386(25):2363–76.
90. Long GV, Hauschild A, Santinami M, et al. Adjuvant dabrafenib plus trametinib in stage III BRAF-MUTATED MELAnoma. N Engl J Med 2017;377(19):1813–23.
91. Moore K, Colombo N, Scambia G, et al. Maintenance olaparib in patients with newly diagnosed advanced ovarian cancer. N Engl J Med 2018;379(26):2495–505.

Understanding the Landscape of Clinically Available Molecular Testing

Julia A. Elvin, MD, PhD

KEYWORDS

- Molecular diagnostics • Precision oncology • Next-generation sequencing (NGS)
- Immunohistochemistry (IHC) • Circulating tumor DNA (ctDNA) • Tumor biomarkers
- Liquid biopsy • Targeted therapy

KEY POINTS

- Molecular diagnostic tests, like other assays provided by medical laboratories, should be selected based on the individual patient's clinical scenario.
- Consider comprehensive genomic profiling (CGP) for rare tumors, when the diagnosis is unclear, and when the clinical presentation is unusual. CGP can also reveal unique combinations of oncogenic drivers in common tumors, aiding in more precise subclassification and personalized treatment selection.
- Recognize that no single molecular test is universally applicable to all clinical situations. Be aware of how pre-analytic variables, such as tissue handling and fixation, can impact assay sensitivity and specificity. Understanding limitations of methodologies can help avoid misinterpretation of test results.

INTRODUCTION

Personalized oncology care is a complex and rapidly evolving field. Traditionally, cancer classification was based on anatomic site, histologic pattern, cytologic features, and staining characteristics observed under the microscope by a trained anatomic pathologist. However, this approach often resulted in significant variation in tumor behavior and therapy responsiveness among patients with the same diagnosis. Cancer is now understood to result from a combination of inherited DNA variants (germline) and accumulated mutations from environmental exposures, replication errors, and aging at the somatic level. These mutations lead to altered gene expression, differentiation, signal transduction, and cell cycle control, among other processes.

Our growing arsenal of molecular diagnostic assays allows us to include changes in DNA sequence and RNA expression, as well as protein composition, quantity, and

Pathology and Diagnostic Medicine, Foundation Medicine, Inc 400 Summer Street, Boston, MA 02210, USA
E-mail address: jelvin@foundationmedicine.com

Surg Oncol Clin N Am 33 (2024) 217–230
https://doi.org/10.1016/j.soc.2023.12.026
1055-3207/24/© 2024 Elsevier Inc. All rights reserved.

cellular compartment location in our tumor categorization. This makes diagnosis more comprehensive and reflective of the underlying biological nature of the disease at the individual patient level. For example, the 2021 WHO Central Nervous System tumor classification system now requires the assessment and integration of molecular findings with anatomic and histopathologic features for a final diagnosis. This includes *IDH1* and *IDH2* gene sequencing, *TERT* promoter methylation, 1p/19q chromosome arm testing for oligodendroglioma and glioblastoma categorization, and methylation signatures to differentiate subtypes of medulloblastomas.[1]

Recently, prognostic differences observed between molecular categories (polymerase E-mutated [*POLEmut*], mismatch repair deficient, nonspecific molecular profile, and P53 abnormal [p53abn]) defined by The Cancer Genome Atlas for endometrial cancer analysis have led to changes in the 2023 International Federation of Gynecology and Obstetrics (FIGO) tumor staging for endometrial cancer.[2] The updated FIGO staging guidelines recommend complete molecular classification in all endometrial cancers for prognostic risk group stratification and as factors that might influence adjuvant and systemic treatment decisions. When molecular classification reveals p53abn or *POLEmut* status in Stages I and II, this results in upstaging to "Stage IICm$_{p53abn}$" or downstaging to "Stage IAm$_{POLEmut}$" based on worse and better molecularly defined prognosis, respectively. As additional tumor types evolve to more precise diagnoses from molecular feature integration, we aim to improve our ability to apply historical experience and clinical trial treatment responses from patients with more biologically similar tumors. This should aid in predicting clinical outcomes and identifying effective therapies or at least in avoiding biologically implausible agents and their side effects.

CLINICAL SCENARIOS FOR MOLECULAR TESTING

Matching the molecular assay to the stage of the patient's cancer journey, the available sample types, and the clinical question at hand is crucial in gathering important data to support the shared decision-making process (**Fig. 1**).

Cancer Detection

Some molecular assays are designed for cancer detection to supplement current screening tests in an asymptomatic, normal-risk population. One example is the polymerase chain reaction (PCR)-based high-risk human papillomavirus (HPV) testing in cervical cancer screening of women 30 to 65 years old, which when negative extends the screening interval to 5 years.[3] Another is the multitarget stool DNA test (tests for six *KRAS* point mutations and methylation of *NDRG4* and *BMP3;* Cologuard, Exact Sciences, WI) for colon cancer screening, which when negative in an average risk adult can be repeated every 3 years in lieu of colonoscopy or annual fecal occult blood testing.[4] In patients with symptoms or radiologic findings highly suggestive of malignancy, but where tissue sampling for diagnosis is risky due to lesion location or the patient's performance status, or when timely access to tissue sampling services is limited, testing peripheral blood plasma for circulating tumor DNA (ctDNA) can be a pragmatic alternative. This approach may allow patients to avoid or delay invasive procedures if diagnostic or targetable mutations are identified in the blood.[5]

Molecularly Specified Diagnosis, Prognosis, and Misdiagnosis

When a tumor biopsy is obtained, testing the tissue for specific molecular markers can support and refine the probable histopathologic diagnosis. For instance, in breast adenocarcinoma (BAC) of any stage, routine molecular tests, such as estrogen receptor (ER) and progesterone receptor (PR) immunohistochemistry (IHC), and human

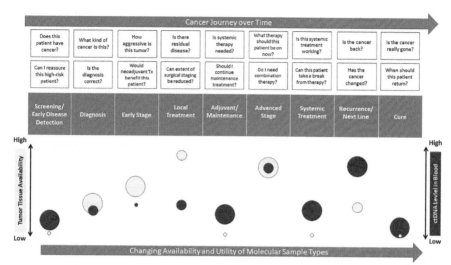

Fig. 1. Timeline of a patient's cancer journey. At each stage of a cancer journey, clinically available molecular assays may provide information to answer evolving clinical questions. The probable availability of tumor tissue appropriate for testing (*orange axis, left*) and the amount of ctDNA present in a patient blood sample (*red axis, right*) also changes at each stage and is reflected by the position of the circle along the vertical axis of graph. The estimated utility of either tumor tissue test (*orange*) or a liquid biopsy (*red*) to answer stage-relevant questions is represented by three different size circles (small circle = low utility; medium circle =moderate utility; large circle = high utility).

epidermal growth factor receptor 2 (HER2) status testing (either via *ERBB2* copy number detection by fluorescent in situ hybridization [FISH] or next-generation sequencing [NGS], or protein expression by IHC), are used to differentiate hormone receptor-positive, HER2-positive, and triple-negative breast cancer (TNBC) subtypes at diagnosis.[6] Commercially available gene expression profiling assays, such as Prosigna PAM-50 (FDA-approved, 50-gene reverse transcription [RT]-PCR with probe hybridization detection, NanoString Tech, Seattle) and BluePrint and MammaPrint (70-gene mRNA expression level by microarray, Agendia, Irvine, CA), can be used in clinically complex cases to further refine the diagnosis into Luminal A, Luminal B, and basal intrinsic subtypes, as each subtype has different prognoses, risks of recurrence, and likely responses to chemotherapy and hormonal therapies.

In early-stage (node-negative) ER+ or ER-positive BAC, gene signature assays generating expression-based recurrence scores (RS), such as Oncotype DX (quantitative RT-PCR assay of 21 genes) and MammaPrint (microarray-based expression levels of 70 genes), are frequently employed to identify patients less likely to benefit from additional chemotherapy to their hormonal therapy. The OncotypeDX RS was prospectively validated in the TAILORx trial and is now included in National Comprehensive Cancer Network (NCCN) and American Society of Clinical Oncology (ASCO) guidelines for ER-positive, HER2-negative, and lymph node-negative patient management. Currently in node-positive ER-positive BAC, these assays have only prognostic value, but their possible utility in treatment decision-making is under investigation.[6]

Molecular test results are crucial in establishing the correct diagnosis when biologically distinct processes have similar clinical or morphologic presentations.

One example where the diagnosis dramatically impacts prognosis and treatment is distinguishing a rare clear cell sarcoma (CCS), typically treated by surgery and radiation, from a more common cutaneous melanoma presenting as a soft tissue mass in an extremity, which may benefit from systemic targeted and/or immunotherapy. Both tumors stain with melanocytic IHC markers, but CCS has a diagnostic fusion involving the *EWSR1* gene, detectable by break-apart FISH or NGS, whereas melanoma may show a high tumor mutation burden (TMB), MEK pathway activating mutations, and an ultraviolet mutational signature (UVsig) from comprehensive genomic profiling (CGP).[7] A recent study of 8143 tumors with UVsig underscores the potential value of CGP, finding that only 51% had a diagnosis consistent with cutaneous origin (skin and adnexal carcinomas and melanomas) and 34% had a diagnosis without a primary site specified (such as "carcinoma of unknown primary") where the UVsig may have helped to specify the primary. Most importantly, 13% had a diagnosis of extracutaneous origin, such as lung, salivary gland, non-salivary head and neck, breast and urothelial cancers, and sarcoma, where knowledge of the presence of a UVsig would likely lead to reclassification, restaging, and alternate therapy selection.

Another example of the diagnostic utility of molecular testing and its impact on conventional treatment selection is highlighted by Eskander and colleagues[8] for distinguishing small cell lung carcinoma (SCLC) and small cell neuroendocrine carcinoma of the cervix (SCNECC) metastatic to the lung. Both can present as aggressive, high-grade carcinomas that stain with neuroendocrine markers, but SCLC is characterized by inactivating mutations in *TP53* (>90%) and *RB1* (>70%) and is responsive to platinum and etoposide chemotherapy. In contrast, more than 85% of SCNECC are positive for HPV16 or HPV18, and nearly half (41%) harbor mutations in the PI3K/AKT/mTOR pathway, and these molecular features may influence first-line and later-line therapy choices.

As molecular information accumulates from testing tumors from millions of patients, additional clinically relevant subtypes of common cancers and new, rare, biologically distinct malignancies are being recognized. This knowledge will continue to impact cancer diagnostic classification and treatment paradigms in the coming decades.

Hereditary Cancer Risk

Inherited genetic changes account for up to 10% of cancer diagnoses. Certain cancer types (such as ovarian, fallopian tube, and peritoneal cancers), early-onset cancers (such as breast, colon, or prostate cancer), multiple sequential cancers, or a strong familial cancer history should prompt consideration of genetic counseling and possible germline genetic testing. Previously, when DNA sequencing was challenging and costly, germline testing typically focused on a few high-yield candidate genes, such as *BRCA1* and *BRCA2*, especially in patients of Ashkenazi Jewish descent. However, when expanded panel testing with greater than 400 cancer-related genes was applied to *mBRCA1/2*-negative families, 44% were found to have deleterious or potentially deleterious variants in other genes.[9] Because of the higher yield, increased availability, and lower cost associated with NGS assays, large germline panels of hundreds of cancer-related genes have become part of the routine cancer diagnostic workup, even when the suspicion for an inherited cancer syndrome is low. One consequence of expanded testing rather than this setting is the frequent identification of variants of unknown significance rather those with clear deleterious functional impact. Patients should be counseled about this possibility, as well as supported in understanding and appropriately reacting to indeterminate results. Tumor testing, while not designed to assess hereditary risk, may detect inherited mutations that are present in both normal and tumor cells, in addition to somatic mutations acquired only by the tumor. Therefore, including trained genetic counselors on molecular tumor boards reviewing tumor molecular testing results can be beneficial for identifying additional patients who may benefit from follow-up germline testing.[10]

Treatment Prediction for Molecularly Matched Therapy

A key driver of increased molecular testing is the opportunity to identify patients eligible for targeted therapies, immunotherapies, and antibody-drug conjugates (ADCs). A recent review of FDA oncology drug approvals from 1998 to 2022 found that one-third were classified as precision oncology drugs, requiring genomic profiling for eligibility. More than 45 genes plus two complex genomic signatures, namely microsatellite instability high and TMB high (TMB > 10 mutations/Mb of DNA), were identified as FDA-recognized biomarkers.[11] Many additional "tumor type + drug + molecular characteristic" combinations are under investigation in clinical trials or currently being reviewed by the FDA.

This new drug approval paradigm highlights the importance of quality and regulatory oversight in molecular diagnostic tests. An FDA-approved companion diagnostic (CDx) is an in vitro diagnostic (IVD) that guides the safe and effective use of a particular therapy and is often a key factor in treatment decisions.[12] To achieve this designation, a diagnostic test developer performs and submits extensive validation studies, often including hundreds or even thousands of samples, to demonstrate analytical performance and clinical validity, and its use in a therapeutic clinical trial establishes clinical utility. When a CDx assay is performed following the manufacturer's technical specifications, any laboratory should be able to achieve comparable analytical performance for the intended use. For this reason, when a laboratory adds a new FDA-approved IVD to its menu, they only need to perform a verification on a set of positive and negative control samples, rather than performing the more extensive analytical validation themselves. IVDs and CDxs result in standardization between laboratories, but limit flexibility, such as accepting alternative specimen types or using alternative reagents or instrumentation. In contrast, laboratory-developed tests (LDTs) can be used for clinical decision-making if they are performed in a Clinical Laboratory Improvement Amendments (CLIA)-certified laboratory and have been approved by the laboratory director for clinical use after the performance of a complete validation according to laboratory accreditation body standards, such as ISO 15189, the American Society of Clinical Pathology, or the College of American Pathologists. Many LDTs are well-designed, well-validated, and accurate. However, LDTs performed by different laboratories to test for the same biomarker, may use different methodologies, reagents, instrumentation, and positive and negative cutoffs, and thus may yield different results on the same patient sample. Inter-laboratory sample exchange and biannual proficiency testing for each assay are employed to minimize differences in test results between LDTs run in different laboratories.[13]

Treatment Response Monitoring and Identification of Resistance Mechanisms

Blood-based, ctDNA assays can be used after diagnosis and alongside radiographic imaging to molecularly monitor treatment response, assess minimal residual disease (MRD), or detect early recurrence.[14] Digital droplet PCR (ddPCR) for the *BRAF* V600 E mutation characteristic of hairy cell leukemia has been used to assess MRD in this disease since 2016. More recently, tissue-informed ctDNA treatment response monitoring (TRM) assays, in which an antecedent tumor-specific mutational profile is used to select a fixed or build a custom PCR assay, have become clinically available for solid tumors. Examples of this type of test include FoundationOneTracker

(Foundation Medicine Inc, MA) and Signatera (Natera, CA), which use a targeted CGP cancer panel or whole exome sequencing tissue baseline to identify 2 to 16 trackable somatic variants and build a patient-specific, highly sensitive PCR assay that measures variants in the plasma at an allele frequency as low as 0.01% (equivalent to one mutant haploid genome in a background of 10,000 normal haploid genomes). In early clinical studies of these assays, decreases of trackable variants correlated with subsequent clinical and radiologic responses to therapy in lung, colon, and breast cancer.[15-17] On recurrence, or when cancer progresses on treatment, molecular profiling performed on a posttreatment specimen can identify additional, acquired mutations causing resistance to therapies. For example, the *EGFR* T790M mutation which conveys resistance to second-generation EGFR inhibitors and *ESR1* ligand binding site mutations that develop in some patients with breast cancer on hormone therapy can be detected in both tissue samples and ctDNA. In this setting, liquid biopsies are extremely valuable, enabling many advanced stage patients to avoid the risk and discomfort of another invasive biopsy procedure.[18-20] Additionally, as patients are diagnosed earlier, survive longer, or appear cured, molecular tests also become crucial for differentiating a second primary malignancy from a recurrence. In turn, this distinction can impact prognosis, management, clinical trial eligibility, and familial risk stratification.

SELECTING THE OPTIMAL MOLECULAR ASSAY

Many factors influence the selection of a molecular assay for a specific clinical question. Key considerations include the assay's size and scope, the patient sample type, the molecular target, and the specific assay methodology.

Assay Scope: Narrow Versus Broad Testing Approaches

The molecular test landscape includes assays that interrogate a single biomarker, those testing multiple biomarkers relevant to a specific tumor type, and pan-tumor assays assessing a wide range of biomarkers. Single-analyte and narrow panels may be preferred for their availability, speed, lower tissue requirements, or cost. In well-characterized cases with few treatment options, single marker tests or small hotspot panels might be appropriate, at least initially. Examples include PCR-based assays for *EGFR*, *ALK*, and *KRAS* in a lung biopsy with non-small cell lung cancer (NSCLC), mismatch repair IHC on a colorectal carcinoma surgical resection, or HER2 FISH on small gastric carcinoma biopsies. While focused assays are suitable when the diagnosis is accurate, and the clinician has a clear hypothesis about the relevant information needed, if the patient has been misdiagnosed, the limited additional molecular information may be misleading and compoud the error.

Broad CGP assays, not limited to common mutations for a particular tumor, reveal the unique "snowflake profile" of oncogenic drivers in each patient. Pan-tumor CGP assays are less sensitive to misdiagnosis and may help reveal a more accurate diagnostic picture, and have tissue-derived DNA or cell-free DNA (cfDNA) input requirements and costs comparable to 5 to 10 single-analyte tests. Moreover, CGP is efficient and economical for identifying low-frequency, highly actionable alterations, such as *NTRK* or *RET* fusions found in less than 1% of all cancers.[21] CGP is particularly helpful for rare tumors, such as cholangiocarcinoma or gastrointestinal neuroendocrine carcinomas, in identifying mutation-matched clinical trials or FDA-approved therapies. For example, anti-RET tyrosine kinase inhibitors were first approved in lung and thyroid carcinomas. Selpercatinib's expanded approval for any RET-mutated cancer was based on a basket-type clinical trial, with many patients identified by CGP.[22] This trial outcome has made testing for *RET* fusions important regardless of the tumor type.

Patient Sample Source: Tumor Tissue Versus Peripheral Blood

Tumor tissue and blood are the most commonly used sample types for molecular testing. The choice between them depends on various factors including availability, timing of testing, treatments received, the extent and location of the disease, patient performance status, and care goals (see **Fig. 1**). Techniques for assessing DNA, RNA, and proteins from formalin-fixed paraffin-embedded (FFPE) tissue samples have improved significantly over the past 20 years. Archival diagnostic biopsies, needle aspirations, and surgical resections often provide a ready substrate for molecular analysis without the risks associated with obtaining fresh tissue. Cell blocks from pleural and peritoneal effusions and direct cytology smears made during rapid onsite assessment of minimally invasive biopsy procedures can also be used for tissue-based molecular assays and are sometimes overlooked as a potential option. It is important for pathologists, proceduralists, and treating physicians to be mindful of tissue utilization at diagnosis, especially when biopsy material is limited, to enable future testing options.

When a suitable tissue sample is not available—for instance, if the diagnostic biopsy has been exhausted, exposed to an incompatible fixative, or lost—testing a blood sample for ctDNA becomes a practical alternative. The plasma component of peripheral blood contains fragments of cfDNA shed from dying cells throughout the body, including normal tissues, bone marrow, and white blood cells.[23] In about 75% of advanced cancers, a small amount of ctDNA is also present. The amount of ctDNA increases with later-stage, higher disease burden, untreated conditions, or progression on therapy. However, even early-stage tumors, especially in high shedding types such as small cell lung, liver, colorectal, bladder, and breast cancers, may have detectable ctDNA.

Unlike tissue testing where tumor nuclei amount can be visually estimated, the ctDNA fraction of total cfDNA is often less than 1% and cannot be predetermined before testing. If a liquid biopsy shows no alterations, it could either accurately reflect an absence of mutations in the tumor, or it could be due to ctDNA levels below the assay's detection limit, resulting in a false negative.[24] Some recent assays quantify the tumor fraction in cfDNA, using aneuploidy and maximum mutant allele frequency as indicators, to gauge the reliability of a negative result. With a ctDNA tumor fraction (%TF) cutoff greater than 1%, the concordance between mutations detected in tissue and concurrent liquid biopsy samples is over 90%. However, this concordance drops below 40% when %TF is less than 1%.[25] Interestingly, ctDNA %TF itself is emerging as a prognostic biomarker in several tumor types, with higher pretreatment percentages associated with poorer prognosis. Conversely, a significant drop in %TF or an undetectable level posttreatment %TF correlates with more substantial radiological changes and a more durable response to therapy.[26,27]

An important complexity associated with liquid biopsy is detection of mutations that arise from clonal hematopoiesis (CH) in the bone marrow, rather than from tumor or germline. CH-associated mutations do not predict tumor responsiveness to targeted therapy and can confound ctDNA TRM applications. CH-associated variants in plasma are very common, with some studies showing they are present in ~25% of liquid biopsy samples and account for up to 50% of identified mutations.[28] When some ctDNA variants in a sample from a patient with a solid tumor occur in myeloid malignancy-associated genes, such as *DNMT3A*, *TET2,* and *ASXL1*, it is more obvious that they are either of CH origin or less commonly indicative of a synchronous myelodysplastic syndrome, myeloproliferative neoplasm, or unrecognized leukemia. Some genes, such as *TP53*, are commonly altered in both solid tumors and CH. One study of paired tumor tissue and peripheral blood mononuclear cells (PBMCs) found up to 15% of *TP53* mutations thought to be tumor-derived were instead identified in the PBMC sample only. Less frequent, but more clinically impactful, are targetable genes which are typically tumor-associated, but may also infrequently occur in CH.[29] One study found that 10% of a prostate cancer cohort had mutations in homologous recombination repair genes associated with PARP inhibitor responsiveness but these were CH-derived rather than originating in their prostate tumor. Another study found 3% of patients with lung cancer had CH-derived *KRAS* variants that could suggest lack of other targetable mutations if lung tumor-derived. Misinterpretation of CH mutations as drivers of a patient's solid tumor could lead to the use of inappropriate, expensive, and potentially toxic therapies. Efforts to improve liquid biopsy technology, such as fragmentomic analysis and paired buffy coat sequencing, are showing promise in differentiating CH and enhancing liquid biopsy specificity.

Molecular Targets and Impact of Sample Quality to DNA, RNA, and Protein-based Assays

DNA analysis in tumor cells allows for the identification of mutations, including base substitutions, insertions or deletions of nucleotides, translocations, and changes in gene copy number. DNA is relatively stable, with a predictable number of chromosome copies in normal cells (typically 2, but up to 4 in cells undergoing mitosis or in normally tetraploid hepatocytes). However, because only about 1% of human genomic DNA is coding (exons) and less than 10% of that is considered cancer-relevant, enrichment strategies are necessary. These strategies focus sequencing resources on high-yield regions, such as exons of cancer-related genes. One such method, hybrid capture, uses synthetic oligonucleotides or "baits" complementary to sequences within genes of interest. Biotin on the baits allows patient DNA-bait hybrids to be captured by streptavidin beads for sequence analysis, whereas unbound DNA fragments are washed away.

Rearrangements often occur within non-coding regions and are challenging to detect via targeted DNA sequencing. Because intronic sequences between coding exons are removed by splicing during gene transcription, RNA-based assays will detect inappropriately adjacent coding sequences, making them more sensitive for gene fusions. In addition, the presence of the fusion transcript itself in the tumor cell provides evidence supporting functional significance.

Finally, most DNA mutations must be translated into aberrant proteins to affect cell function, so proteins are potentially better biomarkers because they are closer to cellular function. However, since currently most clinically available protein assays in oncology, such as IHC, are limited to analyzing one protein at a time, analysis of multiple expressed proteins may not be possible when tissue is limited.

Variability in sample quality due to pre-analytic factors such as biopsy method, fixative type, fixation duration, exposure to low pH, sample age, and storage conditions can impact DNA and RNA yields and quality. These factors may also cause conformational changes in proteins, altering antibody binding in IHC. Adhering to tissue handling best practices is crucial for the success of many molecular tests and precision medicine.[30] Tumor samples always contain a mixture of tumor and normal cells. For assays testing an aggregate of extracted DNA or RNA, the proportion of tumor nuclei (%TN) affects sensitivity. Estimating %TN through microscopic examination and using enrichment techniques to increase %TN are critical for optimizing assay performance.[31]

METHODOLOGIES
Common DNA Analysis Methodologies

Common methodologies in DNA analysis include in situ hybridization (ISH), PCR, and NGS.

In situ hybridization
ISH detects rearrangements, amplifications, and losses at the individual cell level using DNA probes complementary to the target gene segment. FISH, a variant of ISH, uses fluorescently tagged probes, visible under a fluorescence microscope. In gene amplification or loss assessments, the number of fluorescent signals from the gene probe binding is counted and compared with signals from a centromeric reference probe to determine gene copy number. This process distinguishes specific gene amplifications from overall chromosomal gains. For instance, patient responses in trastuzumab clinical trials for breast cancer and the Vysis HER2 FISH CDx established thresholds for both absolute *ERBB2* copy number and the *ERBB2* gene to chromosome 17 centromere ratio.[6] This threshold predicts benefit and has become the benchmark for clinically significant gene amplification.

Polymerase chain reaction in oncology
PCR is a molecular technique widely used in oncology for the sensitive, specific, and rapid amplification of nucleic acid sequences.[32] It can detect genomic alterations in a single gene or serve as a preliminary step for broader analysis. The standard PCR process involves cycles of temperature changes, target-specific forward and reverse oligonucleotide primers, and a heat-stable DNA polymerase that duplicates the target sequence. Each cycle doubles the amount of targeted DNA, leading to exponential amplification.

PCR versatility extends to multiplex PCR, which targets multiple genes simultaneously, and reverse transcriptase PCR, utilized for analyzing RNA transcripts from oncogenes or fusion genes. Real-time PCR combines amplification with simultaneous detection and quantification of the PCR product through fluorescence measurement, and can provide both qualitative and quantitative data on mutant versus wild-type sequences. Digital droplet PCR (ddPCR) further refines this process, enabling more precise quantification of low-abundance nucleic acids. This precision is invaluable in assays for MRD and TRM. However, PCR limitations include the potential to miss alterations outside the amplified regions or within primer-binding sequences, and false positives due to amplification errors that mimic tumor mutations.

Next-generation sequencing
NGS uses "sequencing by synthesis,", a more advanced method than the earlier Sanger sequencing chain termination approach.[33] NGS is faster and more cost-effective per base pair sequenced, allowing for whole genome sequencing within a clinically relevant timeframe. In NGS, millions of short, single-stranded DNA fragments representing overlapping sections of the genes of interest are arrayed on a small glass flow cell surface. During sequencing, fluorescently labeled nucleotides (G, A, T, or C) are introduced sequentially. These nucleotides bind only to complementary sites at the end of the growing fragment. A high-resolution camera captures images of the fluorescent signals across the flow cell, which are compiled to reconstruct each DNA fragment's sequence.

Sophisticated computational algorithms are used in NGS to assemble the overlapping fragments of DNA sequence into entire genes. They also determine the depth of coverage, which is the frequency at which each nucleotide position is sequenced, identify deviations by comparing them to a known reference sequence, and establish the variant allele frequency (VAF). VAF is calculated by dividing the number of reads containing the variant by the total reads at that position. High unique depth of coverage is crucial for assay sensitivity, as it enables true mutations to be detected even when diluted by DNA from non-tumor components in tissue of cfDNA testing.

RNA Analysis and Sequencing

RNA sequencing (RNAseq), a technique similar to DNA sequencing, can provide important complementary information about a patient's tumor. RNA yield from different cell types is more variable than DNA, and the number of copies of each RNA varies widely based on its transcription level and stability. Gene expression of total RNA (which includes coding and noncoding messenger, ribosomal, and transfer RNA) or purified mRNA (ie, polyA RNA selected by oligo(dT)-coated beads), can be analyzed by hybridization to expression microarrays or by whole transcriptome RNAseq (WTS).[34] For RNAseq, reverse transcriptase PCR converts mRNA into a complementary, full-length, single-stranded DNA (cDNA). In WTS, this cDNA library is sequenced in its entirety. When focus on a subset of genes of interest is desired, the cDNA library can be enriched by hybrid capture or amplicon-based methods. RNAseq is capable of identifying the relative abundance of transcripts, splice variants, post-transcriptional modifications, and gene fusions within tumor tissue, which can provide additional insights into the unique biology of the patient's cancer.

Because RNA is degraded rapidly by ubiquitous RNases in tissue until they are inactivated by fixation, prompt placement of tissue in 20% neutral-buffered formalin is a must for successful RNA testing. In addition, RNAseq is even more sensitive than DNAseq to other pre-analytic variables, with prolonged tissue fixation times, exposure to low pH conditions, older sample age, suboptimal storage conditions, and handling of unstained cut sections reducing RNA yield and quality from a given sample. Unfortunately, these factors may result in some tissue samples yielding less RNA than assay input requirements or poor sequencing performance reflected in sample-specific quality control metrics and contribute to a higher RNAseq assay failure rate.

Immunohistochemistry

IHC has been a cornerstone in molecular diagnostics and precision medicine since the early 2000s. It plays a pivotal role in detecting specific proteins, such as ER in breast cancer, which guides hormonal therapies such as exemestane and fulvestrant. Similarly, detecting tyrosine-protein kinase KIT (c-KIT) overexpression in gastrointestinal stromal tumors has been critical for identifying candidates for imatinib therapy. IHC involves using antibodies to target antigens within FFPE tissue sections. The primary antibody binds to the target antigen, and a secondary antibody often linked to a fluorescent tag or an enzyme that catalyzes a chromogenic reaction, is used to detect the primary antibody. This method amplifies the signal, enhancing sensitivity and allowing for a wide variety of primary antibodies. A contrasting counterstain aids a pathologist in interpreting the staining pattern. Scoring IHC can range from a simple "positive," "negative," or "equivocal" qualitative result to a more complex semiquantitative assessment based on staining intensity and the proportion of positive tumor cells.

Programmed cell death ligand 1 immunohistochemistry complexity

Programmed cell death ligand 1 (PD-L1) IHC exemplifies the intricacies encountered when different primary antibody clones and scoring systems are developed for various anti-PD-L1 immunotherapies across cancer types.[35] In NSCLC, the Dako PD-L1 IHC 22C3 pharmDx assay employs a tumor proportion score (TPS), which is the percentage of tumor cells showing any intensity of membranous staining. A TPS over 1% is a criterion for pembrolizumab immunotherapy. The same 22C3 assay, using a combined positive score, is applied in cervical cancer, head and neck squamous cell carcinoma, esophageal squamous cell carcinoma, and TNBC, with varying thresholds for pembrolizumab eligibility. Other clones, such as PD-L1 28-8 and Ventana PD-L1 SP142, are used for different therapies in NSCLC and other cancers, each with unique scoring systems and thresholds. When only a single, generic PD-L1 option is listed on a test menu, it may mean only a single clone is available or that the laboratory will select the most appropriate clone and scoring system from those they offer based on the clinical diagnosis provided. Because these nuances can be crucial for guiding treatment decisions, clarifying your laboratory's approach and discussing cases with uncertain or rare diagnoses with the pathologist is recommended.

Limitations of immunohistochemistry

IHC faces several limitations, including complexities of multiple antibody clones for the same protein for use across the same and different tumor types, intricate scoring systems, the limited availability of reliable multiplex assays, interobserver variability in stain interpretation, and potential pre-analytic variables affecting assay sensitivity and specificity. These limitations have spurred a shift toward nucleic acid-based biomarkers, yet IHC remains a vital tool due to its accessibility, cost-effectiveness, and quick turnaround. Additionally, new IHC CDx assays for immunotherapy agents and ADCs are continuing to be developed and integrated into clinical practice.

SUMMARY

In oncology, the past 3 decades have witnessed a significant shift from the supremacy of the histopathologic diagnosis toward molecularly informed, individualized tumor classification, laying the foundation for more personalized cancer treatment. Advances in technologies such PCR, NGS, and IHC have led to widely available, clinically validated molecular tests, which are deepening our understanding of cancer at the molecular level and unlocking patient access to an increasing number of targeted treatment strategies. Clinicians now have a variety of tools to diagnose cancer and differentiate new subtypes, predict effective therapies, monitor treatment response, detect emergence of treatment resistance, and an opportunity to choose the molecular approach that fits the individual patient-specific clinical situation. Although integrating these molecular insights into clinical practice can be complex, the overarching aim is clear: to improve patient outcomes by making informed, personalized treatment decisions based on each patient's unique cancer molecular profile.

CLINICS CARE POINTS

- Pursue a Personalized Approach to Molecular Testing: Tailor the selection of molecular diagnostic tests to the individual patient's clinical scenario, considering the specific clinical question, disease stage, available samples, prior treatments, overall health status, and care goals. Choose the test that is most likely to be technically successful and will provide the most actionable and relevant information.

- Understand Limitations of Different Methodologies and the Impact of Pre-analytic Variables of Assay Performance: Recognize that no single molecular test is universally applicable to all clinical situations. Be aware of how pre-analytic variables, such as tissue handling and fixation, can impact sensitivity and specificity. Understanding limitations can help avoid misinterpretation of test results.

- Interpret Liquid Biopsy Results Carefully: Liquid biopsies have a significant potential for false negatives, especially when the circulating tumor DNA (ctDNA) fraction is below the assay's detection limit. Variants from clonal hematopoiesis can be misinterpreted as tumor-derived leading to clinical false positives. High levels of ctDNA can be associated with worse prognosis.

- Comprehensive Profiling for Diagnostic Clarity and Rare Tumors: Consider comprehensive genomic profiling (CGP) for rare tumors or when the diagnosis is unclear. CGP can reveal unique "snowflake profiles" of oncogenic drivers, aiding in accurate diagnosis and treatment selection.

DISCLOSURE

J.A. Elvin is an employee of Foundation Medicine, Inc, a wholly owned subsidiary of Roche Holdings, Inc and Roche Finance Ltd; this employee has equity interest in an affiliate of these Roche entities.

REFERENCES

1. Louis DN, Perry A, Wesseling P, et al. The 2021 WHO classification of tumors of the central nervous system: a summary. Neuro Oncol 2021;23(8):1231–51.
2. Berek JS, Matias-Guiu X, Creutzberg C, et al. FIGO staging of endometrial cancer: 2023. Int J Gynaecol Obstet 2023;162(2):383–94.
3. American College of Obstetrics and Gynecology. Updated Cervical Cancer Screening Guidelines, April 2021. Available at: https://www.acog.org/clinical/clinical-guidance/practice-advisory/articles/2021/04/updated-cervical-cancer-screening-guidelines. Accessed November 2023.
4. Jayasinghe M, Prathiraja O, Caldera D, et al. Colon cancer screening methods: 2023 update. Cureus 2023;15(4):e37509.
5. Hirahata T, Ul Quraish R, Quraish AU, et al. Liquid biopsy: a distinctive approach to the diagnosis and prognosis of cancer. Cancer Inform 2022;21. 11769351221076062.
6. Allison KH. Molecular testing in breast cancer. In: Coleman WB, Tsongalis GJ, editors. Diagnostic molecular pathology. 2nd edition. London, UK: Academic Press; 2024.
7. Mata DA, Williams EA, Sokol E, et al. Prevalence of UV mutational signatures among cutaneous primary tumors. JAMA Netw Open 2022;5(3):e223833.
8. Eskander RN, Elvin J, Gay L, et al. Unique genomic landscape of high-grade neuroendocrine cervical carcinoma: implications for rethinking current treatment paradigms. JCO Precis Oncol 2020;4(19):00248.
9. Shahi RB, De Brakeleer S, Caljon B, et al. Identification of candidate cancer predisposing variants by performing whole-exome sequencing on index patients from BRCA1 and BRCA2-negative breast cancer families. BMC Cancer 2019; 19(1):313.
10. Mateo J, Steuten L, Aftimos P, et al. Delivering precision oncology to patients with cancer. Nat Med 2022;28:658–65.
11. Suehnholz SP, Nissan MH, Zhang H, et al. Quantifying the expanding landscape of clinical actionability for patients with cancer. Cancer Discov 2024;14(1):49–65.
12. Valla V, Alzabin S, Koukoura A, et al. Companion diagnostics: state of the art and new regulations. Biomark Insights 2021;16. 11772719211047763.
13. The Role of Lab-Developed Tests in the In Vitro Diagnostics Market, Pew Trusts report, October 22, 2021. Available at: https://www.pewtrusts.org/en/research-and-analysis/reports/2021/10/the-role-of-lab-developed-tests-in-the-in-vitro-diagnostics-market. Accessed November 2023.

14. Chen H, Zhou Q. Detecting liquid remnants of solid tumors treated with curative intent: Circulating tumor DNA as a biomarker of minimal residual disease (Review). Oncol Rep 2023;49(5):106.

15. Assaf ZJF, Zou W, Fine AD, et al. A longitudinal circulating tumor DNA-based model associated with survival in metastatic non-small-cell lung cancer. Nat Med 2023;29(4):859–68.

16. Lonardi S, Nimeiri H, Xu C, et al. Comprehensive genomic profiling (CGP)-informed personalized molecular residual disease (MRD) detection: an exploratory analysis from the predator study of metastatic colorectal cancer (mCRC) patients undergoing surgical resection. Int J Mol Sci 2022;23(19):11529.

17. Vlataki K, Antonouli S, Kalyvioti C, et al. Circulating tumor DNA in the management of early-stage breast cancer. Cells 2023;12:1573.

18. Bidard FC, Hardy-Bessard AC, Dalenc F, et al. Switch to fulvestrant and palbociclib versus no switch in advanced breast cancer with rising ESR1 mutation during aromatase inhibitor and palbociclib therapy (PADA-1): a randomised, open-label, multicentre, phase 3 trial. Lancet Oncol 2022;23(11):1367–77.

19. Zheng D, Ye X, Zhang M, et al. Plasma EGFR T790M ctDNA status is associated with clinical outcome in advanced NSCLC patients with acquired EGFR-TKI resistance. Sci Rep 2016;6:20913.

20. Bayle A, Belcaid L, Palmieri LJ, et al. Circulating tumor DNA landscape and prognostic impact of acquired resistance to targeted therapies in cancer patients: a national center for precision medicine (PRISM) study. Mol Cancer 2023;22:176.

21. Zheng Y, Vioix H, Liu FX, et al. Diagnostic and economic value of biomarker testing for targetable mutations in non-small-cell lung cancer: a literature review. Future Oncol 2022;18(4):505–18.

22. Subbiah V, Wolf J, Konda B, et al. Tumour-agnostic efficacy and safety of selpercatinib in patients with RET fusion-positive solid tumours other than lung or thyroid tumours (LIBRETTO-001): a phase 1/2, open-label, basket trial. Lancet Oncol 2022;23(10):1261–73.

23. Pascual J, Attard G, Bidard F-C, et al. ESMO recommendations on the use of circulating tumour DNA assays for patients with cancer: a report from the ESMO precision medicine working group. Ann Oncol 2022;33(8):750–68.

24. Husain H, Pavlick DC, Fendler BJ, et al. Tumor fraction correlates with detection of actionable variants across > 23,000 circulating tumor DNA samples. JCO Precis Oncol 2022;6:e2200261.

25. Rolfo CD, Madison R, Pasquina LW, et al. Utility of ctDNA tumor fraction to inform negative liquid biopsy (LBx) results and need for tissue reflex in advanced non-small cell lung cancer (aNSCLC). J Clin Oncol 2023;41(16_suppl):9076.

26. Kansara M, Bhardwaj N, Thavaneswaran S, et al. Early circulating tumor DNA dynamics as a pan-tumor biomarker for long-term clinical outcome in patients treated with durvalumab and tremelimumab. Mol Oncol 2023;17(2):298–311.

27. Pellini B, Madison RW, Childress MA, et al. Circulating tumor DNA monitoring on chemo-immunotherapy for risk stratification in advanced non-small cell lung cancer. Clin Cancer Res 2023;29(22):4596–605.

28. Ptashkin RN, Mandelker DL, Coombs CC, et al. Prevalence of clonal hematopoiesis mutations in tumor-only clinical genomic profiling of solid tumors. JAMA Oncol 2018;4(11):1589–93.

29. Marshall CH, Gondek LP, Luo J, et al. Clonal hematopoiesis of indeterminate potential in patients with solid tumor malignancies. Cancer Res 2022;82(22):4107–13.

30. Hussain M, Corcoran C, Sibilla C, et al. Tumor genomic testing for >4,000 men with metastatic castration-resistant prostate cancer in the phase III trial profound (Olaparib). Clin Cancer Res 2022;28(8):1518–30.
31. Mata DA, Harries L, Williams EA, et al. Method of tissue acquisition affects success of comprehensive genomic profiling in lung cancer. Arch Pathol Lab Med 2023;147(3):338–47.
32. Shen CH. Amplification of nucleic acids. In: Coleman WB, Tsongalis GJ, editors. *Diagnostic molecular biology.* 2nd edition. San Diego, CA: Academic Press; 2023.
33. Shiau CJ, Tsao MS. Molecular testing in lung cancer. In: Coleman WB, Tsongalis GJ, editors. *Diagnostic molecular pathology.* 2nd edition. Cambridge, MA: Academic Press; 2024.
34. Shen CH. Genome and transcriptome analysis. In: Coleman WB, Tsongalis GJ, editors. *Diagnostic molecular biology.* 2nd edition. Oxford, UK: Academic Press; 2023.
35. Hayes DF, Herbst RS, Myles JL, et al. Proceedings from the ASCO/college of american pathologists immune checkpoint inhibitor predictive biomarker summit. JCO Precis Oncol 2022;6:e2200454.

Cost-Effectiveness and the Economics of Genomic Testing and Molecularly Matched Therapies

Sudeep Banerjee, MD, MAS

KEYWORDS

- Cost-effectiveness analysis • Clinical decision analysis • Precision medicine
- Next-generation sequencing • Genetic testing • Matched therapy
- Targeted therapy • Personalized therapy

KEY POINTS

- Cost-effectiveness analysis is a rigorous methodology to compare cost, quality of life, and outcomes, including overall survival, among comparable interventions.
- Next-generation sequencing can be cost-effective compared with single gene testing by reducing the need for multiple individual genetic tests and reducing time to diagnosis.
- Genomic profiling can provide information that promotes value-driven therapy, particularly when biomarkers predict poor response to traditional therapies potentially decreasing the use of futile treatments.
- Strongly driven by the high cost associated with newer targeted therapies rather than the cost of genomic profiling, some biomarker-guided matched therapies may not be cost-effective at present.

INTRODUCTION

The pace of cancer drug development is staggering. In 2020, 57 new anticancer drugs or expanded indications received the US Food and Drug Administration (FDA)-approval compared with just 8 approvals in 2009.[1] Along with this, total cancer expenditures continue to increase with estimated cancer drug-related costs of US$18.6 billion in 2015 to US$20.9 billion in 2020 in the United States.[2] Although the increasing cost of treatment is accepted as the inevitable outcome of medical advancement, the question of benefit is increasingly important when considering the future of novel therapeutics. A study of all FDA-approved drugs for solid tumors from 2002 through 2014 found that

Division of Colorectal Surgery, Department of General Surgery, Kaiser Permanente San Jose Medical Center, Kaiser Permanente Northern California, 280 Hospital Parkway, Building B, San Jose, CA 95119, USA
E-mail address: sudeep.banerjee@kp.org
Twitter: @SBanerjeeMD (S.B.)

Surg Oncol Clin N Am 33 (2024) 231–242
https://doi.org/10.1016/j.soc.2023.12.010
1055-3207/24/© 2023 Elsevier Inc. All rights reserved.

surgonc.theclinics.com

median gains in progression-free survival were 2.5 months and overall survival (OS) was 2.1 months.[3] Although this improvement may be statistically significant, the small magnitude of the difference underscores the importance of considering value in oncology.

One major advantage of precision oncology is using biomarker-guided targeted therapy to avoid overtreatment of patients who are unlikely to benefit from a given drug. This paradigm is compelling from a cost standpoint by theoretically minimizing the use of expensive treatment(s) in those least likely to derive benefit. In the last decade, several trials have explored the utility of molecular-guided therapy. In single-agent trials, matching rates ranged widely from 5% to 44% in the MOSCATO (Molecular Screening for Cancer Treatment Optimization (MOSCATO-01) in Pediatric Patients), WINTHER (Worldwide Innovative Network Consortium Trial), and IMPACT (Initiative for Molecular Profiling and Advanced Cancer Therapy) trials.[4–6] A multiagent personalized approach was used in the I-PREDICT (Investigation of Profile-Related Evidence Determining Individualized Cancer Therapy) trial with a match rate of 49%.[7] Despite these promising approaches, the value of precision oncology remains firmly driven by the cost of therapy. As such, it is critically important to identify the clinical scenarios where precision oncology can be considered cost-effective in order to inform future drug development and clinical use.

The objectives of this article are to provide a brief primer on the methodology of cost-effectiveness and its application to molecularly matched therapy. We will examine the cost-effectiveness of traditional single gene testing compared with multigene next-generation sequencing (NGS) panels. We will review the data on cost-effectiveness analysis of targeted therapy emphasizing the clinical situations where molecularly matched therapy provides benefit. Finally, we will consider further avenues of inquiry that may provide insight into ways that cost-effectiveness analysis can influence the delivery of precision oncology.

A PRIMER ON COST EFFECTIVENESS ANALYSIS

Cost-effectiveness analysis (CEA) is a methodological approach that compares relative survival, quality of life, and cost among interventions. There are several important aspects of CEA, which must be defined to understand the state of cost-effectiveness in targeted cancer therapy. Cost-effectiveness is always approached from a particular viewpoint or perspective, which can vary in scope. Examples of these perspectives include the patient, doctor, hospital, payer, or society. The perspective from which CEA is performed will determine the types of costs that are included in the model. For instance, a payer perspective may include reimbursement costs to an insurance company whereas a societal perspective can include costs such as lost productivity from time away from work.

Quality of life in cost-effectiveness is measured in health utility, which ranges from 0 (death) to 1 (perfect health). Health utilities are usually defined by primary studies or empirically through survey data. Quality-adjusted life year (QALY) refers to health utility during 1 year. For example, median literature QALY values after the following health conditions were as follows: myocardial infarction, 0.86; stroke, 0.64; and dialysis, 0.56.[8] Costs included in a model are that of a given intervention as well as costs of downstream consequences such as adverse effects or complications. Additionally, every CEA must be performed with a particular timeline during which QALYs and costs are estimated. This timeline depends on the scope of the model and can be as short as a few months to a lifetime. The length of the timeline generally depends on the risk of a particular outcome and the prognosis associated with a disease. For instance, if a person remains at a high risk for cancer recurrence for a 20-year period, a 5-year horizon may be inadequate for capturing all relevant risks.

Within a CEA model, health states are defined which signify various stages of disease progression. For example, newly diagnosed cancer, remission, and metastasis all represent individual disease states. The relationships between disease states are represented in a state transition diagram (**Fig. 1**). Probabilities of transitioning between disease states are an important aspect of modeling that is extracted from literature values such as clinical trial data. These probabilities include values such as OS, disease-free survival, or probability of an adverse event. Probability of disease state transitions is usually time dependent because the likelihood of disease progression may change in the years following treatment.

Cost-effectiveness modeling is performed through the construction of a decision analytical tree that provides a framework for progression through various disease states. Each model integrates the costs of intervention, risks of transition between disease states, QALYs associated with each disease state and the survival after a particular intervention. There are various approaches in which such a model can be analyzed such as microsimulation, Markov modeling, and probabilistic sensitivity analysis (**Fig. 2**). The details of these are beyond the scope of this discussion but each will provide insight on the relative cost-effectiveness of comparative interventions.

One common metric for measuring value in cost-effectiveness is through a ratio of the difference in QALYs divided by the difference in cost of 2 interventions. This ratio is known as the incremental cost-effectiveness ratio (ICER). Interventions that result in a large improvement in QALYs with a small increase in cost are considered cost-effective (**Fig. 3**). As the cost of health care has increased over time, the generally accepted threshold for a cost-effective intervention has changed. This number is known as the "willingness-to-pay" value and currently, US$100,000/QALY is a well-accepted threshold although some would argue that a higher value is justified based on inflation over time.[9–11]

The outcome of a given CEA model provides important data of whether an intervention may be considered cost-effective. However, sensitivity analyses provide an additional level of granularity about what factors are most important in a certain clinical situation. By varying parameters within the model and evaluating the change to the ICER, a model can reveal the variables that are most impactful. Additionally, unusual sensitivity analysis results may also suggest that assumptions within the model introduced bias or did not accurately reflect the clinical scenario.

COST-EFFECTIVENESS IN PRECISION ONCOLOGY

The major challenge of cost-effectiveness with regard to new therapy is cost. Drug pricing for new therapies must factor in years of research and development as well as risk associated with novel therapeutics. As such, new targeted agents are often

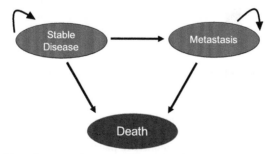

Fig. 1. State transition diagram after new diagnosis of cancer.

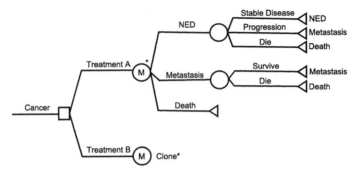

Fig. 2. Representative Markov model decision tree (based on TreeAge Pro). Model for new diagnosis of cancer followed by risk of stable disease (NED: no evidence of disease), disease progression and death after treatment A or treatment B. M-nodes signify Markov nodes. Clone* replicates the referenced tree.

among the most expensive available therapies. The cost effectiveness of targeted therapy is frequently well outside the standard willingness-to-pay threshold.[12] For example, among patients with metastatic colorectal cancer (CRC), regorafenib (approved in patients who have progressed on standard chemotherapy) is associated

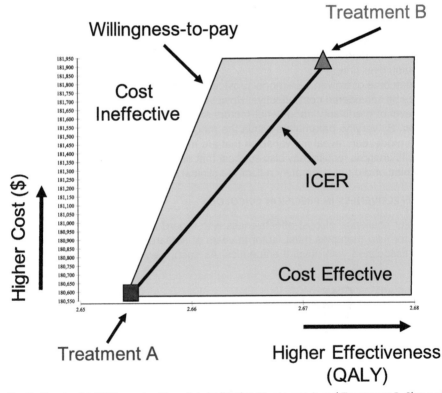

Fig. 3. Graph of QALY by cost with points indicating Treatment A and Treatment B. Slope of the line between Treatment A and Treatment B signifies the ICER. Shaded green area refers to interventions that fall within the willingness-to-pay threshold. The figure has been modified with permission from Dr. James Murphy.

with an ICER of US$900,000/QALY, whereas bevacizumab is associated with an ICER of US$571,240/QALY as first-line therapy.[13,14] Treatment of human epidermal growth factor receptor 2 (HER2)-positive metastatic breast cancer with pertuzumab was associated with an ICER of US$472,668/QALY.[15] Despite these costs, one important benefit of precision oncology is to mitigate these overwhelming costs through a biomarker-informed approach.

There are many aspects of precision oncology that have been examined through the lens of cost-effectiveness, which will be reviewed herein. First, single gene PCR testing is increasingly compared with NGS multigene panels as the preferred diagnostic approach to obtain biomarker data. Next, biomarker-informed matched targeted therapy is compared with standard of care treatment across various cancer types. Finally, the cost-effectiveness of expanded indications for germline genetic testing (ie, in suspected hereditary cancer syndromes or universal testing for any patient with cancer) is compared with no testing or selective testing.

Cost-Effectiveness of Genetic Testing

Options for genetic testing in clinical oncology have rapidly expanded in the last decade. Single gene tests remain frequently used when specific actionable mutations are clinically relevant. Multigene testing refers to genetic panels of relevant genes for a given disease process and use NGS techniques. In some diagnostic approaches, single gene tests can trigger sequential testing, which can dramatically increase the time to diagnosis compared with NGS.[16] Although NGS panels are more expensive, there is increasing evidence that cumulative cost of multiple single gene tests and time required for serial testing favors multigene panels.

In a validated model based on a Spanish referral center population, single gene testing for non-small cell lung carcinoma (NSCLC) was compared with NGS. NGS yielded a higher rate of actionable mutations and had higher QALYs than single gene testing. In this study, the ICER was found to be highly cost-effective at €25,895/QALY. This model was most sensitive to the cost of targeted therapy and the cost of second-line therapy.[17] In another study, a decision analytical model was used to compare various single gene testing strategies to NGS among patients with metastatic NSCLC. Single gene tests included exclusionary, sequential, and hotspot testing approaches. In this model, NGS was faster than exclusionary and sequential testing by 2.7 and 2.8 weeks, respectively. NGS was also found to be cost saving from both Medicare & Medicaid Centers for Medicare & Medicaid Services (CMS) and commercial payers in the United States perspective compared with all single gene testing strategies.[18]

By contrast, Presley and colleagues found that NGS in the community setting did not show an improvement in survival compared with routine epidermal growth factor receptor (EGFR) and/or anaplastic lymphoma kinase (ALK) testing in patients with NSCLC. The authors found that less than 5% of patients who underwent NGS had actionable mutations other than EGFR/ALK. In this study, the authors argued that earlier studies, which found NGS to be cost-effective, did not account for differential immunotherapy between the groups. Immunotherapy treatment is informed by programmed cell death protein 1 (PD-1) expression rather than the results from NGS so it was not considered informed by genomic profiling.[19] Although context dependent, these studies all demonstrate that a higher rate identifying actionable mutations increases the cost-effectiveness of NGS compared with single gene testing.

Cost-Effectiveness of Biomarker-Informed Targeted Therapy

The appeal of precision oncology is to partially alleviate drug cost by tailoring use of targeted therapy to individuals who are most likely to benefit from a given drug. This is accomplished through genomic testing followed by biomarker-guided therapy selection.

In a model of metastatic NSCLC, comprehensive genomic profiling and single gene panel testing were compared with no tumor profiling. Patients who underwent tumor profiling received targeted therapy if an actionable mutation was identified, whereas those who did not undergo profiling received either chemotherapy or immunotherapy. In this model, the ICER associated with single gene testing was US$310,735/QALY, whereas comprehensive molecular testing was even less cost-effective with an ICER of US$445,545/QALY. Threshold analysis showed that 72% and 80% price reductions in both osimertinib and alectinib resulted in cost-effectiveness of single gene testing and comprehensive genomic profiling, respectively.[20]

Another study explored the cost-effectiveness of adjuvant therapy options in *BRAF*-mutated stage III melanoma. The targeted *BRAF* inhibitor dabrafenib-trametinib, was compared with immunotherapy (ipilimumab, nivolumab, or pembrolizumab) or no therapy using a Markov model. This study showed that *BRAF* inhibition was cost-effective compared with no treatment (ICER: US$95,758/QALY) but less cost-effective than the most effective immunotherapy drug (pembrolizumab, ICER: US$285,863/QALY). This model was sensitive to the cost of targeted therapy, which was US$66,000 more expensive than pembrolizumab.[21]

Similarly, in platinum-resistant ovarian cancer, genomic-based testing followed by biomarker-guided therapy was compared with standard of care cytotoxic chemotherapy. *BRCA* altered, *NF1*-mutant, HER2-positive and phosphoinositide 3-kinase (PI3K)/RAS alterations were matched with targeted agents. Through this approach, genomic-based testing and matched therapy was cost-ineffective with an ICER of US$479,303/QALY. The model was sensitive to the cost of targeted therapy and largely unaffected by the cost of genomic testing and the probability of identifying a target alteration. In threshold analysis, a reduction in 56% of the cost of targeted therapy made genomic profiling and matched therapy cost-effective.[22]

Banerjee and colleagues developed a model to examine the cost-effectiveness of genetic testing with tailored first-line therapy compared with empiric low-dose imatinib for all newly diagnosed patients with metastatic gastrointestinal stromal tumor (GIST). The study was predicated on the knowledge that patients with *KIT* exon 9 mutation do not respond to low-dose imatinib, which is frequently the starting treatment of unselected patients. The model found that genetic testing paired with selective use of high-dose imatinib among patients with *KIT* exon 9 mutant GIST was cost effective compared with empiric low-dose imatinib therapy with an ICER of US$92,100/QALY **(Table 1)**.[23]

Overall, biomarker-informed targeted therapy remains beyond typical willingness-to-pay thresholds. This is strongly influenced by the cost of the targeted therapy. Although the use of biomarkers to guide therapy selection improves the value of treatment compared with the unselected approach, there still needs to be improvement in managing drug costs to make this approach favorable from a cost-effectiveness standpoint.

Cost-Effectiveness of Biomarker-Informed Tailored Therapy

Beyond matched targeted therapy, there are several treatment approaches that are modified based on the information gained from genomic profiling. *KRAS* testing in patients with CRC is a prognostic marker for poor response to EGFR inhibitor therapy. Behl and colleagues compared *KRAS/BRAF* testing followed by selective cetuximab use with best supportive care for patients with metastatic CRC and found an ICER of US$648,396/QALY. They also found that anti-EGFR therapy without testing compared

Table 1
Selected cost-effectiveness analyses for biomarker-informed matched therapy

Article	Disease	Intervention	Reference	Horizon	ICER	Outcome
Dong et al,[20] 2022	NSCLC	Comprehensive genomic profiling (CPG) or single gene testing (SGT) followed by anti-EGFR therapy	Chemotherapy or immunotherapy	Lifetime	CGP: US$445,545/QALY SGT: US$310,735/QALY	Matched targeted therapy was not cost-effective. Drug cost reduction of 72%–80% is required to make targeted therapy cost-effective
Mojtahed et al,[21] 2021	Melanoma	BRAF-mutant testing followed by dabrafenib-trametinib	Immunotherapy (ipilimumab, nivolumab, or pembrolizumab)	Lifetime	vs Pembrolizumab: US$285,863/QALY	Matched targeted therapy was not cost-effective compared with best immunotherapy
Wallbillich et al,[22] 2016	Ovarian	NGS followed by BRCA, NF1, HER2, or PI3K/RAS targeted therapy	Chemotherapy	1 y	US$479,303/QALY	Matched targeted therapy was not cost-effective compared with standard of care chemotherapy
Banerjee et al,[23] 2020	GIST	NGS followed by high-dose imatinib (800 mg) for KIT exon 9 mutant GIST	Low-dose imatinib (400 mg)	10 y	US$92,100/QALY	Tailored first-line therapy after genetic testing was cost-effective for newly diagnosed patients with metastatic GIST

Abbreviations: CGP, comprehensive genomic profiling; GIST, gastrointestinal stromal tumor; ICER, incremental cost-effectiveness ratio; NGS, next generation sequencing; NSCLC, non-small cell lung carcinoma; QALY, quality-adjusted life year; SGT, single gene testing.

with *KRAS* testing with selective cetuximab use had an ICER of US$2,932,767/QALY. Although biomarker-informed therapy had superior effectiveness, the increased cost was not within the usual willingness-to-pay threshold.[24] Contrastingly, a systematic review of all studies on *KRAS* testing in metastatic CRC found that 4 out of 6 studies favor cost-effectiveness with ICERs of €62,653/QALY and US$42,701/QALY. ICERs were not reported in the remaining studies.[25–29] The most likely reason that Behl and colleagues found *KRAS* testing to be cost-ineffective is that this model included the cost of resection of metastases and recurrence after resection, which was not included in other studies. Overall, these data support the use of *KRAS/BRAF* testing from a cost-effectiveness perspective.

Another demonstrative example of biomarker-informed therapy is an economic evaluation of surgical and endoscopic therapies for early CRC. In this study, researchers classified early CRC into 6 biomarker profiles based on differential adenomatous polyposis coli (*APC*), *TP53*, and BRAFV600 E mutations. Endoscopic therapy was associated with the highest QALYs and was more cost-effective than open or laparoscopic surgery among the 4 least aggressive risk profiles. In the 2 most aggressive biomarker profiles, laparoscopic colectomy was associated with the highest QALYs but exceeded the cost-effectiveness threshold with ICERs of US$113,290/QALY and US$178,765/QALY. As such, endoscopic treatment was the preferred cost-effective approach for all early stage CRC.[30] Although cost-effective, substantial clinical validation is required before endoscopic treatment of CRC can be considered a safe approach suitable for widespread adoption.

Cost-Effectiveness of Hereditary and Universal Cancer Genetic Testing

A unique application of genetic testing in cancer occurs in the setting of hereditary cancer syndromes. Gallego and colleagues considered the immediate and downstream cost implications of NGS testing compared with routine immunohistochemistry in patients referred to a cancer genetics clinic for evaluation of Lynch syndrome. They found that NGS testing including a panel of highly penetrant genes for colorectal polyposis syndromes was cost-effective with an ICER of US$36,500/QALY. This model was sensitive to the number of relatives at risk for a given proband and the penetrance of CRC among individuals with high-risk genetic mutations. The cost of NGS testing did influence the model but to a far lesser degree than the impact of the downstream familial testing in the model.[31]

Cost-effectiveness of universal germline testing for patients with cancer is a topic of increasing interest as more genetic determinants of cancer are identified. In a study examining universal testing of patients with pancreatic cancer, universal testing was compared with selective, family history-based testing and was associated with ICER of US$121,924/QALY.[32] Interestingly, this study was published 2 years after the National Comprehensive Cancer Network (NCCN) guidelines introduced the recommendation for universal germline testing for patients with pancreatic cancer.[33] CEA of universal *BRCA1/BRCA2/PALB2* testing among new patients with breast cancer compared with only patients with family history of disease showed that universal testing was cost-effective (ICER: US$65,661/QALY from a payer perspective and US$61,618/QALY from the societal perspective).[34]

THE CHALLENGE OF DRUG COST

There are many applications where precision oncology is already cost-effective. However, matched targeted therapy remains highly cost-ineffective and the fundamental challenge is drug cost. The cost of novel therapeutics is increasingly expensive and an often-cited reason is the cost of research and development (R&D) including the cost of failed drugs. However, the true cost of R&D is an elusive value and experts suggest that drug prices are far more strongly driven by usual market forces including the availability of alternatives, value provided to a patient, and what the patient is willing to pay.[35]

Marketing also has an important role in drug price. The development of imatinib was a milestone in the history of targeted therapy and is a life-saving medication. However, the price of Gleevec (imatinib) demonstrates the complexity of drug price. In 2016, the generic version of imatinib was made available. Despite this competitor, the cost of Gleevec remained high and increased for several years after the patent expiration. This was attributed to initial generic market exclusivity that was priced only 30% lower than brand name imatinib. Additionally, the manufacturer of Gleevec (Novartis, Basel, Switzerland) developed a second-generation tyrosine kinase inhibitor, nilotinib, which was heavily marketed to patients with chronic myelogenous leukemia as first-line therapy.[36] Similarly, drug competition between pharmaceutical companies is thought to favor lowering drug prices but, unfortunately, the opposite is often the case. So-called Me-Too drug development has been shown to maintain high drug prices while offering marginal therapeutic benefits.[3]

SUMMARY

In the United States, cost-effectiveness analysis pays a far lesser role in policy than in the other countries with national health systems, such as the United Kingdom. As such, standard-of-care therapies are often well beyond usual willingness-to-pay thresholds. In fact, many NCCN recommendations and widely implemented clinical practices do not meet the stringent criteria of traditional cost-effectiveness analysis. However, the value of cost-effectiveness in the United States is to identify influential factors that can be improved to provide value-based care.

A 2018 study found that the proportion of patients who are eligible for genomic-informed therapy was 15% of which only 5% were expected to benefit from matched therapy.[37] One innovative solution to this problem was described by Lu and colleagues who proposed a "Collaborative Model" for biomarker-dependent drug trials by population screening. In comparison to the current model, where clinical trials use NGS paired with a particular targeted therapy, in the Collaborative Model, population-level trials can capture a larger number of patients and provide biomarker data for multiple trials.[38] Trial design such as this may be one solution to substantially reduce the burden of genomic profiling on a single clinical trial.

Although there are many barriers to the cost-effectiveness of matched therapy, the yield of genomic profiling will only increase as more targeted therapies become available and new biomarkers for existing therapy are identified. Because the health-care system in the United States is placed under increasing economic scrutiny, cost-effectiveness analyses offer valuable insights about how to ensure that value-based therapy is prioritized in the future of precision oncology approaches.

CLINICS CARE POINTS

- Next-generation sequencing panels can provide a cost-effective alternative to single gene tests and should be increasingly considered for biomarker testing.
- Biomarker-informed targeted therapy is frequently cost-ineffective due to the high cost of novel precision therapy drugs.

- Withholding ineffective therapy in a biomarker-informed manner is nearly always cost-effective.
- As more actionable biomarkers are identified in various tumor types, univerisal genetic testing for patient's with cancer is increasingly cost-effective and utilized.

DISCLOSURE

The author has nothing to disclose.

REFERENCES

1. Olivier T, Haslam A, Prasad V. Anticancer drugs approved by the us food and drug administration from 2009 to 2020 according to their mechanism of action. JAMA Netw Open 2021;4(12):e2138793.
2. Mariotto AB, Robin Yabroff K, Shao Y, et al. Projections of the cost of cancer care in the United States: 2010-2020. J Natl Cancer Inst 2011;103(2):117–28.
3. Fojo T, Mailankody S, Lo A. Unintended consequences of expensive cancer therapeutics - the pursuit of marginal indications and a me-too mentality that stifles innovation and creativity: the john conley lecture. JAMA Otolaryngol - Head Neck Surg 2014;140(12):1225–36.
4. Massard C, Michiels S, Ferté C, et al. High-throughput genomics and clinical outcome in hard-to-treat advanced cancers: results of the MOSCATO 01 trial. Cancer Discov 2017;7(6):586–95.
5. Rodon J, Soria JC, Berger R, et al. Genomic and transcriptomic profiling expands precision cancer medicine: the WINTHER trial. Nat Med 2019;25(5): 751–8.
6. Tsimberidou A-M, Hong DS, Ye Y, et al. Initiative for molecular profiling and advanced cancer therapy (IMPACT): an MD anderson precision medicine study. JCO Precis Oncol 2017;1:1–18.
7. Sicklick JK, Kato S, Okamura R, et al. Molecular profiling of cancer patients enables personalized combination therapy: the I-PREDICT study. Nat Med 2019; 25(5):744–50.
8. Institute for Clinical Research and Health Policy Studies. Tufts Medical Center. Center for the Evaluation of Value and Risk in Health. The Cost-Effectiveness Analysis Registry.
9. Schultz BG, Tilton J, Jun J, et al. Cost-effectiveness analysis of a pharmacist-led medication therapy management program: hypertension management. Value Heal 2021;24(4):522–9.
10. Chiang CL, Chan SK, Lee SF, et al. Cost-effectiveness of pembrolizumab as a second-line therapy for hepatocellular carcinoma. JAMA Netw Open 2021;4(1): e2033761.
11. Vijenthira A, Kuruvilla J, Crump M, et al. Cost-effectiveness analysis of frontline polatuzumab-rituximab, cyclophosphamide, doxorubicin, and prednisone and/or second-line chimeric antigen receptor t-cell therapy versus standard of care for treatment of patients with intermediate- to high-risk diffuse large b-cell lymphoma. J Clin Oncol 2023;41(8):1577–89.
12. Aguiar PN, Haaland B, Park W, et al. Cost-effectiveness of osimertinib in the first-line treatment of patients with EGFR-mutated advanced non-small cell lung cancer. JAMA Oncol 2018;4(8):1080–4.

13. Goldstein DA, Chen Q, Ayer T, et al. First- and second-line bevacizumab in addition to chemotherapy for metastatic colorectal cancer:a United States-based cost-effectiveness analysis. J Clin Oncol 2015;33(10):1112–8.

14. Goldstein DA, Ahmad BB, Chen Q, et al. Cost-effectiveness analysis of regorafenib for metastatic colorectal cancer. J Clin Oncol 2015;33(32):3727–32.

15. Durkee BY, Qian Y, Pollom EL, et al. Cost-effectiveness of pertuzumab in human epidermal growth factor receptor 2-positive metastatic breast cancer. J Clin Oncol 2016;34(9):902–9.

16. Payne K, Gavan SP, Wright SJ, et al. Cost-effectiveness analyses of genetic and genomic diagnostic tests. Nat Rev Genet 2018;19(4):235–46.

17. Arriola E, Bernabé R, Campelo RG, et al. Cost-effectiveness of next-generation sequencing versus single-gene testing for the molecular diagnosis of patients with metastatic non–small-cell lung cancer from the perspective of spanish reference centers. JCO Precis Oncol 2023;7. https://doi.org/10.1200/po.22.00546.

18. Pennell NA, Mutebi A, Zhou Z-Y, et al. Economic impact of next-generation sequencing versus single-gene testing to detect genomic alterations in metastatic non–small-cell lung cancer using a decision analytic model. JCO Precis Oncol 2019;3:1–9.

19. Presley CJ, Tang D, Soulos PR, et al. Association of broad-based genomic sequencing with survival among patients with advanced non-small cell lung cancer in the community oncology setting. JAMA 2018;320(5):469–77.

20. Dong OM, Poonnen PJ, Winski D, et al. Cost-effectiveness of tumor genomic profiling to guide first-line targeted therapy selection in patients with metastatic lung adenocarcinoma. Value Heal 2022;25(4):582–94.

21. Mojtahed SA, Boyer NR, Rao SA, et al. Cost-effectiveness analysis of adjuvant therapy for BRAF-mutant resected stage III melanoma in medicare patients. Ann Surg Oncol 2021;28(13):9039–47.

22. Wallbillich JJ, Forde B, Havrilesky LJ, et al. A personalized paradigm in the treatment of platinum-resistant ovarian cancer - A cost utility analysis of genomic-based versus cytotoxic therapy. Gynecol Oncol 2016;142(1):144–9.

23. Banerjee S, Kumar A, Lopez N, et al. Cost-effectiveness analysis of genetic testing and tailored first-line therapy for patients with metastatic gastrointestinal stromal tumors. JAMA Netw Open 2020;3(9):e2013565.

24. Behl AS, Goddard KAB, Flottemesch TJ, et al. Cost-effectiveness analysis of screening for KRAS and BRAF mutations in metastatic colorectal cancer. J Natl Cancer Inst 2012;104(23):1785–95.

25. Unim B, Pitini E, De Vito C, et al. Cost-effectiveness of RAS genetic testing strategies in patients with metastatic colorectal cancer: a systematic review. Value Health 2020;23(1):114–26.

26. Blank PR, Moch H, Szucs TD, et al. KRAS and BRAF mutation analysis in metastatic colorectal cancer: A cost-effectiveness analysis from a Swiss perspective. Clin Cancer Res 2011;17(19):6338–46.

27. Shiroiwa T, Motoo Y, Tsutani K. Cost-effectiveness analysis of KRAS testing and cetuximab as last-line therapy for colorectal cancer. Mol Diagn Ther 2010; 14(6):375–84.

28. Vijayaraghavan A, Efrusy MB, Göke B, et al. Cost-effectiveness of KRAS testing in metastatic colorectal cancer patients in the United States and Germany. Int J Cancer 2012;131(2):438–45.

29. Medical Advisory Secretariat. KRAS Testing for Anti-EGFR Therapy in Advanced Colorectal Cancer: An Evidence-Based and Economic Analysis. Vol 10.; 2010.

http://www.ncbi.nlm.nih.gov/pubmed/23074403%0Ahttp://www.pubmedcentral.nih.gov/articlerender.fcgi?artid=PMC3377508.

30. Jang SR, Truong H, Oh A, et al. Cost-effectiveness Evaluation of Targeted Surgical and Endoscopic Therapies for Early Colorectal Adenocarcinoma Based on Biomarker Profiles. JAMA Netw Open 2020;3(3):e1919963.

31. Gallego CJ, Shirts BH, Bennette CS, et al. Next-generation sequencing panels for the diagnosis of colorectal cancer and polyposis syndromes: a cost-effectiveness analysis. J Clin Oncol 2015;33(18):2084–91.

32. Krepline AN, Geurts JL, George B, et al. Cost-effectiveness analysis of universal germline testing for patients with pancreatic cancer. Surgery 2021;169(3):629–35.

33. Tempero MA. NCCN guidelines updates: pancreatic cancer. J Natl Compr Canc Netw 2019;17(5):603–5.

34. Manchanda R, Sun L, Brentnall A, et al. A cost-effectiveness analysis of multigene testing for all patients with breast cancer. JAMA Oncol 2019;5(12):1718–30.

35. Prasad V, De Jesús K, Mailankody S. The high price of anticancer drugs: Origins, implications, barriers, solutions. Nat Rev Clin Oncol 2017;14(6):381–90.

36. Chen CT, Kesselheim AS. Journey of generic imatinib: a case study in oncology drug pricing. J Oncol Pract 2017;13(6):352–5.

37. Marquart J, Chen EY, Prasad V. Estimation of the percentage of US patients with cancer who benefit from genome-driven oncology. JAMA Oncol 2018;4(8):1093–8.

38. Lu CY, Terry V, Thomas DM. Precision medicine: affording the successes of science. npj Precis Oncol 2023;7(1):1–8.

Tissue-Agnostic Cancer Therapy Approvals

Mohamed A. Gouda, MD, MSc[a], Vivek Subbiah, MD[b],*

KEYWORDS

- Tissue-agnostic • Selpercatinib • Dabrafenib • Trametinib • Pembrolizumab
- Dostarlimab • Entrectinib • Larotrectinib

KEY POINTS

- Tissue-agnostic cancer therapy has been transformative in the way we manage cancer.
- Cancers of different origins with shared biomarkers can be treated with personalized matched therapies independent of histology.
- To date, multiple drugs/regimens have received Food and Drug Administration approval in a tissue-agnostic indication for patients with advanced cancers.
- Early pilot studies have shown the potential benefit of neoadjuvant approaches with tissue-agnostic therapies.

INTRODUCTION

Tissue-agnostic cancer therapy represents a revolutionary paradigm shift in the field of precision oncology. Unlike traditional cancer treatments that primarily target specific tumor types based on their origin (eg, breast cancer, lung cancer, renal cell cancer, etc), tissue-agnostic therapies are histology-independent and focus on the genetic and molecular characteristics of tumors, irrespective of their tissue of origin. This innovative approach offers new hope to cancer patients, as it recognizes that the same genetic aberrations can drive cancer in multiple tissues and locations throughout the body. Over the past few years, several biomarker-driven therapeutics with pancancer tissue-agnostic efficacy have been evaluated in clinical trials and approved by the US Food and Drug Administration (FDA)[1] and the European Medicines Agency (EMA). Such drugs or regimens can be administered to patients with advanced solid tumors regardless of tissue of origin, which represents an evolutionary advance from tumor site-specific therapies that have been standard of care for decades. Those

[a] Department of Investigational Cancer Therapeutics, The University of Texas MD Anderson Cancer Center, 1515 Holcombe Boulevard, Unit 455, Houston, TX, USA; [b] Early-Phase Drug Development, Sarah Cannon Research Institute, 335 24th Avenue North Suite 300, Nashville, TN 37203, USA
* Corresponding author.
E-mail address: Vivek.Subbiah@scri.com
Twitter: @VivekSubbiah (V.S.)

Surg Oncol Clin N Am 33 (2024) 243–264
https://doi.org/10.1016/j.soc.2023.12.001
1055-3207/24/© 2023 Elsevier Inc. All rights reserved.

surgonc.theclinics.com

approvals provide alternative options for patients with advanced cancers and are paradigm shifters, especially in the context of rare malignancies or those that lack effective treatment options.[2]

To date, six drugs/regimens have been approved by the US FDA for use in patients with all solid tumors which harbor one of five biomarkers.[3-9] Herein, we review the current landscape of those tissue-agnostic cancer therapies and elaborate on relevant clinical information which can help surgical oncologists to understand better about those therapies.

CURRENT APPROVALS

The US FDA has approved six drugs/regimens for use in a tissue-agnostic manner **(Fig. 1)**. Those include larotrectinib or entrectinib in patients with *NTRK* fusions, dabrafenib plus trametinib in patients with *BRAF* V600E mutations, selpercatinib in patients with *RET* fusions, pembrolizumab in patients with high tumor mutation burden (TMB) or deficient mismatch repair (dMMR), and dostarlimab in patients with dMMR. In the following sections, we will elaborate on each of those approved drugs/regimens from a clinical perspective, recognizing that with improved theraepeutic potential, patients previously believed to be biologically or technically unresectable (or borderline resection) may have new options that can allow for multimodal treatment.

DABRAFENIB PLUS TRAMETINIB

Dabrafenib is an inhibitor of BRAF and trametinib is a MEK inhibitor, which when combined together lead to synergistic activity blocking aberrant BRAF signaling.[10]

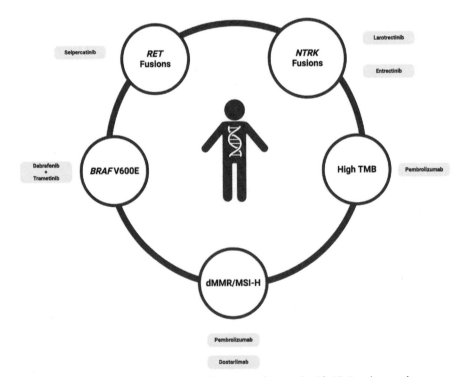

Fig. 1. Currently approved tissue-agnostic targets. (Created with BioRender.com.)

Dabrafenib plus trametinib combination is currently approved by the US FDA for the treatment of patients with advanced unresectable or metastatic solid tumors whose tumors harbor *BRAF* V600E mutations and have progressed following prior treatment with no satisfactory alternative treatment options, with the exception of patients with colorectal cancer (CRC) as discussed in a later section.[4,5] In addition to its tissue-agnostic indication, dabrafenib plus trametinib combination is approved in multiple other disease-specific indications including melanoma, non–small-cell lung cancer (NSCLC), anaplastic thyroid cancer (ATC), and pediatric low-grade glioma (LGG) **(Table 1)**.

Alteration of Interest

BRAF V600E is a MAPK pathway pathogenic alteration that leads to uncontrolled cellular growth and differentiation which is independent on upstream activation.[11,12] A prior study suggested that *BRAF* V600E is present in nearly 3% of patients in the American Association for Cancer Research (AACR) GENIE (Genomics Evidence Neoplasia Information Exchange) database pan-cancer cohort. The highest frequency of *BRAF* V600E mutation was observed in patients with thyroid cancer (40.2%), melanoma (20.3%), histiocytosis (17.3%), and CRC (7.9%). A long list of other tumor types that harbored *BRAF* V600E mutations was identified by investigators suggesting that *BRAF* V600E mutations are not infrequent.[2]

Detection of Biomarker

BRAF V600E can be detected using immunohistochemistry, polymerase chain reaction (PCR)–based technologies, and sequencing-based technologies including sanger sequencing and next-generation sequencing (NGS).[13–15] Each method will have its own advantages and disadvantages; cost-effectiveness may also play a role in assay selection especially in low-resource settings. Nevertheless, patients with advanced solid tumors should be tested for *BRAF* V600E, as such testing may confer sensitivity to a targeted therapeutic option, especially at the time of progression.[10,16]

Clinical Evidence

Registrational studies leading to approval of dabrafenib plus trametinib combination in the tissue-agnostic indications included a pooled analysis of the Rare Oncology Agnostic Research (ROAR) basket trial (NCT02034110), National Cancer Institute's Molecular Analysis for Therapy Choice (NCI-MATCH) Arm H (NCT02465060), Study X2101 (NCT02124772), and Study G2201 (NCT02684058).[4,5,17–20] The safety and effectiveness of this treatment were assessed in a group of 131 adult patients enrolled in 2 open-label basket trials known as BRF117019 (NCT02034110) and NCI-MATCH (NCT02465060), as well as in 36 pediatric patients participating in CTMT212 × 2101 (NCT02124772). These results were further substantiated by findings from the COMBI-d, COMBI-v, and BRF113928 studies which tested the combination in patients with melanoma and NSCLC. BRF117019 focused on adult patients with *BRAF* V600E mutation-positive solid tumors, which encompassed a range of conditions such as biliary tract cancers (ie, gallbladder cancer and intrahepatic/extrahepatic cholangiocarcinoma), adenocarcinoma of the small intestine, gastrointestinal stromal tumor, and ATC, as well as high-grade glioma (HGG) and LGG. Meanwhile, the NCI-MATCH Subprotocol H examined adult patients with *BRAF* V600E mutation-positive solid tumors, excluding melanoma, thyroid cancer, or CRC. In CTMT212 × 2101 trial, parts C and D of the study involved 36 pediatric patients with *BRAF* V600–refractory or *BRAF* V600–recurrent LGG or HGG.[19] The primary measure of effectiveness in these trials was the overall response rate (ORR), evaluated using standard response criteria.

Table 1
Food and Drug Administration–approved indications for tissue-agnostic drugs as of Food and Drug Administration packaging labels on October 2023

Dabrafenib and trametinib	• Patients with unresectable or metastatic melanoma with *BRAF* V600E or V600K mutations as detected by an FDA-approved test.
	• The adjuvant treatment of patients with melanoma with *BRAF* V600E or V600K mutations, as detected by an FDA-approved test, and involvement of lymph node(s), following complete resection.
	• Patients with metastatic NSCLC with *BRAF* V600E mutation as detected by an FDA-approved test.
	• Patients with locally advanced or metastatic anaplastic thyroid cancer with *BRAF* V600E mutation and with no satisfactory locoregional treatment options.
	• Adult and pediatric patients 1 year of age and older with unresectable or metastatic solid tumors with *BRAF* V600E mutation who have progressed following prior treatment and have no satisfactory alternative treatment options.
	• Pediatric patients 1 year of age and older with low-grade glioma with a *BRAF* V600E mutation who require systemic therapy.
Selpercatinib	• Adult patients with locally advanced or metastatic NSCLC with a *RET* gene fusion, as detected by an FDA-approved test.
	• Adult and pediatric patients 12 years of age and older with advanced or metastatic MTC with a *RET* mutation, as detected by an FDA-approved test, who require systemic therapy.
	• Adult and pediatric patients 12 years of age and older with advanced or metastatic thyroid cancer with a *RET* gene fusion, as detected by an FDA-approved test, who require systemic therapy and who are radioactive iodine-refractory (if radioactive iodine is appropriate)
	• Adult patients with locally advanced or metastatic solid tumors with a *RET* gene fusion that have progressed on or following prior systemic treatment or who have no satisfactory alternative treatment options.

Entrectinib

- Adult patients with ROS1-positive metastatic NSCLC as detected by an FDA-approved test.
- Adult and pediatric patients older than 1 month of age with solid tumors that have a NTRK gene fusion, as detected by an FDA-approved test without a known acquired resistance mutation, are metastatic or where surgical resection is likely to result in severe morbidity and have progressed following treatment or have no satisfactory alternative therapy.

Larotrectinib

- Adult and pediatric patients with solid tumors that have a NTRK gene fusion without a known acquired resistance mutation are metastatic or where surgical resection is likely to result in severe morbidity and have no satisfactory alternative treatments or that have progressed following treatment.

Pembrolizumab

- Melanoma
  - For the treatment of patients with unresectable or metastatic melanoma.
  - For the adjuvant treatment of adult and pediatric (12 years and older) patients with stage IIB, IIC, or III melanoma following complete resection.
- NSCLC
  - In combination with pemetrexed and platinum chemotherapy, as first-line treatment of patients with metastatic nonsquamous NSCLC, with no EGFR or ALK genomic tumor aberrations.
  - In combination with carboplatin and either paclitaxel or paclitaxel protein-bound, as first-line treatment of patients with metastatic squamous NSCLC.
  - As a single agent for the first-line treatment of patients with NSCLC expressing PD-L1 (TPS ≥1%) as determined by an FDA-approved test, with no EGFR or ALK genomic tumor aberrations, and is stage III, where patients are not candidates for surgical resection or definitive chemoradiation, or metastatic.
  - As a single agent for the treatment of patients with metastatic NSCLC whose tumors express PD-L1 (TPS ≥1%) as determined by an FDA-

(continued on next page)

Table 1
(continued)

approved test, with disease progression on or after platinum-containing chemotherapy. Patients with *EGFR* or *ALK* genomic tumor aberrations should have disease progression on FDA-approved therapy for these aberrations prior to receiving pembrolizumab.

○ For the treatment of patients with resectable (tumors ≥4 cm or node positive) NSCLC in combination with platinum-containing chemotherapy as neoadjuvant treatment, and then continued as a single agent as adjuvant treatment after surgery.

○ As a single agent, for adjuvant treatment following resection and platinum-based chemotherapy for adult patients with stage IB (T2a ≥4 cm), II, or IIIA NSCLC.

• HNSCC

○ In combination with platinum and FU for the first-line treatment of patients with metastatic or with unresectable, recurrent HNSCC.

○ As a single agent for the first-line treatment of patients with metastatic or with unresectable, recurrent HNSCC whose tumors express PD-L1 (CPS ≥1) as determined by an FDA-approved test.

○ As a single agent for the treatment of patients with recurrent or metastatic HNSCC with disease progression on or after platinum-containing chemotherapy.

• cHL

○ For the treatment of adult patients with relapsed or refractory cHL.

○ For the treatment of pediatric patients with refractory cHL, or cHL that has relapsed after 2 or more lines of therapy.

• PMBCL

○ For the treatment of adult and pediatric patients with refractory PMBCL, or who have relapsed after 2 or more prior lines of therapy.

• Urothelial carcinoma

○ In combination with enfortumab vedotin, for the treatment of adult patients with locally advanced or metastatic urothelial carcinoma who are not eligible for cisplatin-containing chemotherapy.

○ As a single agent for the treatment of patients with locally advanced or metastatic urothelial carcinoma who are not eligible for any platinum-containing chemotherapy, or who have disease progression during or following platinum-containing chemotherapy or within 12 months of neoadjuvant or adjuvant treatment with platinum containing chemotherapy.

○ As a single agent for the treatment of patients with Bacillus Calmette-Guerin-unresponsive, high-risk, non-muscle invasive bladder cancer with carcinoma in situ with or without papillary tumors who are ineligible for or have elected not to undergo cystectomy.

• MSI-H or dMMR cancer

○ For the treatment of adult and pediatric patients with unresectable or MSI-H or dMMR solid tumors, as determined by an FDA-approved test, that have progressed following prior treatment and who have no satisfactory alternative treatment options.

• MSI-H or dMMR CRC

○ For the treatment of patients with unresectable or metastatic MSI-H or dMMR CRC as determined by an FDA-approved test.

• Gastric cancer

○ In combination with trastuzumab, fluoropyrimidine-containing chemotherapy, and platinum-containing chemotherapy, for the first-line treatment of patients with locally advanced unresectable or metastatic HER2-positive gastric or GEJ adenocarcinoma.

• Esophageal cancer

○ For the treatment of patients with locally advanced or metastatic esophageal or GEJ (tumors with epicenter 1–5 cm above the GEJ) carcinoma that is not amenable to surgical resection or definitive chemoradiation either in combination with platinum-based and fluoropyrimidine-based chemotherapy, or as a single agent after one or more prior lines of systemic therapy for patients with tumors of squamous cell histology that express PD-L1 (CPS $\geq$10) as determined by an FDA-approved test.

• Cervical cancer

(continued on next page)

Table 1
(continued)

- o In combination with chemotherapy, with or without bevacizumab, for the treatment of patients with persistent, recurrent, or metastatic cervical cancer whose tumors express PD-L1 (CPS ≥1) as determined by an FDA-approved test.
- o As a single agent for the treatment of patients with recurrent or metastatic cervical cancer with disease progression on or after chemotherapy whose tumors express PD-L1 (CPS ≥1) as determined by an FDA-approved test.

- HCC
  - o For the treatment of patients with HCC who have been previously treated with sorafenib.

- MCC
  - o For the treatment of adult and pediatric patients with recurrent locally advanced or metastatic MCC.

- RCC
  - o In combination with axitinib, for the first-line treatment of adult patients with advanced RCC.
  - o In combination with lenvatinib, for the first-line treatment of adult patients with advanced RCC.
  - o For the adjuvant treatment of patients with RCC at intermediate-high or high risk of recurrence following nephrectomy, or following nephrectomy and resection of metastatic lesions.

- Endometrial carcinoma
  - o In combination with lenvatinib, for the treatment of patients with advanced endometrial carcinoma that is mismatch repair proficient as determined by an FDA-approved test or not MSI-H, who have disease progression following prior systemic therapy in any setting and are not candidates for curative surgery or radiation.
  - o As a single agent, for the treatment of patients with advanced endometrial carcinoma that is MSI-H or dMMR, as determined by an FDA-approved test who have disease progression following prior

systemic therapy in any setting and are not candidates for curative surgery or radiation.

- TMB-H Cancer
  o For the treatment of adult and pediatric patients with unresectable or metastatic TMB-H ($\geq$10 mutations/megabase) solid tumors, as determined by an FDA-approved test, that have progressed following prior treatment and who have no satisfactory alternative treatment options.
- cSCC
  o For the treatment of patients with recurrent or metastatic cSCC or locally advanced cSCC that is not curable by surgery or radiation.
- TNBC
  o For the treatment of patients with high-risk early-stage TNBC in combination with chemotherapy as neoadjuvant treatment, and then continued as a single agent as adjuvant treatment after surgery.
  o In combination with chemotherapy, for the treatment of patients with locally recurrent unresectable or metastatic TNBC whose tumors express PD-L1 (CPS $\geq$10) as determined by an FDA approved test.
- Adult classical Hodgkin lymphoma and adult primary mediastinal large b-cell lymphoma: Additional dosing regimen of 400 mg every 6 weeks
  o For use at an additional recommended dosage of 400 mg every 6 weeks for classical Hodgkin lymphoma and primary mediastinal large b-cell lymphoma in adults.

(continued on next page)

Table 1
(continued)

Dostarilmab

- Endometrial cancer
  - In combination with carboplatin and paclitaxel, followed by dostarlimab as a single agent for the treatment of adult patients with primary advanced or recurrent endometrial cancer that is dMMR, as determined by an FDA-approved test, or MSI-H.
  - As a single agent for the treatment of adult patients with dMMR recurrent or advanced endometrial cancer, as determined by an FDA-approved test, that has progressed on or following prior treatment with a platinum-containing regimen in any setting and are not candidates for curative surgery or radiation.
- dMMR recurrent or advanced solid tumors
  - As a single agent for the treatment of adult patients with dMMR recurrent or advanced solid tumors, as determined by an FDA-approved test, that have progressed on or following prior treatment and who have no satisfactory alternative treatment options.

Abbreviations: cHL, classical Hodgkin lymphoma; CPS, combined positive score; CRC, colorectal cancer; cSCC, cutaneous squamous cell carcinoma; dMMR, mismatch repair deficient; EGFR, epidermal growth factor receptor; FDA, Food and Drug Administration; GEJ, gastroesophageal junction; HCC, hepatocellular carcinoma; HNSCC, head and neck squamous cell cancer; MCC, Merkel cell carcinoma; MSI-H, microsatellite instability-high; MTC, medullary thyroid cancer; NSCLC, non-small-cell lung cancer; NTRK, neurotrophic tyrosine receptor kinase; PD-L1, programmed cell death-ligand 1; PMBCL, primary mediastinal large b-cell lymphoma; RCC, renal cell carcinoma; RET, rearranged during transfection; TMB-H, tumor mutational burden-high; TNBC, triple-negative breast cancer; TPS, Tumor Proportion Score.

Among the 131 adult patients, 41% (with a 95% confidence interval [CI] of 33% to 50%) achieved an objective response. The patient pool included 24 different tumor types. Notably, for specific tumor types, the ORR was 46% (95% CI: 31% to 61%) for biliary tract cancers, 33% (95% CI: 20% to 48%) for HGG (combined), and 50% (95% CI: 23% to 77%) for LGG (combined). As for the 36 pediatric patients, they achieved an ORR of 25% (95% CI: 12% to 42%). Moreover, 78% of these patients had a duration of response (DOR) lasting at least 6 months, and an impressive 44% experienced a DOR of at least 24 months. The accumulating evidence from all those studies has shown pan-cancer activity of dabrafenib plus trametinib in multiple cancer types.[16] It is notable that due to low response rates to BRAF and MEK inhibitor therapy, patients with CRC harboring BRAF V600 mutation were excluded in the FDA indication. Lack of response is in part due to an adaptive/innate mechanism of resistance with epidermal growth factor receptor (EGFR) activation which can be addressed by the addition of EGFR inhibitor therapy.[4,5,21,22] Therefore, BRAF V600 may still be actionable in CRC with the addition of cetuximab. In fact, another BRAF inhibitor (encorafenib) in combination with cetuximab is approved for CRC.[22]

Side Effects

Common side effects with dabrafenib and trametinib include fatigue, fever, nausea, vomiting, diarrhea, constipation, rash, chills, headache, hemorrhage, cough, myalgia, arthralgia, and edema. Less frequent but more serious side effects include secondary malignancies, gastrointestinal perforation, venous thromboembolic events, cardiomyopathy, ocular toxicities, pneumonitis, serious febrile reactions, hyperglycemia, and hemophagocytic lymphohistiocytosis.[4,5] Management with preventive measures, supportive care, and treatment modification might be warranted given the high rates of adverse events with combination therapy.[16]

Dosage

In adult patients, dabrafenib is approved for use at a dose of 150 mg orally twice daily while trametinib is approved at a dose of 2 mg orally once daily. Both drugs should be taken at the same time each day at least 1 hour before or 2 hours after a meal.[4,5] In pediatrics, dosing should be based on body weight, and oral suspension formulations are available.[4,5] Dosing modifications maybe necessary as guided by possible toxicities.[16]

SELPERCATINIB

Selpercatinib is a highly potent selective RET inhibitor that is currently approved by the US FDA for treatment of patients with advanced solid tumors with *RET* fusions who have progressed on or following prior systemic therapy or have no satisfactory alternative treatment options. In addition to its tissue-agnostic indication, selpercatinib is approved in patients with advanced NSCLC and *RET* fusion, medullary thyroid carcinoma with *RET* mutation, and advanced thyroid cancer with *RET* fusion (see **Table 1**).[3,23,24]

Alteration of Interest

RET fusions are chromosomal rearrangement of the *RET* gene which have been suggested to drive oncogenesis in a variety of tumor types.[25–30] In a prior study, *RET* fusions were identified in 1.5% of samples that were tested for structural variants and only 0.3% of the pan-cancer cohort, which highlights the importance of testing on identification of an important biomarker. *RET* fusions were most common in patients with thyroid cancer (36%) and NSCLC (5.7%), among other cancer types.[2]

Detection of Biomarker

RET fusions can be detected using immunohistochemistry, PCR-based technologies, or NGS-based technologies.[31–40] Multiple factors including cost-effectiveness, assay's sensitivity and/or specificity, and the ability to detect fusion partner may weigh in while deciding the optimum diagnostic method.[41] Nevertheless, patients with advanced solid tumors should be tested for *RET* fusions as such testing may confer sensitivity to a targeted therapeutic option, especially at the time of progression.

Clinical Evidence

LIBRETTO-001 (NCT03157128) was the registrational study leading to tissue-agnostic approval of selpercatinib.[3,42] The study was a multi-cohort study that showed pan-cancer efficacy of selpercatinib consistent with initial positive results seen in patients with *RET* fusion positive thyroid cancer and NSCLC.[42–45] The ORR was 61% in previously treated NSCLC, 84% in treatment-naïve NSCLC, 79% in previously treated thyroid cancer, and 100% in treatment-naïve thyroid cancer.[3] The ORR in cancers other than lung and thyroid was 44%. Among the tumor types enrolled, the ORR in tumor types reported included pancreatic cancer (n = 11; 55%), CRC (n = 10; 20%), and salivary gland (n = 4, 50%), among others.[42]

Side Effects

Common side effects with selpercatinib include nausea, diarrhea, constipation, edema, fatigue, dry mouth, hypertension, abdominal pain, rash, and headache. Less frequent but more serious side effects include hepatotoxicity, pneumonitis, QT interval prolongation, hemorrhagic events, hypersensitivity, tumor lysis syndrome, impaired wound healing, and hypothyroidism.[3] Recommendations for management of adverse events related to selective RET inhibitors, including selpercatinib, have been published.[46]

Dosage

Selpercatinib is approved for use at a dose of 160 mg orally twice daily in patients 50 kg or greater and 120 mg orally twice daily in patients less than 50 kg. Specific dose modifications might be necessary especially in patients with severe hepatic impairment.[3]

ENTRECTINIB

Entrectinib is a multikinase inhibitor with primary activity against TRK, ROS1, and ALK.[47] Entrectinib is currently FDA approved for adult and pediatric patients with advanced or metastatic solid tumors that harbor *NTRK* gene fusion, which have progressed following treatment or have no satisfactory alternative therapy.[9] In addition, disease-specific indication is approved in patients with NSCLC with tumors positive for ROS1 (see **Table 1**).

Alteration of Interest

NTRK fusions result from chromosomal rearrangement between one of the NTRK genes (*NTRK1*, *NTRK2*, or *NTRK3*) and a second gene, resulting in aberrant activation signal that leads to promotion of cellular growth and survival.[48–50] *NTRK* fusions are estimated to be present in nearly 1.6% of cancer specimens based on an analysis of a pan-cancer cohort in the AACR GENIE database.[2] The highest frequency of *NTRK* fusions was observed in thyroid cancer (n = 46; 17.2%) and salivary gland cancer (n = 29; 15.3%), among other cancers.[2]

Detection of Biomarker

Similar to *RET* fusions, different technologies are available for the detection of *NTRK* fusions including immunohistochemistry, fluorescence in situ hybridization, PCR-based technologies, and NGS-based technologies. Several factors may help to select the optimum approach including assay's availability, cost, turnaround time, and analytical characteristics.[51] Regardless of the method, it is important to emphasize the need to test patients with advanced solid tumors to *NTRK* fusions as those may confer sensitivity to approved TRK inhibitors.

Clinical Evidence

Data on tissue agnostic-activity of entrectinib in adults come from a pooled analysis of 3 phase 1-2 trials: ALKA-372 to 001, STARTRK-1 (NCT02097810), and STARTRK-2 (NCT02568267); while in pediatrics, data originate from STARTRK-NG (NCT02650401) and TAPISTRY (NCT04589845) trials.[9,52] Given the relatively high and durable response rate (ORR of 59% in adults and 70% in children) which was seen in patients with multiple tumor types including brain tumors and infantile fibrosarcoma, entrectinib is currently approved for patients with advanced solid tumors regardless of histology.[9]

Side Effects

The most common side effects observed with entrectinib are fatigue, nausea, vomiting, diarrhea, constipation, dysgeusia, edema, dizziness, dysesthesia, dyspnea, myalgia, cognitive impairment, increased weight, cough, pyrexia, arthralgia, and vision problems. Other less frequent but serious side effects include congestive heart failure, central nervous system (CNS) side effects, skeletal fractures, hepatotoxicity, hyperuricemia, and QT prolongation.[9]

Dosage

The currently approved dose of entrectinib is 600 mg orally once daily in adult patients while age-specific and body weight–specific dosing may be required in pediatrics.[9] Dosing modifications may be required in cases of toxicities.

LAROTRECTINIB

Larotrectinib is another small-molecule tyrosine kinase inhibitor with activity against TRK. It is currently approved for treatment of patients with advanced solid tumors which have *NTRK* gene fusion without a known resistance mutation who have progressed after prior therapy or have no satisfactory alternative treatment options.[8]

Alteration of Interest and Biomarker Detection

As discussed in the section on entrectinib, *NTRK* fusions are estimated to be prevalent in nearly 1.6% of patients with cancer. Variable methods for detection are available with different advantages and disadvantages, although testing should be done in all patients with solid tumors.[2,51]

Clinical Evidence

The pan-cancer efficacy of larotrectinib has been demonstrated in LOXO-TRK-14001 (NCT02122913), SCOUT (NCT02637687), and NAVIGATE (NCT02576431) trials. With an ORR of 75% in a pooled analysis of 55 patients with *NTRK* fusions, the FDA issued approval for the use of larotrectinib in patients with advanced solid tumors.[53,54] Intracranial activity has also been reported.

Side Effects

The most common side effects observed with larotrectinib are increased aspartate transaminase, increased alanine transaminase, increased alkaline phosphatase, anemia, leukopenia, neutropenia, lymphopenia, musculoskeletal pain, fatigue, hypoalbuminemia, cough, constipation, diarrhea, dizziness, hypocalcemia, nausea, vomiting, pyrexia, and abdominal pain. Less frequent but possibly serious side effects include CNS adverse reactions and skeletal fractures.[8]

Dosage

The recommended dose of larotrectinib is 100 mg orally twice daily. In patients with a body surface of less than 1 m^2, the dose should be adjusted to 100 mg/m^2 orally twice daily. Dose adjustment may be needed in case of toxicity.[8]

PEMBROLIZUMAB

Pembrolizumab is a monoclonal anti-programmed death receptor-1 (PD-1) antibody which blocks interaction between PD-1 receptor and PD-L1 ligand normally leading to the suppression of T-cell function; hence, enhancing immune response against cancer cells.[55] Pembrolizumab is currently approved for multiple disease indications including melanoma, NSCLC, head and neck squamous cell carcinoma, classic Hodgkin lymphoma, primary mediastinal large B-cell lymphoma, urothelial carcinoma, CRC, gastric cancer, esophageal cancer, cervical cancer, hepatocellular carcinoma (HCC), Merkel cell carcinoma, renal cell carcinoma, endometrial carcinoma, cutaneous squamous cell carcinoma, and triple-negative breast cancer (see **Table 1**). In addition, it is currently the only drug regimen with 2 tissue-agnostic indications in patients with advanced solid tumors. These include tumors with high TMB defined as greater than 10 mutations per megabase of DNA or microsatellite instability-high (MSI-H)/dMMR status.[6]

Alterations of Interest

TMB is a reflection of the magnitude of genomic instability defined by burden of mutation across the genome. Data suggest that tumors with high burden of mutations may respond better to therapies activating the immune system.[56] In a pan-cancer cohort, 20.3% of samples had high TMB status (defined as ≥10 mutations per megabase which is the current cutoff used for pembrolizumab tissue-agnostic approval). Cancers with highest frequency of high-TMB status are melanoma (49.1%), bladder cancer (38.8%), non-melanoma skin cancer (36.9%), small-cell lung cancer (35.8%), and small bowel cancer (35.3%), among other cancers.[2]

Mismatch repair (MMR) is a process for repair of DNA damage that maintains genomic integrity. Cancers deficient in MMR accumulate genetic mutations which can drive oncogenesis and associate with poor prognosis. Such hypermutational status and dMMR can also lead to missed correction of repeated multinucleotide sequences, also called microsatellites which have been implicated in the development of cancer.[57,58] It is estimated that MSI-H status is present in nearly 3% of pan-cancer samples according to meta-analysis data.[59] Highest frequencies are expected in patients with endometrial cancer and gastrointestinal cancers.[58,59]

Detection of Biomarker

TMB status can be identified based on a calculation of the number of mutations per megabase as detected in NGS. Cutoffs used for defining high, intermediate, and low status vary, although the pembrolizumab approval was based on data suggesting that tumors with TMB of 10 or more would show favorable response to treatment with immunotherapy.[6,56,60,61]

MSI/MMR status can be detected using either testing for relevant genetic alterations in MMR genes (eg, *MSH2*, *MLH1*, *PMS2*, and *MSH6*) via NGS, although complex, or, more commonly, indirect detection of protein expression using immunohistochemistry or PCR-based detection. Other methods may be available although less frequently applied in clinical practice.[57,62,63]

Clinical Evidence

The pan-cancer efficacy of pembrolizumab in patients with TMB high cancers was demonstrated based on data from the KEYNOTE-158 trial (NCT02628067) which showed an ORR of 29% across multiple tumor types when using cutoff of 10 mutations per megabase. Similarly, the pan-cancer efficacy of pembrolizumab in patients with MSI-H/dMMR cancers was demonstrated based on data from multiple trials including KEYNOTE-164 (NCT02460198), KEYNOTE-158 (NCT02628067), and KEYNOTE-051 (NCT02332668). The ORR in pooled analysis was 33.3% with a median DOR of 63.2 months.[6]

Side Effects

The most common side effects observed with pembrolizumab monotherapy are fatigue, musculoskeletal pain, rash, pruritis, nausea, diarrhea, constipation, pyrexia, dyspnea, cough, decreased appetite, pain including abdominal pain, and hypothyroidism. Guidelines for management of immune-related adverse events have been published by different societies.[64–66]

Dosage

Pembrolizumab is given in intravenous infusion of 200 mg every 3 weeks or 400 mg every 6 weeks. In pediatric patients with TMB-high cancers, the dose is 2 mg/kg (up to 200 mg) every 3 weeks.[6] Dosing modifications might be needed.

DOSTARLIMAB

Dostarlimab is an anti-PD-1 monoclonal antibody that promotes immune response against cancer cells by blocking the PD-1/PD-L1 interaction.[67] Dostarlimab is currently approved as a single agent for treatment of adult patients who have dMMR recurrent or advanced solid tumors which have progressed after prior therapy and have no alternative satisfactory treatment options. In addition to its tissue-agnostic indication, dostarlimab have a disease-specific indication for patients with advanced dMMR endometrial cancer[7] (see **Table 1**).

Alteration of Interest and Detection of Biomarker

As discussed with pembrolizumab, the most common methods for detection of dMMR status are immunohistochemistry and PCR. Other methods may be available although less established.[57,62,63]

Clinical Evidence

The pan-cancer efficacy of dostarlimab was demonstrated as part of the GARNET trial (NCT02715284) which showed an ORR of 41.6% in 209 patients with advanced solid tumors that had dMMR.[7,68]

Side Effects

The most common side effects observed with dostarlimab are fatigue, anemia, diarrhea, and nausea. Immune-mediated side effects have been reported, and guidelines exist for their management.[64–66]

Dosage

The current approved dose for dostarlimab is 500 mg every 3 weeks for 4 doses followed by 1000 mg every 6 weeks given as intravenous infusion over 30 minutes.[7] Dosing modifications might be needed in patients with toxicities.

EMERGING TISSUE-AGNOSTIC THERAPIES

The current approvals only represent the beginning of the revolution in tissue-agnostic precision therapies for cancer. For example, promising pan-cancer efficacy data were reported recently with adagrasib in patients with KRAS G12C cancers.[69] Similarly, erdafitinib showed responses across 16 distinct tumor types with FGFR alterations.[70] Trastuzumab deruxtecan showed tissue-agnostic activity in patients with HER2-overexpressing tumors.[71] In addition, zenocutuzumab showed activity across patients with different types of NRG fusion positive cancers.[72] TP53 Y220 C mutations appear as a possible additional tissue-agnostic target with responses seen with PC14586, a small molecule corrector of Y220 C mutant p53.[73] ALK fusions are also potentially tissue-agnostic targets given cumulative evidence from multiple trials with ALK inhibitors[74]

Belzutifan, a hypoxia-inducible factor inhibitor, was approved in adult patients with germline von Hippel-Lindau (VHL)–driven positive malignancies that could arguably be called tumor agnostic in the germline setting.[75] VHL disease is known to be linked with the development of both benign and malignant neoplasms, encompassing conditions such as clear-cell renal cell carcinoma, pancreatic neuroendocrine tumors, as well as hemangioblastomas found in the CNS and retina. In addition, pemigatinib has been approved for FGFR1-rearranged myeloid neoplasms which is a hematological tissue–agnostic targeted therapy.[76,77]

SURGICAL CONSIDERATIONS

As highlighted in prior sections, some complications of tissue-agnostic therapies may require surgical interventions (eg, perforations and skeletal fractures). Those complications should be managed according to standard surgical management algorithms given the lack of specific recommendations.

Wound healing may be a concern during the use of dabrafenib/trametinib combination or selpercatinib due to the antiangiogenic effects of trametinib and/or selpercatinib. The recommendation for selpercatinib is to hold the drug for 5 to 7 days prior to and 2 weeks after a planned major surgical procedure.[46] In the case of dabrafenib/trametinib, trametinib may need to be held 5 to 7 days prior to surgery while dabrafenib can be continued until the day of surgery.[78]

NEOADJUVANT USE OF TISSUE-AGNOSTIC THERAPIES

The use of tissue-agnostic therapies in the neoadjuvant setting might have a compelling rationale. Primarily, immunotherapy fosters a more robust immune response against a diverse array of antigens, enhancing the tumor-antigen load. Its efficacy is heightened by circumventing immunosuppression, preventing potential impediments such as postsurgical glucocorticoid secretion, which may otherwise compromise immune cell dynamics.[79] The intact structure of the lymphatic system under neoadjuvant conditions facilitates superior interaction between immune cells and the tumor microenvironment. Moreover, neoadjuvant immunotherapy proves cost-effective with fewer doses required, diminishing the possibility of resistance due to limited exposure. Its patient-friendly regimen enhances compliance, and it serves as a platform for biomarker development and a deeper comprehension of the underlying mechanisms of action, marking a paradigm shift in cancer therapeutics. Pembrolizumab, administered neoadjuvantly in cancers characterized by dMMR or MSI-H, has demonstrated both safety and remarkable outcomes.[80] The neoadjuvant intervention yielded high rates of pathologic, radiographic, and endoscopic response, thereby presenting significant considerations for the implementation of organ-sparing therapeutic approaches.[80]

Beyond immunotherapy, neoadjuvant therapy with other tissue-agnostic agents have been explored in some pilot studies and this is an emerging area, given that patients are sequenced earlier at diagnosis. It offers several advantages such as those discussed earlier. For example, neoadjuvant dabrafenib/trametinib regimen has been used in patients with *BRAF* V600E–mutated anaplastic thyroid carcinoma and has demonstrated feasibility of complete resection, decreased need for tracheostomy, high pathologic response rates, and durable locoregional control with symptom amelioration.[78] Similarly, selpercatinib has been used as a neoadjuvant therapy in patients with advanced thyroid cancer with *RET* alterations.[81,82] The use of larotrectinib has also been reported in the neoadjuvant setting of children with locally advanced *TRK* fusion positive sarcomas.[83] For children with locally advanced *TRK* fusion sarcomas, the prospect of surgical resection posttreatment with the selective TRK inhibitor, larotrectinib, emerges as an exciting option offering hope. This alternative avenue not only showcases promising outcomes but also offers a potential reprieve from the substantial morbidity associated with existing modalities. The findings from the neoadjuvant study with larotrectinib underscore the feasibility and efficacy of utilizing larotrectinib as a presurgical therapeutic intervention for children with newly diagnosed *TRK* fusion sarcomas. The implication of this approach goes beyond mere treatment; it signals a paradigm shift in the management of such pediatric malignancies (and adults), suggesting a path that holds promise for both clinical efficacy and a reduction in the adverse impacts of conventional treatments.

SUMMARY

The current approvals represent only the beginning of the era of tissue-agnostic precision therapies. The genomic revolution has led to an increased understanding of oncogenic alterations, cancer biology, and molecular pathways. It is increasingly evident that biomarkers are shared across multiple tumor types and are not restricted to one histology. Simultaneously, the exponential increase in the discovery of targeted therapies, immunotherapies, and antibody-drug conjugates to target these aberrant pathways across tumor types opens up options to expand therapeutic choices and expedite drug development. Tissue-agnostic drug development is also increasingly important for rare cancers that would otherwise not have access to alternative therapies. Early anecdotal and pilot studies have shown the potential benefit of neo-adjuvant approaches with tissue-agnostic therapies. As more biomarkers are unraveled and more drugs are developed, the field is poised for further expansion. Finally, in diseases where drugs were generally ineffective or where surgical interventions had limited roles, it remains to be determined whether these new and highly active drugs will have roles in the neoadjuvant setting to convert unresectable to resectable disease or in the adjuvant setting to decrease the risk of recurrence. Further trials are warranted to investigate these unanswered questions.

DISCLOSURE

MG declares no conflicts of interest. VS reports Scientific Advisory board participation (Funding to institution) Relay therapeutics, Pheon therapeutics, Incyte, Novartis, Eli Lilly/ Loxo Oncology, Roche, Pfizer, Bayer, ABBVIE, Regeneron, Clinical Care Communications, PERS (CME fees for education).

REFERENCES

1. Zettler ME. FDA approvals of oncology drugs for tissue-agnostic indications. Target Oncol 2023;18(5):777–92.
2. Gouda MA, Nelson BE, Buschhorn L, et al. Tumor-Agnostic Precision Medicine from the AACR GENIE Database: Clinical Implications. Clin Cancer Res 2023; 29(15):2753–60.
3. RETEVMO® (selpercatinib) capsules, for oral use: FDA Packaging Insert.
4. TAFINLAR® (dabrafenib) capsules, for oral use. FDA Packaging Insert; 2022.
5. MEKINIST® (trametinib) tablets, for oral use. FDA Packaging Insert; 2022.
6. KEYTRUDA® (pembrolizumab) injection, for intravenous use. FDA Packaging insert; 2022.
7. JEMPERLI (dostarlimab-gxly) injection, for intravenous use. FDA Packaging Insert; 2022.
8. VITRAKVI® (larotrectinib) capsules, for oral use. FDA Packaging Insert; 2022.
9. ROZLYTREK (entrectinib) capsules, for oral use. FDA Packaging Insert; 2022.
10. Gouda MA, Subbiah V. Precision Oncology for BRAF Mutant Cancers with BRAF and MEK inhibitors: From Melanoma to Tissue-agnostic therapy. ESMO Open 2023;8:100788.
11. Ascierto PA, Kirkwood JM, Grob JJ, et al. The role of BRAF V600 mutation in melanoma. J Transl Med 2012;10:85.
12. Davies H, Bignell GR, Cox C, et al. Mutations of the BRAF gene in human cancer. Nature 2002;417(6892):949–54.
13. Martins-de-Barros AV, Anjos RSD, Silva CCG, et al. Diagnostic accuracy of immunohistochemistry compared with molecular tests for detection of BRAF V600E mutation in ameloblastomas: Systematic review and meta-analysis. J Oral Pathol Med 2022;51(3):223–30.
14. Vanni I, Tanda ET, Spagnolo F, et al. The Current State of Molecular Testing in the BRAF-Mutated Melanoma Landscape. Front Mol Biosci 2020;7:113.
15. Zhao J, Liu P, Yu Y, et al. Comparison of diagnostic methods for the detection of a BRAF mutation in papillary thyroid cancer. Oncol Lett 2019;17(5):4661–6.
16. Gouda MA, Subbiah V. Expanding the Benefit: Dabrafenib/Trametinib as Tissue-Agnostic Therapy for BRAF V600E-Positive Adult and Pediatric Solid Tumors. Am Soc Clin Oncol Educ Book 2023;43:e404770. https://doi.org/10.1200/EDBK_404770.

17. Salama AKS, Li S, Macrae ER, et al. Dabrafenib and Trametinib in Patients With Tumors With BRAF(V600E) Mutations: Results of the NCI-MATCH Trial Subprotocol H. J Clin Oncol 2020;38(33):3895–904.

18. Geoerger B, Bouffet E, Whitlock JA, et al. Dabrafenib plus trametinib combination therapy in pediatric patients with BRAF V600-mutant low-grade glioma: Safety and efficacy results. J Clin Oncol 2020;38(15).

19. FDA grants accelerated approval to dabrafenib in combination with trametinib for unresectable or metastatic solid tumors with BRAF V600E mutation. https://www.fda.gov/drugs/resources-information-approved-drugs/fda-grants-accelerated-approval-dabrafenib-combination-trametinib-unresectable-or-metastatic-solid.

20. Bouffet E, Geoerger B, Moertel C, et al. Efficacy and safety of trametinib monotherapy or in combination with dabrafenib in pediatric BRAF V600-mutant low-grade glioma. J Clin Oncol 2022. https://doi.org/10.1200/JCO.22.01000. JCO2201000.

21. Tian J, Chen JH, Chao SX, et al. Combined PD-1, BRAF and MEK inhibition in BRAF(V600E) colorectal cancer: a phase 2 trial. Nat Med 2023. https://doi.org/10.1038/s41591-022-02181-8.

22. BRAFTOVI® (encorafenib) capsules, for oral use. FDA Packaging Insert; 2022.

23. Brandhuber B, Haas J, Tuch B, et al. The development of a potent, KDRNEGFR2-sparing RET kinase inhibitor for treating patients with RET-dependent cancers. European Journal of Cancer 2016;69:S144.

24. Subbiah V, Velcheti V, Tuch BB, et al. Selective RET kinase inhibition for patients with RET-altered cancers. Ann Oncol 2018;29(8):1869–76.

25. Drilon A, Hu ZI, Lai GGY, et al. Targeting RET-driven cancers: lessons from evolving preclinical and clinical landscapes. Nat Rev Clin Oncol 2018;15(3):151–67.

26. Arighi E, Borrello MG, Sariola H. RET tyrosine kinase signaling in development and cancer. Cytokine Growth Factor Rev Aug-Oct 2005;16(4–5):441–67.

27. Jhiang SM. The RET proto-oncogene in human cancers. Oncogene 2000;19(49):5590–7.

28. Donis-Keller H, Dou S, Chi D, et al. Mutations in the RET proto-oncogene are associated with MEN 2A and FMTC. Hum Mol Genet 1993;2(7):851–6.

29. Hofstra RM, Landsvater RM, Ceccherini I, et al. A mutation in the RET proto-oncogene associated with multiple endocrine neoplasia type 2B and sporadic medullary thyroid carcinoma. Nature 1994;367(6461):375–6.

30. Mulligan LM, Kwok JB, Healey CS, et al. Germ-line mutations of the RET proto-oncogene in multiple endocrine neoplasia type 2A. Nature 1993;363(6428):458–60.

31. Belli C, Penault-Llorca F, Ladanyi M, et al. ESMO recommendations on the standard methods to detect RET fusions and mutations in daily practice and clinical research. Ann Oncol 2021;32(3):337–50.

32. Lipson D, Capelletti M, Yelensky R, et al. Identification of new ALK and RET gene fusions from colorectal and lung cancer biopsies. Nat Med 2012;18(3):382–4.

33. Wang R, Hu H, Pan Y, et al. RET fusions define a unique molecular and clinicopathologic subtype of non-small-cell lung cancer. J Clin Oncol 2012;30(35):4352–9.

34. Platt A, Morten J, Ji Q, et al. A retrospective analysis of RET translocation, gene copy number gain and expression in NSCLC patients treated with vandetanib in four randomized Phase III studies. BMC Cancer 2015;15:171.

35. Tsuta K, Kohno T, Yoshida A, et al. RET-rearranged non-small-cell lung carcinoma: a clinicopathological and molecular analysis. Brit J Cancer 2014;110(6):1571–8.

36. Go H, Jung YJ, Kang HW, et al. Diagnostic method for the detection of KIF5B-RET transformation in lung adenocarcinoma. Lung Cancer 2013;82(1):44–50.

37. Cheng TY, Cramb SM, Baade PD, et al. The International Epidemiology of Lung Cancer: Latest Trends, Disparities, and Tumor Characteristics. J Thorac Oncol. Oct 2016;11(10):1653–71.

38. Nikiforov YE. Thyroid carcinoma: molecular pathways and therapeutic targets. Mod Pathol. May 2008;21(Suppl 2):S37–43.

39. Mizukami T, Shiraishi K, Shimada Y, et al. Molecular mechanisms underlying oncogenic RET fusion in lung adenocarcinoma. J Thorac Oncol. May 2014;9(5):622–30.

40. Ferrara R, Auger N, Auclin E, et al. Clinical and Translational Implications of RET Rearrangements in Non-Small Cell Lung Cancer. J Thorac Oncol. Jan 2018;13(1):27–45.

41. Gouda MA, Subbiah V. Precision oncology with selective RET inhibitor selpercatinib in RET-rearranged cancers. Ther Adv Med Oncol 2023;15. https://doi.org/10.1177/17588359231177015. 17588359231177015.

42. Subbiah V, Wolf PJ, Konda B, et al. Tumour-agnostic efficacy and safety of selpercatinib in patients with RET fusion-positive solid tumours other than lung or thyroid tumours (LIBRETTO-001): a phase 1/2, open-label, basket trial. Lancet Oncol 2022. https://doi.org/10.1016/s1470-2045(22)00541-1.

43. Drilon A, Oxnard GR, Tan DSW, et al. Efficacy of Selpercatinib in RET Fusion-Positive Non-Small-Cell Lung Cancer. New Engl J Med 2020;383(9):813–24.

44. Drilon A, Subbiah V, Gautschi O, et al. Selpercatinib in patients with RET fusion-positive non-small-cell lung cancer: updated safety and efficacy from the registrational LIBRETTO-001 phase I/II Trial. J Clin Oncol 2022. https://doi.org/10.1200/JCO.22.00393. JCO2200393.

45. Wirth LJ, Sherman E, Robinson B, et al. Efficacy of selpercatinib in RET-altered thyroid cancers. New Engl J Med 2020;383(9):825–35.

46. Nardo M, Gouda MA, Nelson BE, et al. Strategies for Mitigating Adverse Events Related to Selective RET Inhibitors in Patients with RET-altered Cancers. Cell Reports Medicine 2023. in press.

47. Khotskaya YB, Holla VR, Farago AF, et al. Targeting TRK family proteins in cancer. Pharmacol Therapeut 2017;173:58–66.

48. Cocco E, Scaltriti M, Drilon A. NTRK fusion-positive cancers and TRK inhibitor therapy. Nat Rev Clin Oncol 2018;15(12):731–47.

49. Knezevich SR, McFadden DE, Tao W, et al. A novel ETV6-NTRK3 gene fusion in congenital fibrosarcoma. Nat Genet 1998;18(2):184–7.

50. Amatu A, Sartore-Bianchi A, Siena S. NTRK gene fusions as novel targets of cancer therapy across multiple tumour types. ESMO Open 2016;1(2):e000023.

51. Nguyen MA, Colebatch AJ, Van Beek D, et al. NTRK fusions in solid tumours: what every pathologist needs to know. Pathology 2023;55(5):596–609.

52. Doebele RC, Drilon A, Paz-Ares L, et al. Entrectinib in patients with advanced or metastatic NTRK fusion-positive solid tumours: integrated analysis of three phase 1-2 trials. Lancet Oncol 2020;21(2):271–82.

53. Hong DS, DuBois SG, Kummar S, et al. Larotrectinib in patients with TRK fusion-positive solid tumours: a pooled analysis of three phase 1/2 clinical trials. Lancet Oncol 2020;21(4):531–40.

54. Scott LJ. Larotrectinib: First Global Approval. Drugs 2019;79(2):201–6.

55. Kwok G, Yau TC, Chiu JW, et al. Pembrolizumab (Keytruda). Hum Vaccin Immunother 2016;12(11):2777–89.
56. Fusco MJ, West HJ, Walko CM. Tumor Mutation Burden and Cancer Treatment. JAMA Oncol 2021;7(2):316.
57. Li K, Luo H, Huang L, et al. Microsatellite instability: a review of what the oncologist should know. Cancer Cell Int 2020;20:16.
58. Bonneville R, Krook MA, Kautto EA, et al. Landscape of Microsatellite Instability Across 39 Cancer Types. JCO Precis Oncol 2017;2017doi. https://doi.org/10.1200/PO.17.00073.
59. Kang YJ, O'Haire S, Franchini F, et al. A scoping review and meta-analysis on the prevalence of pan-tumour biomarkers (dMMR, MSI, high TMB) in different solid tumours. Sci Rep-Uk 2022;12(1):20495.
60. Galuppini F, Dal Pozzo CA, Deckert J, et al. Tumor mutation burden: from comprehensive mutational screening to the clinic. Cancer Cell Int 2019;19:209.
61. Subbiah V, Solit DB, Chan TA, et al. The FDA approval of pembrolizumab for adult and pediatric patients with tumor mutational burden (TMB) >/=10: a decision centered on empowering patients and their physicians. Ann Oncol 2020;31(9):1115–8.
62. Dedeurwaerdere F, Claes KB, Van Dorpe J, et al. Comparison of microsatellite instability detection by immunohistochemistry and molecular techniques in colorectal and endometrial cancer. Sci Rep-Uk 2021;11(1):12880.
63. Gilson P, Merlin JL, Harle A. Detection of Microsatellite Instability: State of the Art and Future Applications in Circulating Tumour DNA (ctDNA). Cancers 2021;24(7):13.
64. Schneider BJ, Naidoo J, Santomasso BD, et al. Management of Immune-Related Adverse Events in Patients Treated With Immune Checkpoint Inhibitor Therapy: ASCO Guideline Update. J Clin Oncol 2021;39(36):4073–126.
65. Pavlick AC, Ariyan CE, Buchbinder EI, et al. Society for Immunotherapy of Cancer (SITC) clinical practice guideline on immunotherapy for the treatment of melanoma, version 3.0. J Immunother Cancer 2023;(10):11. https://doi.org/10.1136/jitc-2023-006947.
66. Haanen J, Obeid M, Spain L, et al. Management of toxicities from immunotherapy: ESMO Clinical Practice Guideline for diagnosis, treatment and follow-up. Ann Oncol 2022;33(12):1217–38.
67. Costa B, Vale N. Dostarlimab: A Review. Biomolecules 2022;12(8). https://doi.org/10.3390/biom12081031.
68. FDA grants accelerated approval to dostarlimab-gxly for dMMR advanced solid tumors. https://www.fda.gov/drugs/resources-information-approved-drugs/fda-grants-accelerated-approval-dostarlimab-gxly-dmmr-advanced-solid-tumors.
69. Bekaii-Saab TS, Yaeger R, Spira AI, et al. Adagrasib in Advanced Solid Tumors Harboring a KRAS(G12C) Mutation. J Clin Oncol 2023;41(25):4097–106.
70. Pant S, Schuler M, Iyer G, et al. Erdafitinib in patients with advanced solid tumours with FGFR alterations (RAGNAR): an international, single-arm, phase 2 study. Lancet Oncol 2023;24(8):925–35.
71. Meric-Bernstam F, Makker V, Oaknin A, et al. Efficacy and Safety of Trastuzumab Deruxtecan in Patients With HER2-Expressing Solid Tumors: Primary Results From the DESTINY-PanTumor02 Phase II Trial. J Clin Oncol 2023. https://doi.org/10.1200/JCO.23.02005. 101200JCO2302005.
72. Schram AM, Goto K, Kim D-W, et al. Efficacy and safety of zenocutuzumab, a HER2 x HER3 bispecific antibody, across advanced NRG1 fusion (NRG1+) cancers. J Clin Oncol 2022;40(16_suppl):105.

73. Dumbrava EE, Johnson ML, Tolcher AW, et al. First-in-human study of PC14586, a small molecule structural corrector of Y220C mutant p53, in patients with advanced solid tumors harboring a TP53 Y220C mutation. J Clin Oncol 2022; 40(16_suppl):3003.

74. Shreenivas A, Janku F, Gouda MA, et al. ALK fusions in the pan-cancer setting: another tumor-agnostic target? npj Precis Oncol 2023;7(1):101.

75. FDA approves belzutifan for cancers associated with von Hippel-Lindau disease. https://www.fda.gov/drugs/resources-information-approved-drugs/fda-approves-belzutifan-cancers-associated-von-hippel-lindau-disease.

76. FDA approves pemigatinib for relapsed or refractory myeloid/lymphoid neoplasms with FGFR1 rearrangement.

77. Gotlib J, Kiladjian J-J, Vannucchi A, et al. A Phase 2 Study of Pemigatinib (FIGHT-203; INCB054828) in Patients with Myeloid/Lymphoid Neoplasms (MLNs) with Fibroblast Growth Factor Receptor 1 (FGFR1) Rearrangement (MLN FGFR1). Blood 2021;138(Supplement 1):385.

78. Wang JR, Zafereo ME, Dadu R, et al. Complete Surgical Resection Following Neoadjuvant Dabrafenib Plus Trametinib in BRAF(V600E)-Mutated Anaplastic Thyroid Carcinoma. Thyroid 2019;29(8):1036–43.

79. Bilusic M. What are the advantages of neoadjuvant immunotherapy over adjuvant immunotherapy? Expert Rev Anticancer Ther 2022;22(6):561–3.

80. Ludford K, Ho WJ, Thomas JV, et al. Neoadjuvant Pembrolizumab in Localized Microsatellite Instability High/Deficient Mismatch Repair Solid Tumors. J Clin Oncol 2023;41(12):2181–90.

81. Contrera KJ, Gule-Monroe MK, Hu MI, et al. Neoadjuvant Selective RET Inhibitor for Medullary Thyroid Cancer: A Case Series. Thyroid 2023;33(1):129–32.

82. Jozaghi Y, Zafereo M, Williams MD, et al. Neoadjuvant selpercatinib for advanced medullary thyroid cancer. Head Neck 2021;43(1):E7–12.

83. DuBois SG, Laetsch TW, Federman N, et al. The use of neoadjuvant larotrectinib in the management of children with locally advanced TRK fusion sarcomas. Cancer 2018;124(21):4241–7.

Immuno-Oncology
New Insights into Targets and Therapies

Shiruyeh Schokrpur, MD, PhD[a], Michael G. White, MD, MSc[b],
Christina L. Roland, MD, MS[c], Sandip Pravin Patel, MD[a],*

KEYWORDS

- Immunotherapy • Perioperative therapy • Cancer vaccine • Cytokine therapy
- Viral therapy

KEY POINTS

- Neoadjuvant and adjuvant immune checkpoint blockade has demonstrated efficacy in several cancer types and has been implemented into treatment guidelines.
- Emerging agents have been designed to target additional immune checkpoints on various lymphocyte populations in order to enhance immunotherapy responses.
- Vaccines delivered through mRNA, dendritic cells, or through peptides, cytokines, and cellular therapies are additional areas of promising investigation.
- More studies and innovative treatment approaches are needed for advancing the intersection of immunotherapy and surgical oncology.

INTRODUCTION

Over a decade since the first reports of the clinical efficacy of immune checkpoint inhibitors, these immune-based treatments continue to disrupt the oncology space for medical and surgical oncologists alike. Initially applied to patients with metastatic disease, responses to immunotherapy across select cancer histologies have been impressive and continue to improve. As we begin to better understand the biology of these various disease processes, we can also better predict those tumors that will respond to therapy. As such, immunotherapy regimens have been increasingly studied and applied to curative intent surgical procedures. This has come with, at times, impressive response rates, including many patients demonstrating a complete response at the time of surgical resection.[1–6] Moreover, neoadjuvant or window of opportunities treatment strategies offer important clinical insights into the mechanisms of

[a] Division of Hematology/Oncology, Department of Medicine, University of California, San Diego, 3855 Health Sciences Drive, La Jolla, CA 92037, USA; [b] Department of Colon & Rectal Surgery, The University of Texas MD Anderson Cancer Center, 1400 Pressler Street, Unit 1401, Houston, TX 77030, USA; [c] Department of Surgical Oncology, The University of Texas MD Anderson Cancer Center, 1400 Pressler St, Unit 1401, Houston, TX 77030, USA
* Corresponding author.
E-mail address: patel@ucsd.edu

Surg Oncol Clin N Am 33 (2024) 265–278
https://doi.org/10.1016/j.soc.2023.12.006
1055-3207/24/© 2023 Elsevier Inc. All rights reserved.

action of these medications. They also provide opportunities to identify biomarkers for better patient selection for enrollment in these trials, as well as future adoption of standard or care therapies.

The initial targets of these therapies that "take the brakes off the body's immune response" included the inhibition of programmed death ligand 1 (PD-L1) and cytotoxic T-lymphocyte associated protein 4 (CTLA-4). Both of these allowed for immune killing of tumor cells identified as nonself that previously evaded normal immune surveillance. These therapies have since been paired with cytotoxic chemotherapies, radiation therapy, anticancer vaccines, and other novel treatment modalities. Because the utilization of these tools becomes more ubiquitous, new agents, and new combinatorial therapies are becoming increasingly used in the neoadjuvant and adjuvant settings to augment curative intent surgical resection. The first iteration of these therapies has been approved by the US Food and Drug Administration (FDA) and well integrated into clinical guidelines such as those of the National Comprehensive Cancer Network. However, a new wave of these studies are either reaching completion or actively accruing surgical oncology patients. Here, we review ongoing efforts to define optimal immuno-oncology treatment paradigms for these patients including the use of novel therapies or combination approaches. This study will provide a contemporary guide for surgical oncologists looking to understand the landscape of these trials and drug mechanisms of action under active investigation.

EXISTING APPROVED PERIOPERATIVE IMMUNOTHERAPIES

Although most immunotherapies have been studied in the metastatic setting, the success of these trials has led to the study and approval of several agents in the perioperative setting. To date these approved uses are limited, in large part, due to the challenge of demonstrating improved efficacy of surgical resection. Nevertheless, efficacy and approval has been achieved in select patients with non-small cell lung cancer (NSCLC), renal cell carcinoma (RCC), urothelial carcinoma, melanoma, triple negative breast cancer (TNBC), colon cancer including mismatch repair deficient (dMMR), or esophageal/esophagogastric junction cancer (**Table 1**).

Importantly, the use of immunotherapies in curative intent procedures such as primary tumor resections, multivisceral resections of locally advanced disease, or in patients undergoing curative intent metastasectomy must be weighed against the potential for disease progression while on these therapies, as well as the potential for toxicities that could limit their ability to safely tolerate an operation. As such, a clear benefit to these patient populations must be demonstrated. Similarly, although neoadjuvant therapy has been increasingly adopted due to noted benefits in defining disease response to therapy, downsizing tumors, and/or improving disease-specific survival in several therapies, identification of which patients will benefit from adjuvant therapy after surgery is not completely understood, especially in patients whom all measurable disease has been resected. As an example, in a study on the use of adjuvant atezolizumab in urothelial carcinoma, patients noted to have positive circulating tumoral DNA (ctDNA) after resection did show a benefit with the addition of adjuvant atezolizumab, whereas there was no clear benefit found in the overall cohort following curative intent resection.[7] The use of adjuvant immunotherapies, as is true with all adjuvant therapies, should be prescribed in a thoughtful and patient-directed manner. Given the success of these agents in the perioperative setting, several ongoing studies are underway studying novel approaches to further improve responses in resected solid tumors. Moreover, existing and future biomarkers will play an important role in these treatment decisions.

Table 1
Food and Drug Administration-approved perioperative immunotherapy regimens

Perioperative	Tumor Type	Phase	Trial	Drug	Stage/Risk
Adjuvant (Completely resected disease)	NSCLC	III	KEYNOTE-091[43]	Pembrolizumab	IB–IIIA
	NSCLC	III	IMPower10[44]	Atezolizumab	IB–IIIA
	RCC	III	KEYNOTE-564[45]	Pembrolizumab	Intermediate-high or high-risk s/p nephrectomy/metastectomy
	Urothelial carcinoma	III	CheckMate-274[46]	Nivolumab	High-risk
	Melanoma	III	KEYNOTE-716[47]	Pembrolizumab	IIB–IIC
	Melanoma	III	CheckMate-238[48]	Nivolumab	Lymph nodes involvement or metastatic disease
	Melanoma	III	CheckMate-76K[49]	Nivolumab	IIB–IIC
	Melanoma	II	IMMUNED[50]	Nivolumab + Ipilimumab	Metastatic
	Melanoma	III	CheckMate-238[48,51]	Nivolumab	IIIB–IIIC or IV
	Melanoma	III	KEYNOTE-054[52,53]	Pembrolizumab	III
	Esophageal or GEJ	III	CheckMate-577[54]	Nivolumab	Residual pathologic disease following chemoradiation
Neoadjuvant (Completely resectable disease)	NSCLC	III	CheckMate 816[55]	Nivolumab + chemotherapy	IB–IIIA
	TNBC	III	KEYNOTE-522[56]	Pembrolizumab + chemotherapy	II–III
	Melanoma	II	SWOG1801[57]	Pembrolizumab	High-risk IIIB–IV without brain metastases
	Melanoma	IB/II	OpACIN[58] OpACIN-neo[58] PRADO[59]	Nivolumab + Ipilimumab	III (macroscopic)
	Colon cancer	II	NICHE[60]	Nivolumab + Ipilimumab	I–III
	Colon cancer	II	NICHE-2[61]	Nivolumab + Ipilimumab	I–III (dMMR)

Colors denoted different categories within a column, such as tumor type, trial phase, or treatment.

NEWER CHECKPOINT INHIBITORS

With the success of agents targeting the PD-1 and CTLA-4 immune checkpoints, there has been a drive to seek additional opportunities to unleash the adaptive immune response. Agents targeting additional checkpoints, such as lymphocyte activation gene 3 (LAG-3), T cell immunoreceptor with Ig and ITIM domains (TIGIT), and killer Ig-like receptor 2DL1/2L3 (KIR2DL1/2L3), are actively being explored in the adjuvant, neoadjuvant, and/or perioperative space.

Lymphocyte Activation Gene 3

LAG-3 is a transmembrane protein found on various lymphocytes, including CD8+, CD4+, natural killer (NK), natural killer T, and regulatory T cells.[8] LAG-3 binds major histocompatibility complex class II (MHC-II) and inhibits the activation of lymphocytes through the interaction of MHC-II and CD4/T cell receptor complex (TCR), thereby preventing lymphocyte activation.[9] Its expression in tumors is associated with tumor progression and poor prognosis in numerous tumor types, implicating it as a viable immune checkpoint to target clinically.[10–12] Notably, combined targeting of the LAG-3 and PD-1 immune checkpoints has shown to have a synergistic effect in an in vitro assay of interleukin-2 (IL-2) production, with levels 5-fold higher than either agent alone.[13] The addition of LAG-3 inhibition to PD-1 blockade improved responses in several murine cancer models.[14,15] In line with these findings, relatlimab, a monoclonal antibody targeting LAG-3, has been approved in the treatment of metastatic melanoma in combination with nivolumab based on its demonstrated improvement in progression-free survival (PFS) compared with nivolumab monotherapy in the RELATIVITY-047 trial.[16] The efficacy of this combination is now being evaluated in the adjuvant setting following resection of stage III-IV melanoma (RELATIVITY-098, NCT05002569). This phase III trial randomized patients to receive either relatlimab plus nivolumab or nivolumab alone following complete surgical resection of their disease. The primary endpoint for this study is PFS and is actively recruiting patients.

Relatlimab is also being assessed in the neoadjuvant management of NSCLC in an ongoing trial.[17] This phase II trial randomizes stage IB-IIIA patients to receive either relatlimab plus nivolumab or nivolumab alone as neoadjuvant therapy. The primary endpoint was the number of patients who underwent curative resection within 43 days of initiation of systemic treatment. All 60 patients were able to undergo surgery within this time frame. Ninety-five percent of patients achieved an R0 resection. Complete or major histopathological response was observed in 30% of the combination group and 27% of the monotherapy group. Overall survival (OS) at 12 months was 96% (95% CI, 83%–99%) in both arms. Future assessment of this survival will reveal if there is a benefit of adding LAG-3 inhibition in this context.

T Cell Immunoglobin and Immunoreceptor Tyrosine-based Inhibitory Motif Domain

TIGIT is another transmembrane protein expressed on various lymphocyte populations, including activated CD4+, CD8+, NK, and Treg cells.[18] Antigen presenting cells, such as dendritic cells, express poliovirus receptor, or CD155, which binds TIGIT. This binding leads to diminished TCR expression, increased IL-10, and reduced IL-12p40, mediating an immunosuppressive effect.[19] Furthermore, TIGIT expression in Treg cells inhibits Th1 and Th17 responses important for effective antitumor immunity.[20] Preclinical studies support a synergistic antitumor effect of blocking TIGIT and PD-1 immune checkpoints.[21] Neoadjuvant tiragolumab, a monoclonal antibody targeting TIGIT, is being studied in combination with atezolizumab in a phase II study in patients with resected head and neck squamous cell carcinoma (HNSCC, NCT03708224). In this nonrandomized, open label study, patients will receive either neoadjuvant tirago-lumab with atezolizumab, neoadjuvant atezolizumab alone, or neoadjuvant atezolizu-mab and adjuvant atezolizumab. The primary outcomes are percent of patients with a greater than 40% increase in CD3 counts and R0 resection rate. This study is currently enrolling patients.

Killer Ig-like Receptor 2DL1/2L3

Killer Ig-like receptors (KIRs) are human leukocyte antigen (HLA) class I-specific inhib-itory receptors found on NK cells.[22] Exploiting this interaction has provided another opportunity to exploit an immune checkpoint to promote immunotherapy. Lirilumab targets NK cells by targeting KIR2DL1/2L3. A phase I/II study of this agent in combi-nation with nivolumab in advanced HN cancer showed an objective response rate (ORR) of 24% and disease control rate (DCR), including patients with responses ranging from stable disease to complete response, of 52%.[23] It is now being studied in the perioperative management of recurrent, resectable HNSCC. In a phase II study, patients received neoadjuvant lirilumab and nivolumab for one dose before surgery, then 6 cycles of adjuvant treatment.[24] The primary endpoint, disease-free survival (DFS) was 55.2% (95% CI, 34.8%–71.7%) at 1 year. One-year OS was 85.7% (95% CI, 66.3%–94.4%). Pathologic responses were seen in 43% of the 28 patients treated. Notably, 2-year OS of these responding patients was 80%. Future reports will reveal the durability of this approach.

CANCER VACCINES

Adjuvant and perioperative use of cancer vaccines have been developed as a prom-ising avenue to prevent tumor recurrence following surgical resection. To date, several different techniques for these vaccines including mRNA, dendritic cell, peptide, and whole cell vaccines have been evaluated. These have been used in combination with existing immunotherapies with or without additional adjunctive therapies, such as cytotoxic therapies. In this subsection, we will describe myriad vaccine technolo-gies that hold future promise to improve cure rates and extend disease-free intervals for surgical oncology patients, recognizing that we are still in early days of studying these approaches.

Messenger RNA Vaccines

One of the most notable of these recent studies has been the integration of lipid nano-particle delivered mRNA as vaccine technology. Its use in the adjuvant setting in pancre-atic cancer was reported in a recent study.[25] Autogene cevumeran, an individualized mRNA vaccine based on uridine mRNA–lipoplex nanoparticles with up to 20 neoanti-gens from the patient, was delivered intravenously in combination with adjuvant atezo-lizumab and chemotherapy (mFOLFIRINOX). Sixteen patients were treated in this phase I trial. Of these, 8 demonstrated induction of high-magnitude neoantigen specific T cells. The median PFS for these patients at 18 months was not reached, compared with 13.4 months for those patients that did not demonstrate a T cell response ($P = .003$). These promising findings will be expanded in future clinical trials with this agent.

Expanding on initial successes in melanoma, the KEYNOTE-942 trial, enrolled pa-tients with resected high-risk stage IIIB-D and stage IV melanoma and randomized them to receive mRNA-4157, a personalized cancer vaccine with up to 34 individual-ized tumor-specific neoantigens, in combination with pembrolizumab versus pembro-lizumab alone. Results of this phase II trial were recently reported at the American

Society of Clinical Oncology 2023 Annual Meeting.[26] A total of 157 patients were randomized, with 107 receiving combination adjuvant therapy. The primary endpoint was investigator-assessed recurrence-free survival (RFS). At a median follow-up of 23 and 24 months, respectively, 22.4% of combination patients and 40% of monotherapy patients experienced recurrence. The RFS at 18 months was 78.6% (95% CI, 69%–85.6%) versus 62.2% (95% CI, 46.9%–74.3%). The hazard ratio (HR) for distant metastasis-free survival was 0.347 (95%CI, 0.145–0.828, $P = .0063$). These data suggest adjuvant personalized mRNA vaccines may be a valuable addition to adjuvant immune therapy for resected, high-risk melanoma.

Dendritic Cell Vaccines

Dendritic cell-based vaccines have demonstrated a role in the castration-resistant, metastatic prostate cancer. However, there is no approval for these in the neoadjuvant or adjuvant setting in any cancer. The recently reported results of DCVax-L, an autologous lysate-loaded dendritic cell vaccine for patients with resected glioblastoma starts to pave the way in the nonmetastatic setting.[27] In this phase III trial, patients with newly diagnosed or recurrent glioblastoma were treated with DCVax-L plus temozolomide (standard of care chemotherapy) as compared with matched external control patients treated with temozolomide plus placebo for newly diagnosed glioblastoma or approved therapies for the recurrent patients with glioblastoma. The primary end point was OS in newly diagnosed patients with glioblastoma. Overall, 331 patients were enrolled in the trial, with 232 randomized to the group receiving temozolomide plus the vaccine. Median OS for these patients was 19.3 (95% CI, 17.5–21.3) months from randomization compared with 16.5 (95% CI, 16–17.5) months for those receiving temozolomide plus placebo. The HR was 0.80 (98% CI, 0.00–0.94, $P = .002$). OS at 5 years was 13.0% versus 5.7%, respectively. These encouraging results suggest that dendritic-cell based vaccines may be a promising addition to standard of care for glioblastoma and likely hold promise in other cancers. Another phase II trial evaluating the benefit of GlioVax, or lysate-loaded dendritic cells, as an adjuvant therapy with standard of care chemoradiation for glioblastoma will likely offer further insights into the benefit of this approach.

A similar phase I/II trial is underway evaluating the efficacy of autologous *WT1* mRNA-loaded dendritic cells in addition to standard temozolomide chemotherapy as adjuvant treatment of glioblastoma following total or subtotal resection (ADDIT-GLIO, NCT02649582). In this protocol, leukocytes are removed before standard chemoradiation. They are loaded with the *WT1* mRNA, then injected intradermally weekly for 3 weeks. Subsequently, they are started on standard of care temozolomide treatment with the addition of dendritic cell vaccination on day 21 ± 3 of every 4-week cycle. This study is currently recruiting with an anticipated study completion date in December 2024.

A neoantigen dendritic cell vaccine in combination with nivolumab in patients with hepatocellular carcinoma or liver metastases from colorectal cancer (CRC) will be tested in a phase II clinical trial currently recruiting patients (NCT04912765). This single-arm study includes blood and resected tumor genomic sequencing followed by neoantigen prediction and production. About 3 to 5 million dendritic cells loaded with predicted neoantigens will be delivered once every 2 weeks for 10 doses along with adjuvant nivolumab.

The ENSURE trial is a phase I study involving the generation of autologous dendritic cells loaded with allogeneic tumor lysate as neoadjuvant and adjuvant treatment in resectable epithelioid malignant pleural mesothelioma (NCT05304208). Before standard of care chemotherapy, a leukapheresis to obtain monocytes for dendritic cell differentiation will be performed. These dendritic cells will be loaded with tumor lysate and injected 3 weeks following the completion of chemotherapy, 2 times every other week. At 4 weeks following the initial injection, patients will receive extrapleural pleurectomy/decortication followed by 3 biweekly injections of the dendritic cell vaccine starting 4 weeks following surgery. The primary endpoints will be the number of patients living and completing the 5 doses of dendritic cell vaccine plus surgery, evidence of progression, and persistent grade 3 to 4 adverse events. This trial is actively enrolling patients.

Peptide Vaccines

Peptide vaccines are sequences of amino acids derived from part of a protein that are intended to stimulate an immunogenic humoral or cellular response. In the context of cancer, these tend to be taken from tumor-associated or tumor-specific antigens.[28] Peptide vaccines have been used alone or in combination with adjuvants or other approaches to enhance immune responses and are an area of active investigation.

The use of a human epidermal growth factor receptor 2 (HER2)/*neu* vaccine using GP2, a 9-amino acid peptide of the protein, in combination of granulocyte-macrophage colony-stimulating factor (GM-CSF), known as GLSI-100, is being explored in the FLAMINGO-01 phase III trial in patients with breast cancer.[29] Patients with HER2/*neu* positive with residual disease or high-risk pathologic complete response (pCR) postneoadjuvant therapy are eligible. In a prior phase IIb study, no recurrences were observed in the HER2-positive population for those that were given the experimental treatment, survived, and were tracked for more than 6 months. The phase III trial will randomize patients to receive 6 intradermal injections of GLSI-100 or placebo following 1 year of trastuzumab-based therapy. This study is currently enrolling.

Another phase II trial is looking to combine GM-CSF treatment with a multiepitope HER2 vaccine TPIV100 (NCT04197687). TPIV100 is derived from a pool of 4 HER2-derived HLA-DR epitopes. This agent has been shown to activate CD4 helper T cells in combination with sargramostim, another form of GM-CSF. Patients with stage II-III HER2-positive breast cancer will receive standard of care neoadjuvant chemotherapy. Patients with residual disease will be randomized to receive TPIV100 plus sargramostim every 3 weeks for up to 6 cycles, or placebo, with standard maintenance trastuzumab. Booster injections of TPIV100 and sargramostim are given 3 and 12 months following completion of trastuzumab maintenance. The primary endpoint is invasive DFS.

The AMPLIFY-7P phase I/II trial seeks to determine if ELI-002 7P, a 7-peptide formulation vaccine targeted toward 7 common *KRAS* mutations accounting for 25% of all solid tumors (NCT05726864). This trial is open to patients with pancreatic ductal adenocarcinoma (PDAC), CRC, or NSCLC harboring *KRAS* G12 A/C/D/R/S/V, *KRAS* G13D, or *NRAS* G12 C/D/R/S/V.

A multicenter phase I trial is evaluating the use of a peptide vaccine for patients with H3-mutated gliomas (INTERCEPT-H3, NCT04808245). Patients enrolling in the study will have K27M-mutant histone-3.1 (H3.1K27 M) or histone-3.3 (H3.3K27 M) diffuse midline gliomas. Only treatment-naïve patients other than surgical resection will be enrolled. They will receive H3K27 M peptide vaccine subcutaneously for a total of 11 doses with topical imiquimod that serves as an adjuvant treatment. In addition, they will receive 14 doses of atezolizumab. The primary endpoints are safety and immunogenicity of this regimen.

Another recently described adjuvant vaccine trial reported results in the annual AACR Annual Meeting 2023.[30] EVX-02, a personalized neoantigen vaccine based on a proprietary artificial intelligence-based target platform called PIONEER, was tested in a phase I/IIa clinical trial. They found that all patients receiving the treatment tolerated the drug well, with only mild adverse events. Neoantigen-induced activation of both CD4$^+$ and CD8$^+$ T cells were robust and long lasting. These findings suggest efficacy that may be directly tested in future clinical trials.

Tumor Cell Vaccine

Clinical trial NCT02451982 aims to evaluate the use of combination immunotherapy including GVAX, a GM-CSF gene transduced tumor cell autologous PDAC vaccine. This is being explored in combinations in neoadjuvant and adjuvant courses with cyclophosphamide, nivolumab, and urelumab (agonistic CD137 monoclonal antibody). This phase II study is currently enrolling with an estimated completion at the end of 2024.

CYTOKINES

The benefit of cytokines in the stimulation of immune responses in advanced cancers has been known for some time. High-dose IL-2 leads to cancer regression in a subset of patients with advanced metastatic melanoma and RCC. However, the response rates to this therapy have been low, with only 10% to 20% responding.[31,32] Based on these findings, new studies are currently evaluating additional cytokine agents as potentially effective additions in mobilizing the immune system for surgical oncology patients. Below, we will describe trials that are actively investigating this approach.

A phase II randomized, open-label study seeks to determine if adding pegfilgrastim, a long-acting formulation of GM-CSF to trastuzumab and paclitaxel shows benefit in the neoadjuvant setting (BREASTIMMU02, NCT03571633). Patients with operable HER2-positive breast cancer with previous treatment with 4 cycles of adriamycin and cyclophosphamide are randomized to received either weekly paclitaxel plus trastuzumab every 3 weeks with or without pegfilgrastim every 3 weeks. They intend to enroll 90 patients with a primary endpoint of pCR rate. This study is currently enrolling with an estimated completion date of April 2024.

Bempegaldesleukin (bempeg), a CD122-preferential IL-2 agonist engineered to drive this pathway in a controlled, sustained manner will be studied in the perioperative setting in cisplatin ineligible patients with muscle-invasive bladder cancer (NCT04209114). Patients will be randomized to receive either neoadjuvant nivolumab plus or minus bempeg followed by radical cystectomy, and adjuvant nivolumab plus or minus bempeg. A third group will receive standard of care treatment with radical cystectomy alone. The primary endpoints of this study are pCR rate and event-free survival of the combination therapy compared with radical cystectomy alone. This trial is completed, pending results. It is notable that the PIVOT-12 trial evaluating this agent in the adjuvant setting in melanoma was stopped early following failure of its combination with nivolumab to improve PFS or ORR in patients with metastatic melanoma.

T CELL THERAPY

There has been great excitement in recent years for the use of tumor infiltrating lymphocytes and chimeric antigen receptor T (CAR T) cells as immunotherapeutic approaches in advanced and metastatic solid tumors. These cells are generated by isolating a patient's T cells from the peripheral blood and modifying them by fusing an antibody portion known to react with a particular antigen with an intracellular signaling domain that drives T cell activation. In this way, they can recognize tumors based on specific ligands and generate a cytotoxic antitumor response. These techniques may also hold promise in the perioperative treatment setting for resectable surgical oncology patients.

A phase I study seeks to determine if IL13Ralpha2-CAR T cells are effective in combination with immune checkpoint blockade (ICB) in patients with resectable recurrent glioblastoma (NCT04003649). The IL13 Rα2-CAR T cells are IL13 Rα2-specific Hinge optimized 4-1BB-co-stimulatory CAR/Truncated CD19-expressing autologous naive and memory T cells, which include naive T cells, central memory T cells, and stem cell memory T cells. Of note, to qualify for participation, patients must have IL13Ralpha2 expression by IHC on the primary tumor or recurrent tumor sample. Treatment arms include neoadjuvant ipilimumab plus nivolumab followed by adjuvant CAR T cell treatment with nivolumab, just adjuvant CAR T cell treatment with nivolumab, or adjuvant CAR T cell treatment as monotherapy. The primary endpoints for this study include incidence of adverse events, dose-limiting toxicity, feasibility of neoadjuvant therapy with ipilimumab and nivolumab, feasibility of adjuvant therapy with CAR T cells plus nivolumab, and OS. This trial is currently enrolling patients.

VIRAL THERAPY

After initial excitement of the utilization of viral therapies, these have been largely eclipsed by the utilization of ICB. Nevertheless, their utility in difficult to treat localized tumors and those refractory to systemic therapy. This has created interest in applying these therapies to potentially augment checkpoint blockade response in refractory patients.

Talimogene laherparepvec (T-VEC) is an oncolytic viral immunotherapy with approval for use in the local treatment of unresectable metastatic melanoma. Its direct injection leads to tumor cell lysis and activation of tumor-specific effector T cells (NCT02923778). A multicenter cooperative group study, run through the Experimental Therapeutics Clinical Trials Network (ETCTN) recently completed accrual of a phase II trial evaluating pathologic response rate to T-VEC plus preoperative radiation therapy in patients with localized soft tissue sarcoma. The primary endpoint was pathologic complete necrosis rate ($\geq$95% necrosis) with exploratory endpoints evaluating the impact of T-VEC with radiation on tumor infiltrating and circulating immune cells. Reported results exploring changes in the microenvironment demonstrated an increase in infiltrating immune cells, with specific increases in M2 macrophages, B cells, and CD4$^+$ T cells after neoadjuvant treatment.[33] Of note, a favorable pathologic response ($\geq$90% necrosis) correlated with increased monocytes in the tumor.

A phase II study is evaluating the efficacy of combination treatment with neoadjuvant T-VEC and nivolumab in patients with resectable, early metastatic melanoma with injectable disease (NIVEC, NCT04330430). Patients in the study will receive 4 T-VEC doses and nivolumab starting with the second T-VEC dose. The primary endpoint for this neoadjuvant study is pathologic response. This is currently recruiting.

To date, a completed trial of T-VEC with pembrolizumab has demonstrated an adequate safety profile; however, the results of a double-blind randomized control trial of T-VEC with pembrolizumab versus placebo with pembrolizumab in 692 patients with advanced melanoma failed to demonstrate an improvement in PFS or OS.[34] As such, the use of T-VEC in conjunction with immunotherapies is largely used currently in the setting of future clinical trials.

BIOMARKERS AND INDIVIDUALIZED TREATMENT

As part of many of the phase II and III clinical trials leading to the adoption of neoadjuvant immunotherapy regimens, many clinicians designing these trials had the foresight to incorporate tissue, circulating serum, and microbial collections that have allowed for correlative associations with response. Initially, these biomarkers were limited to tumor mutational burden, microsatellite instability, and PD-L1 staining associations with response to therapy. Although these have clear utilization in the clinic currently, we are also beginning to understand the importance of additional biomarkers.

The role of the tumor immune infiltrate in driving response to immunotherapy cannot be overstated. Although many of these mechanisms are inherently T-cell related and subpopulations of T-cells have correlated with response, this study has also led to the recognition that many cell types must develop a coordinated response to develop an anticancer immune response. This is perhaps best demonstrated by associations of organized B-cell infiltrates termed tertiary lymphoid structures that have been associated with response to immunotherapy in melanoma, RCC, NSCLC, and soft tissue sarcoma.[5,35–38] Although these have been correlated with response, their definition, and adoption in clinical practice continues to be a work in progress.

Beyond tumor-specific markers of response, markers of response to adjuvant immunotherapy have allowed for the thoughtful use of immunotherapies in the adjuvant setting. Importantly, ICB regimens require disease to prime the immune system. As such, we see that the adjuvant use of ICB has primarily shown a benefit in the setting of minimal residual disease (MRD) after resection. In the case of esophageal adenocarcinoma or squamous cell carcinoma, this is defined as a pathologic R1 resection or node positive disease.[39] However, in the case of adjuvant atezolizumab in urothelial carcinomas, ICB failed to show an improvement in outcomes.[7] A subset analysis of this study, however, demonstrated that patients with MRD, defined by positive bespoke ctDNA, did see an improvement in RFS when treated with adjuvant ICB. As such, there is an increased recognition of the importance of judicious use of adjuvant ICB.

Finally, these biomarkers not only present useful clinical tools but also provide insight into the biology of the interface between a tumor, the host immune system, and immunomodulatory therapies. Currently, several groups are studying whether these biomarkers are modifiable and if those modifications can improve response to therapy. Given correlative associations between response to ICB and the gut or tumoral microbiome, a few groups have studied the potential to modulate the gut microbiome in improving response to therapy. Currently, the ability to modulate the microbiome to improve response has been demonstrated in preclinical models of ICB therapy.[40] Whereas pilot studies of fecal transplant have shown the ability to induce a response to ICB in melanoma nonresponders.[41,42] Moreover, further trials are ongoing in MSI-H CRC (NCT04729322).

SUMMARY

Ultimately, the intersection of clinical and translational science will need to continue to be mined to identify the best path to optimal and personalized immunotherapy treatments for our patients. As the number of indications and agents using immunotherapies in treating cancer multiply, it is increasingly important for oncologists to remain abreast of current and upcoming therapies and biomarkers of likelihood of response.

CLINICS CARE POINTS

- Neoadjuvant, adjuvant, and perioperative immunotherapy have been adopted into current clinical management of several tumor types, including NSCLC, melanoma, RCC, and more.

- Robust ongoing clinical trials seek to expand the role of immunotherapy to new approaches and tumor types.
- Clinicians must maintain awareness of the latest findings, as the pace of immunotherapy integration into the management of surgical patients may accelerate.

FUNDING

Dr Patel receives scientific advisory income from: Amgen, AstraZeneca, BeiGene, Bristol-Myers Squibb, Certis, Eli Lilly, Jazz, Genentech, Illumina, Merck, Pfizer, Signatera, Tempus; Dr. Patel's university receives research funding from: Amgen, AstraZeneca/MedImmune, A2bio, Bristol-Myers Squibb, Eli Lilly, Fate Therapeutics, Gilead, Iovance, Merck, Pfizer, Roche/Genentech.

DISCLOSURE

The authors have nothing to disclose.

REFERENCES

1. Kothari A, White MG, Peacock O, et al. Pathological response following neoadjuvant immunotherapy in mismatch repair-deficient/microsatellite instability-high locally advanced, non-metastatic colorectal cancer. Br J Surg 2022;109(6): 489–92.
2. Cercek A, Lumish M, Sinopoli J, et al. PD-1 Blockade in Mismatch Repair–Deficient, Locally Advanced Rectal Cancer. N Engl J Med 2022;386(25):2363–76.
3. Amaria RN, Postow M, Burton EM, et al. Neoadjuvant relatlimab and nivolumab in resectable melanoma. Nature 2022;611(7934):155–60.
4. Ganguly S, Gogia A, Dent R. Pembrolizumab in Early Triple-Negative Breast Cancer. N Engl J Med 2022;386(18):1771.
5. Cascone T, William WN, Weissferdt A, et al. Neoadjuvant nivolumab or nivolumab plus ipilimumab in operable non-small cell lung cancer: the phase 2 randomized NEOSTAR trial. Nat Med 2021;27(3):504–14.
6. Keung EZ, Lazar AJ, Torres KE, et al. Phase II study of neoadjuvant checkpoint blockade in patients with surgically resectable undifferentiated pleomorphic sarcoma and dedifferentiated liposarcoma. BMC Cancer 2018;18:913.
7. Powles T, Assaf ZJ, Davarpanah N, et al. ctDNA guiding adjuvant immunotherapy in urothelial carcinoma. Nature 2021;595(7867):432–7.
8. Maruhashi T, Sugiura D, Okazaki I mi, et al. LAG-3: from molecular functions to clinical applications. J Immunother Cancer 2020;8(2):e001014.
9. Hannier S, Tournier M, Bismuth G, et al. CD3/TCR complex-associated lymphocyte activation gene-3 molecules inhibit CD3/TCR signaling. J Immunol Baltim Md 1950 1998;161(8):4058–65.
10. Chen J, Chen Z. The effect of immune microenvironment on the progression and prognosis of colorectal cancer. Med Oncol Northwood Lond Engl 2014;31(8):82.
11. Deng WW, Mao L, Yu GT, et al. LAG-3 confers poor prognosis and its blockade reshapes antitumor response in head and neck squamous cell carcinoma. OncoImmunology 2016;5(11):e1239005.
12. Giraldo NA, Becht E, Pagès F, et al. Orchestration and Prognostic Significance of Immune Checkpoints in the Microenvironment of Primary and Metastatic Renal Cell Cancer. Clin Cancer Res 2015;21(13):3031–40.

13. Bhagwat B, Cherwinski H, Sathe M, et al. Establishment of engineered cell-based assays mediating LAG3 and PD1 immune suppression enables potency measurement of blocking antibodies and assessment of signal transduction. J Immunol Methods 2018;456:7–14.

14. Goding SR, Wilson KA, Xie Y, et al. Restoring immune function of tumor-specific CD4+ T cells during recurrence of melanoma. J Immunol Baltim Md 1950 2013; 190(9):4899–909.

15. Huang RY, Eppolito C, Lele S, et al. LAG3 and PD1 co-inhibitory molecules collaborate to limit CD8 + T cell signaling and dampen antitumor immunity in a murine ovarian cancer model. Oncotarget 2015;6(29):27359–77.

16. Tawbi HA, Schadendorf D, Lipson EJ, et al. Relatlimab and Nivolumab versus Nivolumab in Untreated Advanced Melanoma. N Engl J Med 2022;386(1):24–34.

17. Aigner C, Du Pont B, Hartemink K, et al. Surgical outcomes of patients with resectable non-small-cell lung cancer receiving neoadjuvant immunotherapy with nivolumab plus relatlimab or nivolumab: Findings from the prospective, randomized, multicentric phase II study NEOpredict-Lung. J Clin Oncol 2023; 41(16_suppl):8500.

18. Rousseau A, Parisi C, Barlesi F. Anti-TIGIT therapies for solid tumors: a systematic review. ESMO Open 2023;8(2):101184.

19. Yu X, Harden K, Gonzalez LC, et al. The surface protein TIGIT suppresses T cell activation by promoting the generation of mature immunoregulatory dendritic cells. Nat Immunol 2009;10(1):48–57.

20. Joller N, Lozano E, Burkett PR, et al. Treg cells expressing the coinhibitory molecule TIGIT selectively inhibit proinflammatory Th1 and Th17 cell responses. Immunity 2014;40(4):569–81.

21. Johnston RJ, Comps-Agrar L, Hackney J, et al. The immunoreceptor TIGIT regulates antitumor and antiviral CD8(+) T cell effector function. Cancer Cell 2014; 26(6):923–37.

22. Pende D, Falco M, Vitale M, et al. Killer Ig-Like Receptors (KIRs): Their Role in NK Cell Modulation and Developments Leading to Their Clinical Exploitation. Front Immunol 2019;10. Available at: https://www.frontiersin.org/articles/10.3389/fimmu.2019.01179. Accessed August 31, 2023.

23. Althammer S, Steele K, Rebelatto M, et al. 31st Annual Meeting and Associated Programs of the Society for Immunotherapy of Cancer (SITC 2016): late breaking abstracts. J Immunother Cancer 2016;4(2):91.

24. Hanna GJ, O'Neill A, Shin KY, et al. Neoadjuvant and Adjuvant Nivolumab and Lirilumab in Patients with Recurrent, Resectable Squamous Cell Carcinoma of the Head and Neck. Clin Cancer 2022;28(3):468–78.

25. Rojas LA, Sethna Z, Soares KC, et al. Personalized RNA neoantigen vaccines stimulate T cells in pancreatic cancer. Nature 2023;618(7963):144–50.

26. Khattak A, Weber JS, Meniawy T, et al. Distant metastasis-free survival results from the randomized, phase 2 mRNA-4157-P201/KEYNOTE-942 trial. J Clin Oncol 2023;41(17_suppl):LBA9503.

27. Liau LM, Ashkan K, Brem S, et al. Association of autologous tumor lysate-loaded dendritic cell vaccination with extension of survival among patients with newly diagnosed and recurrent glioblastoma: a phase 3 prospective externally controlled cohort trial. JAMA Oncol 2023;9(1):112–21.

28. Abd-Aziz N, Poh CL. development of peptide-based vaccines for cancer. J Oncol 2022;2022:9749363.

29. Patel SS, Thompson JL, Patel MS, et al. Abstract CT064: phase III study to evaluate the efficacy and safety of GLSI-100 (GP2 + GM-CSF) in breast cancer

patients with residual disease or high-risk PCR after both neo-adjuvant and post-operative adjuvant anti-HER2 therapy. Flamingo-01. Cancer Res 2023; 83(8_Supplement):CT064.

30. Kleine-Kohlbrecher D, Petersen NV, Pavlidis MA, et al. Abstract LB199: A personalized neoantigen vaccine is well tolerated and induces specific T-cell immune response in patients with resected melanoma. Cancer Res 2023; 83(8_Supplement):LB199.

31. Yang JC, Sherry RM, Steinberg SM, et al. Randomized Study of High-Dose and Low-Dose Interleukin-2 in Patients With Metastatic Renal Cancer. J Clin Oncol 2003;21(16):3127–32.

32. Davar D, Ding F, Saul M, et al. High-dose interleukin-2 (HD IL-2) for advanced melanoma: a single center experience from the University of Pittsburgh Cancer Institute. J Immunother Cancer 2017;5(1):74.

33. Goff PH, Riolobos L, LaFleur BJ, et al. Neoadjuvant Therapy Induces a Potent Immune Response to Sarcoma, Dominated by Myeloid and B Cells. Clin Cancer Res 2022;28(8):1701–11.

34. Chesney JA, Ribas A, Long GV, et al. Randomized, Double-Blind, Placebo-Controlled, Global Phase III Trial of Talimogene Laherparepvec Combined With Pembrolizumab for Advanced Melanoma. J Clin 2023;41(3):528–40.

35. Petitprez F, de Reyniès A, Keung EZ, et al. B cells are associated with survival and immunotherapy response in sarcoma. Nature 2020;577(7791):556–60.

36. Helmink BA, Reddy SM, Gao J, et al. B cells and tertiary lymphoid structures promote immunotherapy response. Nature 2020;577(7791):549–55.

37. Cabrita R, Lauss M, Sanna A, et al. Tertiary lymphoid structures improve immunotherapy and survival in melanoma. Nature 2020;577(7791):561–5.

38. Meylan M, Petitprez F, Becht E, et al. Tertiary lymphoid structures generate and propagate anti-tumor antibody-producing plasma cells in renal cell cancer. Immunity 2022;55(3):527–41.e5.

39. Patel MA, Kratz JD, Lubner SJ, et al. Esophagogastric Cancers: Integrating Immunotherapy Therapy Into Current Practice. J Clin Oncol 2022;40(24): 2751–62.

40. Gopalakrishnan V, Helmink BA, Spencer CN, et al. The Influence of the Gut Microbiome on Cancer, Immunity, and Cancer Immunotherapy. Cancer Cell 2018; 33(4):570–80.

41. Baruch EN, Youngster I, Ben-Betzalel G, et al. Fecal microbiota transplant promotes response in immunotherapy-refractory melanoma patients. Science 2021;371(6529):602–9.

42. Davar D, Dzutsev AK, McCulloch JA, et al. Fecal microbiota transplant overcomes resistance to anti-PD-1 therapy in melanoma patients. Science 2021; 371(6529):595–602.

43. O'Brien M, Paz-Ares L, Marreaud S, et al. Pembrolizumab versus placebo as adjuvant therapy for completely resected stage IB–IIIA non-small-cell lung cancer (PEARLS/KEYNOTE-091): an interim analysis of a randomised, triple-blind, phase 3 trial. Lancet Oncol 2022;23(10):1274–86.

44. Wakelee HA, Altorki NK, Zhou C, et al. IMpower010: Primary results of a phase III global study of atezolizumab versus best supportive care after adjuvant chemotherapy in resected stage IB–IIIA non-small cell lung cancer (NSCLC). J Clin Oncol 2021;39(15_suppl):8500.

45. Choueiri TK, Tomczak P, Park SH, et al. Adjuvant Pembrolizumab after Nephrectomy in Renal-Cell Carcinoma. N Engl J Med 2021;385(8):683–94.

46. Bajorin DF, Witjes JA, Gschwend JE, et al. Adjuvant Nivolumab versus Placebo in Muscle-Invasive Urothelial Carcinoma. N Engl J Med 2021;384(22):2102–14.
47. Luke JJ, Rutkowski P, Queirolo P, et al. Pembrolizumab versus placebo as adjuvant therapy in completely resected stage IIB or IIC melanoma (KEYNOTE-716): a randomised, double-blind, phase 3 trial. Lancet 2022;399(10336):1718–29.
48. Weber J, Mandala M, Del Vecchio M, et al. Adjuvant Nivolumab versus Ipilimumab in Resected Stage III or IV Melanoma. N Engl J Med 2017;377(19):1824–35.
49. Long GV, Vecchio MD, Weber J, et al. Adjuvant therapy with nivolumab versus placebo in patients with resected stage IIB/C melanoma (CheckMate 76K). SKIN J Cutan Med 2023;7(2):s163.
50. Livingstone E, Zimmer L, Hassel JC, et al. Adjuvant nivolumab plus ipilimumab or nivolumab alone versus placebo in patients with resected stage IV melanoma with no evidence of disease (IMMUNED): final results of a randomised, double-blind, phase 2 trial. Lancet 2022;400(10358):1117–29.
51. Larkin J, Del Vecchio M, Mandalá M, et al. Adjuvant Nivolumab versus Ipilimumab in Resected Stage III/IV Melanoma: 5-Year Efficacy and Biomarker Results from CheckMate 238. Clin Cancer Res 2023;29(17):3352–61.
52. Eggermont AMM, Blank CU, Mandala M, et al. Adjuvant Pembrolizumab versus Placebo in Resected Stage III Melanoma. N Engl J Med 2018;378(19):1789–801.
53. Eggermont AMM, Kicinski M, Blank CU, et al. 804P Pembrolizumab versus placebo after complete resection of high-risk stage III melanoma: 5-year results of the EORTC 1325-MG/Keynote-054 double-blinded phase III trial. Ann Oncol 2022;33:S912–3.
54. Kelly RJ, Ajani JA, Kuzdzal J, et al. Adjuvant Nivolumab in Resected Esophageal or Gastroesophageal Junction Cancer. N Engl J Med 2021;384(13):1191–203.
55. Forde PM, Spicer J, Lu S, et al. Neoadjuvant Nivolumab plus Chemotherapy in Resectable Lung Cancer. N Engl J Med 2022;386(21):1973–85.
56. Schmid P, Cortes J, Pusztai L, et al. Pembrolizumab for Early Triple-Negative Breast Cancer. N Engl J Med 2020;382(9):810–21.
57. Patel SP, Othus M, Chen Y, et al. Neoadjuvant–Adjuvant or Adjuvant-Only Pembrolizumab in Advanced Melanoma. N Engl J Med 2023;388(9):813–23.
58. Versluis JM, Menzies AM, Sikorska K, et al. Survival update of neoadjuvant ipilimumab plus nivolumab in macroscopic stage III melanoma in the OpACIN and OpACIN-neo trials. Ann Oncol 2023;34(4):420–30.
59. Reijers ILM, Menzies AM, van Akkooi ACJ, et al. Personalized response-directed surgery and adjuvant therapy after neoadjuvant ipilimumab and nivolumab in high-risk stage III melanoma: the PRADO trial. Nat Med 2022;28(6):1178–88.
60. Chalabi M, Fanchi LF, Dijkstra KK, et al. Neoadjuvant immunotherapy leads to pathological responses in MMR-proficient and MMR-deficient early-stage colon cancers. Nat Med 2020;26(4):566–76.
61. Chalabi M, Verschoor YL, Berg J van den, et al. LBA7 Neoadjuvant immune checkpoint inhibition in locally advanced MMR-deficient colon cancer: The NICHE-2 study. Ann Oncol 2022;33:S1389.

Targeted Therapies, Biologics, and Immunotherapy in the Neoadjuvant and Adjuvant Settings: Perioperative Risks

Daisuke Nishizaki, MD[a],*, Ramez N. Eskander, MD[b]

KEYWORDS

- Immune checkpoint inhibitors • Molecular targeted therapy • Biological products
- Neoadjuvant therapy • Intraoperative complications

KEY POINTS

- Advances in systemic therapy have revolutionized cancer treatment, facilitating the combination of systemic therapy and surgical interventions.
- As neoadjuvant therapies expand, understanding potential perioperative implications is crucial for surgical oncologists.
- This article aims to highlight surgical considerations associated with immune checkpoint inhibitors, targeted therapies, and biologics.

BACKGROUND

Over the past 2 decades, advances in systemic therapy, including molecularly targeted treatments and immune checkpoint inhibitors (ICIs), have transformed the therapeutic landscape and improved the outcomes for several cancer types. In the field of surgical oncology, the combination of surgery and such systemic therapies has been employed in an effort to improve oncologic outcomes. Adjuvant therapy was first investigated in the 1970s, with the aim of controlling locoregional recurrences after complete surgical resection in multiple cancer types.[1] The term "neoadjuvant" refers to the use of systemic treatment before surgery. Initially, neoadjuvant therapy was

[a] Division of Hematology and Oncology, Department of Medicine, Center for Personalized Cancer Therapy, University of California San Diego, Moores Cancer Center, 3855 Health Sciences Drive, La Jolla, CA 92037, USA; [b] Division of Gynecologic Oncology, Department of Obstetrics, Gynecology and Reproductive Sciences, Center for Personalized Cancer Therapy, University of California San Diego, Moores Cancer Center, La Jolla, CA, USA
* Corresponding author.
E-mail address: dnishizaki@health.ucsd.edu

Surg Oncol Clin N Am 33 (2024) 279–291
https://doi.org/10.1016/j.soc.2023.12.002
1055-3207/24/© 2023 Elsevier Inc. All rights reserved.

employed to treat inoperable, locally advanced breast cancer.[2] Subsequently, the use of neoadjuvant therapy was investigated and expanded for the treatment of operable solid tumors. Chemotherapy or chemoradiotherapy with anticancer cytotoxic agents has been utilized for neoadjuvant and adjuvant therapy in various malignancies. While these therapies are successful in reducing tumor burden, they are also associated with potential treatment-related adverse events and higher perioperative implications in surgical patients.[3] Nonetheless, the idea of reducing tumor burden in primary lesions or metastatic lesions has been widely adopted in clinical practice.

The emergence of ICIs has further transformed the treatment landscape of multiple solid tumors, with utilization in both the neoadjuvant and adjuvant settings. Melanoma and non–small-cell lung cancer (NSCLC) are among the "immunogenic" tumors and, as such, have been investigated as targets for neoadjuvant therapy using ICIs.[4–6] Recent trials exploring the efficacy of neoadjuvant immunotherapy in patients with advanced melanoma have reported promising results, demonstrating improved event-free survival after surgery and an increased rate of pathologic complete response.[7,8] Even for generally less "immunogenic" tumors, like hepatocellular carcinoma (HCC), neoadjuvant immunotherapy has recently been employed.[9] There are multiple active clinical trials examining the utility of ICIs in the neoadjuvant space, with melanoma, glioblastoma, and head and neck cancer as the primary targets (see article by Schokrpur, Patel and colleagues).

With the growth of neoadjuvant therapeutic interventions in the cancer arena, an increased interest in understanding the surgical implications of such drugs has emerged. But, there remains a lack of scientifically robust information about which drugs/agents are more likely to be associated with surgical complications if administered in the perioperative window. Advancements in systemic therapy have also introduced uncertainty regarding the potential interactions between drugs and operative interventions, with surgical oncologists keen to understand how to circumvent complications related to these therapeutic agents. Furthermore, clinical trials are additionally exploring off-label uses of Food and Drug Administration (FDA)–approved drugs that are typically not utilized for certain solid tumors. This dynamic treatment landscape necessitates that surgical oncologist understand the nuanced relationships between novel drugs and surgery, as well as potential complications.

This article aims to outline potential surgical considerations associated with systemic agents, including ICIs, targeted agents, and biologics used in the neoadjuvant and adjuvant settings. It also discusses drugs that could potentially influence complications and are likely to be administered concurrently to cancer patients. Throughout this review, the term 'targeted therapy' includes small-molecule drugs and monoclonal antibodies, as defined by the National Comprehensive Cancer Network (NCCN).[10]

WHAT DRUGS ARE RELATED TO SURGICAL COMPLICATIONS?

Perioperative surgical complications include, but are not limited to, clotting (coagulation) complications, postoperative bleeding, wound-healing disturbances (including fistulas), and surgical site infections.

Drugs Associated with Thrombotic Complications

Cancer patients are at risk of developing venous thrombosis, with a reported in-hospital incidence following major cancer surgery of 1.3%.[11] There are multiple factors influencing clotting risk including perioperative medications, cancer stage, and specific cancer treatments. Pelvic and abdominal surgeries are also established risk factors for venous thrombosis.[12] Moreover, cancer itself results in a hypercoagulation effect.[13]

The incorporation of new anticancer therapies in the management of metastatic disease, including targeted therapy and immunotherapy, has also been associated with increased risk of venous thromboembolism[14]; however, it remains unclear whether immunotherapy and target therapy directly induce thromboembolism.

Drugs that target vascular endothelial growth factor (VEGF) are recognized as risk factors for arterial thromboembolic events. According to a meta-analysis, the risk of arterial thromboembolic events associated with bevacizumab combined with chemotherapy was 1.63 times higher than control, a difference of 1.2% (equivalent to an increase of 7 patients per 1000).[15] Another study reported that baseline cardiovascular risk factors, including hypertension, diabetes, atrial fibrillation, and the absence of statin therapy, are associated with cardiovascular hospitalization related to bevacizumab.[16] Meanwhile, ramucirumab, another anti-VEGF monoclonal antibody, did not demonstrate a definite increased risk of thromboembolic events.[17] Aflibercept, while not a monoclonal antibody, inhibits VEGF by trapping VEGF-A and VEGF-B, as well as placental growth factor (PlGF)-1 and PlGF-2.[18] Approved for colorectal cancer (CRC) in combination with FOLFIRI, a trial of aflibercept reported the frequencies of arterial and venous thromboembolic events to be 2.6% and 9.3%, respectively. These rates were 1.1% and 2.0% higher, respectively, than those in the placebo group.[19] Lenvatinib, a multikinase inhibitor that inhibits VEGF receptors was also reported to have arterial thromboembolic events (any grade, 5.4%) and venous thromboembolic events (any grade, 5.4%).[20] Overall, the incidence of arterial and venous thrombosis is slightly higher when using anti-VEGF agents. Although the efficacy of prolonged thromboprophylaxis with low–molecular weight heparin for abdominal or pelvic surgery is established,[21] it remains to be seen whether this is also effective for patients who receive anti-VEGF agents prior to surgical intervention.

Drugs Associated with Bleeding Complications

Preoperative thrombocytopenia, defined as platelet counts of $\leq 150 \times 10^9$/L, may occur as a result of anticancer therapy and is associated with a higher risk of blood transfusion and death.[22] Patients with hematological malignancies or solid tumors generally have a higher risk of thrombocytopenia; therefore, caution should be exercised regarding perioperative platelet counts. Interestingly, however, platelet counts do not linearly correlate with the frequency of bleeding complications.[23] While the rate of spontaneous bleeding is high in patients with platelet counts $\leq 10 \times 10^9$/L, the rate of clinically significant major bleeding does not appear to be correlated. Mokart and colleagues[24] also reported that neither neutropenia nor thrombocytopenia was associated with prognosis in patients with hematologic malignancies who underwent abdominal surgery due to acute abdominal complications. They noted that 69% [40/58] of patients survived and that preoperative septic shock and the use of dialysis were associated with higher in-hospital mortality. However, they did not report the frequency of surgical bleeding. It remains unclear whether thrombocytopenia itself influences complication rates or whether the underlying conditions leading to thrombocytopenia or the procedures undertaken to address it, such as blood transfusions, contribute to these complications. Given the unpredictable bleeding risk in thrombocytopenic patients who undergo surgery, surgical teams must be prepared for potential bleeding events. The decision to proceed with platelet transfusion is also nuanced due to potential transfusion-related complications and thus should be carefully considered.

Table 1
Examples of targeted drugs associated with thrombocytopenia that may be used in the treatment for solid tumors

Drugs	Primary Targets	Indications	Frequency of Thrombocytopenia
Dasatinib	SRC, PDGFR	CML, ALL, GIST	19%[61]
Lenvatinib	VEGFR 1–3, FGFR 1–4, PDGFR	Thyroid carcinoma, HCC	25% (≥grade 3)[33]
Pazopanib	PDGFR, VEGEFR, KIT	RCC, sarcoma	41% (all grades); 4% (grade ≥3)[31]
Regorafenib	PDGFR, KIT	GIST, CRC	42% (all grades); 5% (grade ≥3)[62]
Sunitinib	PDGFR, KIT, FLT3, RET, VEGFR	GIST, RCC, NET	21%–78% (all grades); 6%–22% (grade ≥3)[31,32]
Niraparib	BRCA1, BRCA2	Ovarian cancer, peritoneal cancer	61% (all grades); 34% (grade ≥3)[25]
Olaparib	BRCA1, BRCA2, ATM, BARD1	Breast cancer, ovarian cancer, prostate cancer	11% (all grades)
Rucaparib	BRCA1, BRCA2	Ovarian cancer	28% (all grades); 5% (grade ≥3)[26]
Abemaciclib	CDK4/6, CDKN2A, PIK3CA	Breast cancer	19% (all grades)[63]
Palbociclib	CDK4/6, CDKN2A	Breast cancer	10% (grade 3–4)[64]
Trastuzumab	ERBB2	Breast cancer	6.6% (4.4–10.0)[65]

Abbreviations: ALL, acute lymphoblastic leukemia; CML, chronic myeloid leukemia; CRC, colorectal cancer; GIST, gastrointestinal stromal tumor; HCC, hepatocellular carcinoma; NET, neuroendocrine tumor; RCC, renal cell carcinoma.

Targeted therapy can potentially lower platelet counts. **Table 1** shows targeted therapies that may potentially result in thrombocytopenia. Niraparib, an oral poly-ADP-ribose-polymerase inhibitor (PARPi), had higher incidence of thrombocytopenia, with 34% grade ≥3 thrombocytopenia in randomized clinical trials.[25] Two alternate PARPi, rucaparib and olaparib, have also been shown to result in thrombocytopenia, although both less frequently and to a lesser degree.[26,27] Thrombocytopenia linked to PARPi is attributed to a reversible decline in proliferation and maturation of megakaryocytes.[28] A perioperative withholding period is not specifically designated for PARPi, but experts recommended discontinuing olaparib several days before major surgery (**Table 2**).[29]

Overall, a meta-analysis indicated that platelet-derived growth factor receptor (PDGFR) inhibitors significantly increased the risks of both all grade and grade ≥3 thrombocytopenia, with an approximately 5-fold increased risk.[30] Thrombocytopenia with the use of combined VEGFR and PDGFR inhibitors, pazopanib and sunitinib, is also relatively common, with 41%[31] and 78%[32] incidences in prior studies, respectively. The reported incidence of thrombocytopenia with sunitinib varies amongst trials,[31] although it remains important to evaluate platelet counts. The reported incidence of thrombocytopenia with lenvatinib, which inhibits PDGFR, amongst other tyrosine kinases, varies amongst studies. One randomized study in patients with thyroid cancer did not report the incidence of thrombocytopenia, but another phase 2 observational study reported a 50% rate of thrombocytopenia in patients with

Table 2 Current information on perioperative withholding period	
Drug	**Quote and Reference**
Bevacizumab	"Discontinue at least 28 d prior to elective surgery. Do not initiate Avastin for at least 28 d after surgery and until the surgical wound is fully healed." https://www.accessdata.fda.gov/drugsatfda_docs/label/2014/125085s301lbl.pdf
Lenvatinib	"Withhold Lenvima for at least 1 wk before elective surgery. Do not administer for at least 2 wk following major surgery and until adequate wound healing." https://www.lenvima.com/-/media/Project/EISAI/Lenvima/PDF/prescribing-information.pdf
Olaparib	"To stop olaparib for several days prior to surgery and not recommence olaparib until wound healing has occurred."[29]
Pazopanib	"Withhold Votrient for at least 1 wk prior to elective surgery. Do not administer for at least 2 wk following major surgery and until adequate wound healing." https://www.accessdata.fda.gov/drugsatfda_docs/label/2020/022465s029lbl.pdf
Ramucirumab	"A randomized clinical trial excluded patients with major surgery within 28 d" "Withhold Cyramza prior to surgery." https://www.accessdata.fda.gov/drugsatfda_docs/label/2014/125477s002lbl.pdf
Regorafenib	"Treatment with regorafenib should be stopped at least 2 wk prior to scheduled surgery. The decision to resume regorafenib after surgery should be based on clinical judgment of adequate wound healing. Regorafenib should be discontinued in patients with wound dehiscence." https://www.accessdata.fda.gov/drugsatfda_docs/label/2017/203085s007lbl.pdf
Sunitinib	"Withhold Sutent for at least 3 wk prior to elective surgery. Do not administer for at least 2 wk following major surgery and until adequate wound healing." https://www.accessdata.fda.gov/drugsatfda_docs/label/2020/021938s037lbl.pdf

unresectable biliary tract cancer. Platelet-derived growth factor ligand, by binding to PDGFR, facilitates the restoration of platelets. Thus, blocking of PDGFR by lenvatinib (as well as other PDGFR inhibitors) may lead to thrombocytopenia.[33] It is recommended that lenvatinib be held for at least 1 week before elective surgery (see **Table 2**).

Bevacizumab and ramucirumab have a direct effect on vessel formation; therefore, bleeding complications may occur even in the absence of platelet dysfunction.[34] In a clinical trial, bleeding events of any grade, including gastrointestinal bleeding, were more common in patients who received ramucirumab (42% vs 18%), albeit with a relatively low rate of grade ≥ 3 bleeding (4.3% vs 2.4%). Neoadjuvant ramucirumab for resectable esophagogastric cancer did not show a difference in the incidence of postoperative bleeding.[35]

Imatinib, which is used to treat gastrointestinal stromal tumor (GIST), does inhibit PDGFR and is known to cause bleeding from tumors.[36] In a phase III trial comparing various dosages of imatinib, 5% and 11% of patients who received 400 mg and 800 mg, respectively, developed grade ≥ 3 hemorrhage.[37] Hemorrhage was not associated with thrombocytopenia,[38] and the incidence of grade ≥ 3 thrombocytopenia in the treatment of GIST was reported at around 1%.[39] Patients with bulky GIST should be monitored closely during the first few weeks after treatment initiation for potential hemorrhagic events, which may be related to rapid and dramatic tumor responses to treatment.

Despite a lower frequency, ICIs may also be associated with thrombocytopenia. A multicenter study reported 17 cases of immune-related thrombocytopenia (grade ≥2) among 7626 registered patients.[40] Another single-center retrospective study, which investigated sequential cancer patients treated with ICIs, reported a grade ≥3 thrombocytopenia rate of 8.6%; of these, 1.7% was attributed to ICIs.[41] Notably, this study revealed that patients who developed ICI-related thrombocytopenia had worse overall survival compared to those who developed thrombocytopenia unrelated to ICIs. Although the incidence of immune-related thrombocytopenia appears low, surgeons should pay close attention to this potential complication.

Drugs Associated with Wound-Healing Issues

Anti-VEGF monoclonal antibodies inhibit angiogenesis, which may have an impact on postoperative wound healing. The FDA recommends that bevacizumab be held at least 28 days prior to major surgery and resumed no earlier than 28 days after surgery (see **Table 2**). A meta-analysis of randomized controlled trials comparing bevacizumab-containing regimens to standard chemotherapy revealed that the risk of wound-healing disruption (≥grade 3) was significantly increased in patients treated with a bevacizumab-containing regimen (risk ratio 3.55, 95% confidence interval [CI] 1.09–11.59).[42] A Cochrane review reported that chemotherapy with bevacizumab in recurrent platinum-resistant epithelial ovarian cancer may slightly increase rates of bowel fistula/perforation (grade ≥2), although the certainty of the evidence is low.[43] Holding the medication for a period of time prior to surgery is hypothesized to reduce the complication rate, but there is a dearth of information concerning the optimal period of perioperative hold period for bevacizumab. A randomized clinical trial that investigated the efficacy of bevacizumab plus chemotherapy for patients with operable esophagogastric adenocarcinoma had at least 8 weeks between the last dose of preoperative bevacizumab and surgical resection.[44] This study showed that wound-healing complications in patients who received bevacizumab plus chemotherapy were more prevalent compared to patients who did not receive bevacizumab (12% vs 7%), but the study investigators concluded the overall incidence of life-threatening complications was similar in both groups. A population-based study that followed patients with CRC who received bevacizumab revealed that approximately one-third of patients who underwent surgery subsequent to bevacizumab exposure encountered a substantial incidence of postoperative complications (36%), which included wound complications (12.5%).[45] Of note, the frequency of postoperative complications was not related to the timing of the last bevacizumab exposure in this study, suggesting that recent bevacizumab exposure is not an absolute contraindication to surgery. Several studies advocate that preoperative bevacizumab is not associated with increased morbidity and mortality in various clinical settings including cytoreductive surgery[46] and implanted port placement.[47] Taken together, recent exposure to bevacizumab is not an absolute contraindication to surgical intervention, although surgeons should be mindful of potential wound-healing complications.

Neoadjuvant ramucirumab was examined in patients with resectable esophagogastric adenocarcinoma in a randomized study where surgery was performed 4 to 6 weeks after the last dose of ramucirumab.[35] Adding ramucirumab to chemotherapy was compared to chemotherapy alone, and the incidence of wound-healing complications was 1% versus 3%, respectively. However, the incidence of postoperative complications, including hemorrhage, abscess formation, multiorgan failure, and sepsis, was higher among patients who received ramucirumab (41% vs 32%). Of note, the investigators of the trial reported that use of ramucirumab in patients with Siewert type I tumors undergoing transthoracic esophagectomy with intrathoracic anastomosis may be associated with increased risk of anastomotic leakage, and thus enrollment of patients with Siewert type I tumors was stopped after the interim analysis. Taken together, perioperative VEGF-pathway inhibitors may not be a contraindication for surgery; however, the use of ramucirumab should be avoided for patients with Siewert type I gastroesophageal cancer if they are candidates for curative resection.

Drugs Associated with Infectious and Other Complications

Biologics, including infliximab, vedolizumab, golimumab, and adalimumab, are associated with a lower risk of inflammatory bowel disease (IBD)–associated cancer in patients with ulcerative colitis (UC).[48] Biologics are widely used to control mucosal inflammation and may result in a reduction of cases of IBD-associated cancer. However, surgical oncologists are commonly faced with difficult clinical situations mandating surgery in patients with UC who are on treatment with these biologics. Indeed, the use of biologics, such as those targeting tumor necrosis factor (TNF)-α, may have uncertain effects on perioperative morbidity. A database analysis showed that preoperative anti-TNF therapy was not associated with increased complications among patients who underwent bowel resection alone. Meanwhile, among patients who underwent ileal pouch-anal anastomosis (IPAA), the use of anti-TNF therapy within 90 days prior to surgery was associated with a higher morbidity.[49] A meta-analysis suggested that the complication rate among UC patients did not increase with the use of anti-TNF agents, while a slight increase in the rate of infectious complications was seen with the use of anti-TNF agents in patients with Crohn's disease.[50]

The aforementioned TNF-α inhibitors are also commonly used to control immune-related adverse events (irAEs). Tocilizumab, an anti-interleukin 6 receptor, which was originally used for rheumatoid arthritis and known to be associated with an increased risk of developing diverticulitis and diverticulitis-related intestinal perforation,[51] is also used for treating irAEs. Although surgical oncologists sometimes encounter a case of diverticulitis or perforation after administration of tocilizumab among patients with rheumatoid arthritis,[52] it remains unclear if this is the case among patients with irAEs treated with tocilizumab. The incidence of such drug-related adverse events among patients with irAE is unknown. But, it is prudent for surgeons to be aware of potential complications related to drug usage, given the possible perioperative implications. Further, guidelines regarding irAE list immune-related cholecystitis as a potential gastrointestinal toxicity.[53] In case of immune-related cholecystitis, the recommended treatment is surgical intervention (ie, cholecystectomy), rather than steroid administration.

WHEN SHOULD IMMUNE CHECKPOINT INHIBITORS, TARGETED AGENTS, AND BIOLOGICS BE STOPPED BEFORE SURGERY, AND WHEN CAN THEY SAFELY BE STARTED AFTER SURGERY?

To date, there is limited information on when drugs, including ICI, targeted agents, and biologics, should be stopped before surgery and when they can be safely resumed after surgery. **Table 2** summarizes currently available information on perioperative withholding periods for the agents reviewed this far. As mentioned earlier, anti-VEGF antibodies are empirically held 4 to 6 weeks before surgery and anti-TNF drugs within 90 days prior to surgery may increase the complication rate after IPAA procedures among patients with UC. However, limited to no data are available defining a safe perioperative window for other targeted drugs and ICIs. The clinical relevance of this data is more pronounced in the neoadjuvant setting. A study of neoadjuvant cemiplimab for resectable HCC reported a 10% rate of perioperative adverse events, with little data available regarding surgical complications.[9] The NCCN guidelines state that imatinib can be discontinued right before surgery and restarted if the patient can tolerate oral medication. Indeed, a phase II study of neoadjuvant imatinib for advanced GIST reported that the median time from imatinib discontinuation to surgery was 2 days. Amongst patients without surgical complications, the median time from surgery to imatinib resumption was 24 days.[54] The NCCN guidelines for GIST also recommend stopping sunitinib, regorafenib, ripretinib, and avapritinib at least 1 week prior to surgery.[55]

There has been ongoing discussion regarding the appropriate period after implantation of a totally implanted port (TIP) before initiating anticancer drugs. TIPs are widely used devices for delivering systemic therapy due to their cost-effectiveness and safety.[56] However, clear guidelines about the timing of implantation surgery prior to the administration of systemic therapy are lacking. Although implantation does not usually require general anesthesia and is often considered a minor surgery, complications associated with foreign body implantation can be severe. These include bloodstream infections, which can occur more than 30 days after implantation and are potentially life-threatening for immunocompromised patients. Some sources suggest that immediate use after implantation is safe,[57] while others recommend waiting 6 to 8 days to minimize complications.[58,59] Notably, certain patients with oncologic emergencies may need immediate systemic therapy and port implantation, where the urgent benefits would outweigh any potential risks associated with early use. Furthermore, the previously mentioned studies did not evaluate the impact of immunotherapy or targeted agents on post-TIP placement complications, likely due to the timeframes in which they were conducted. A recent single-center study reported that bevacizumab exposure shortly after port implantation did not increase the complication rate.[47] Larger studies are needed to confirm this finding.

FUTURE PERSPECTIVES

Currently, numerous clinical trials are underway to examine the efficacy of neoadjuvant approaches using novel drugs in the cancer space. Studies in the NSCLC and melanoma arenas are leading the way, with some data presently available.[8,60] Generally, randomized controlled trials offer the highest level of evidence for treatment efficacy. However, due to the strict eligibility criteria of such trials, the prevalence of adverse events might be underestimated compared to what is observed in daily practice. Therefore, observational or registry studies, which have the potential to capture the reality of daily practice, should be utilized for a more accurate understanding of perioperative complications related to the use of targeted therapy, ICIs, and biologics. It is important to try and identify biomarkers that effectively predict response to neoadjuvant immunotherapy. By doing so, we can avoid administering ICIs to patients who are unlikely to benefit from ICIs, thereby avoiding unnecessary irAEs.

CLINICS CARE POINTS

- To date, limited data are available on the optimal timing for stopping and resuming cancer drugs, including immune checkpoint inhibitors (ICIs), targeted drugs, and biologics, around surgery.

> • Recent exposure to certain cancer drugs is not necessarily an absolute contraindication for surgery. However, surgical oncologists should be aware of and monitor potential complications.
>
> • Perioperative risks associated with ICIs, targeted drugs, and biologics should be assessed on a patient-by-patient basis, utilizing as much of the best available evidence as possible.

DISCLOSURE

D. Nishizaki has nothing to disclose. R.N. Eskander reports research funding (institutional) from Clovis Oncology, United States, GlaxoSmithKline (GSK), Merck, United States, AstraZeneca; consulting fees (including participation on Data Safety Monitoring Board or Advisory Board) from AstraZeneca, Clovis, Eisai, GSK, Immunogen, Mersana, Myriad, Novocure, Onconova, Elevar Therapeutics, Daiichi Sankyo, IMV, Natera, Novartis, ORIC; payment for presentations/writing/educational events from Astra Zeneca, GSK, Immunogen, Merck, Medscape, CURIO, Great Debates and Updates; role as GOG P Associate Clinical Trial Advisor; role as Scientific and Medical Advisor to Clearity Foundation.

REFERENCES

1. DeVita VT Jr, Chu E. A history of cancer chemotherapy. Cancer Res 2008;68(21): 8643–53.
2. Korde LA, Somerfield MR, Carey LA, et al. Neoadjuvant chemotherapy, endocrine therapy, and targeted therapy for breast cancer: ASCO guideline. J Clin Oncol 2021;39(13):1485–505.
3. Zhao J, van Mierlo KMC, Gómez-Ramírez J, et al. Systematic review of the influence of chemotherapy-associated liver injury on outcome after partial hepatectomy for colorectal liver metastases. Br J Surg 2017;104(8):990–1002.
4. Blank CU, Rozeman EA, Fanchi LF, et al. Neoadjuvant versus adjuvant ipilimumab plus nivolumab in macroscopic stage III melanoma. Nat Med 2018;24(11): 1655–61.
5. Cascone T, William WN Jr, Weissferdt A, et al. Neoadjuvant nivolumab or nivolumab plus ipilimumab in operable non-small cell lung cancer: the phase 2 randomized NEOSTAR trial. Nat Med 2021;27(3):504–14.
6. Forde PM, Spicer J, Lu S, et al. Neoadjuvant nivolumab plus chemotherapy in resectable lung cancer. N Engl J Med 2022;386(21):1973–85.
7. Patel S, Othus M, Prieto V, et al. LBA6 Neoadjvuant versus adjuvant pembrolizumab for resected stage III-IV melanoma (SWOG S1801). Ann Oncol 2022;33: S1408.
8. Amaria RN, Postow M, Burton EM, et al. Neoadjuvant relatlimab and nivolumab in resectable melanoma. Nature 2022;1–6.
9. Marron TU, Fiel MI, Hamon P, et al. Neoadjuvant cemiplimab for resectable hepatocellular carcinoma: a single-arm, open-label, phase 2 trial. Lancet Gastroenterology & hepatology 2022;7(3):219–29.
10. National Cancer Institute. Targeted Therapy to Treat Cancer. https://www.cancer.gov/about-cancer/treatment/types/targeted-therapieshttps://www.cancer.gov/about-cancer/treatment/types/targeted-therapies. Accessed May 16, 2023.
11. Trinh VQ, Karakiewicz PI, Sammon J, et al. Venous thromboembolism after major cancer surgery: temporal trends and patterns of care. JAMA Surg 2014; 149(1):43–9.

12. Rausa E, Kelly ME, Asti E, et al. Extended versus conventional thromboprophy-laxis after major abdominal and pelvic surgery: Systematic review and meta-analysis of randomized clinical trials. Surgery 2018;164(6):1234–40.

13. Varki A. Trousseau's syndrome: multiple definitions and multiple mechanisms. Blood 2007;110(6):1723–9.

14. Guntupalli SR, Spinosa D, Wethington S, et al. Prevention of venous thromboem-bolism in patients with cancer. BMJ (Clinical research ed) 2023;381:e072715.

15. Alahmari AK, Almalki ZS, Alahmari AK, et al. Thromboembolic events associated with bevacizumab plus chemotherapy for patients with colorectal cancer: a meta-analysis of randomized controlled trials. Am Health Drug Benefits 2016;9(4): 221–32.

16. Ngo DTM, Williams T, Horder S, et al. Factors associated with adverse cardiovas-cular events in cancer patients treated with bevacizumab. J Clin Med 2020;9(8): 2664.

17. Arnold D, Fuchs CS, Tabernero J, et al. Meta-analysis of individual patient safety data from six randomized, placebo-controlled trials with the antiangiogenic VEGFR2-binding monoclonal antibody ramucirumab. Ann Oncol 2017;28(12): 2932–42.

18. Ciombor KK, Berlin J, Chan E. Aflibercept. Clin Cancer Res 2013;19(8):1920–5.

19. Van Cutsem E, Tabernero J, Lakomy R, et al. Addition of aflibercept to fluoro-uracil, leucovorin, and irinotecan improves survival in a phase III randomized trial in patients with metastatic colorectal cancer previously treated with an oxaliplatin-based regimen. J Clin Oncol 2012;30(28):3499–506.

20. Schlumberger M, Tahara M, Wirth LJ, et al. Lenvatinib versus placebo in radioiodine-refractory thyroid cancer. N Engl J Med 2015;372(7):621–30.

21. Felder S, Rasmussen MS, King R, et al. Prolonged thromboprophylaxis with low molecular weight heparin for abdominal or pelvic surgery. Cochrane Database Syst Rev 2018;11(11):Cd004318.

22. Glance LG, Blumberg N, Eaton MP, et al. Preoperative thrombocytopenia and postoperative outcomes after noncardiac surgery. Anesthesiology 2014;120(1): 62–75.

23. Nagrebetsky A, Al-Samkari H, Davis NM, et al. Perioperative thrombocytopenia: evidence, evaluation, and emerging therapies. Br J Anaesth 2019;122(1):19–31.

24. Mokart D, Penalver M, Chow-Chine L, et al. Surgical treatment of acute abdom-inal complications in hematology patients: outcomes and prognostic factors. Leuk Lymphoma 2017;58(10):2395–402.

25. Mirza MR, Monk BJ, Herrstedt J, et al. Niraparib maintenance therapy in platinum-sensitive, recurrent ovarian cancer. N Engl J Med 2016;375(22): 2154–64.

26. Coleman RL, Oza AM, Lorusso D, et al. Rucaparib maintenance treatment for recurrent ovarian carcinoma after response to platinum therapy (ARIEL3): a rand-omised, double-blind, placebo-controlled, phase 3 trial. Lancet (London, En-gland) 2017;390(10106):1949–61.

27. Pujade-Lauraine E, Ledermann JA, Selle F, et al. Olaparib tablets as maintenance therapy in patients with platinum-sensitive, relapsed ovarian cancer and a BRCA1/2 mutation (SOLO2/ENGOT-Ov21): a double-blind, randomised, placebo-controlled, phase 3 trial. Lancet Oncol 2017;18(9):1274–84.

28. LaFargue CJ, Dal Molin GZ, Sood AK, et al. Exploring and comparing adverse events between PARP inhibitors. Lancet Oncol 2019;20(1):e15–28.

29. Friedlander M, Banerjee S, Mileshkin L, et al. Practical guidance on the use of ola-parib capsules as maintenance therapy for women with BRCA mutations and

platinum-sensitive recurrent ovarian cancer. Asia Pac J Clin Oncol 2016;12(4): 323–31.

30. Liu Y, Sun W, Li J. Risk of thrombocytopenia with platelet-derived growth factor receptor kinase inhibitors in cancer patients: a systematic review and meta-analysis of phase 2/3 randomized, controlled trials. J Clin Pharmacol 2021; 61(11):1397–405.

31. Motzer RJ, Hutson TE, Cella D, et al. Pazopanib versus sunitinib in metastatic renal-cell carcinoma. N Engl J Med 2013;369(8):722–31.

32. Ravaud A, Motzer RJ, Pandha HS, et al. Adjuvant sunitinib in high-risk renal-cell carcinoma after nephrectomy. N Engl J Med 2016;375(23):2246–54.

33. Zhu C, Ma X, Hu Y, et al. Safety and efficacy profile of lenvatinib in cancer therapy: a systematic review and meta-analysis. Oncotarget 2016;7(28):44545–57.

34. Watson N, Al-Samkari H. Thrombotic and bleeding risk of angiogenesis inhibitors in patients with and without malignancy. J Thromb Haemost 2021;19(8):1852–63.

35. Goetze TO, Hofheinz RD, Gaiser T, et al. Perioperative FLOT plus ramucirumab for resectable esophagogastric adenocarcinoma: A randomized phase II/III trial of the German AIO and Italian GOIM. Int J Cancer 2023;153(1):153–63.

36. Demetri GD, von Mehren M, Blanke CD, et al. Efficacy and safety of imatinib mesylate in advanced gastrointestinal stromal tumors. N Engl J Med 2002;347(7): 472–80.

37. Blanke CD, Rankin C, Demetri GD, et al. Phase III randomized, intergroup trial assessing imatinib mesylate at two dose levels in patients with unresectable or metastatic gastrointestinal stromal tumors expressing the kit receptor tyrosine kinase: S0033. J Clin Oncol 2008;26(4):626–32.

38. Demetri GD, von Mehren M, Antonescu CR, et al. NCCN Task Force report: update on the management of patients with gastrointestinal stromal tumors. J Natl Compr Cancer Netw 2010;8(Suppl 2):S1–41, quiz S42-44.

39. Verweij J, Casali PG, Zalcberg J, et al. Progression-free survival in gastrointestinal stromal tumours with high-dose imatinib: randomised trial. Lancet (London, England) 2004;364(9440):1127–34.

40. Kramer R, Zaremba A, Moreira A, et al. Hematological immune related adverse events after treatment with immune checkpoint inhibitors. Eur J Cancer 2021; 147:170–81.

41. Haddad TC, Zhao S, Li M, et al. Immune checkpoint inhibitor-related thrombocytopenia: incidence, risk factors and effect on survival. Cancer Immunol Immunother 2022;71(5):1157–65.

42. Wu YS, Shui L, Shen D, et al. Bevacizumab combined with chemotherapy for ovarian cancer: an updated systematic review and meta-analysis of randomized controlled trials. Oncotarget 2017;8(6):10703–13.

43. Gaitskell K, Rogozińska E, Platt S, et al. Angiogenesis inhibitors for the treatment of epithelial ovarian cancer. Cochrane Database Syst Rev 2023;4(4):Cd007930.

44. Cunningham D, Stenning SP, Smyth EC, et al. Peri-operative chemotherapy with or without bevacizumab in operable oesophagogastric adenocarcinoma (UK Medical Research Council ST03): primary analysis results of a multicentre, open-label, randomised phase 2-3 trial. Lancet Oncol 2017;18(3):357–70.

45. Baxter NN, Fischer HD, Richardson DP, et al. A population-based study of complications after colorectal surgery in patients who have received bevacizumab. Dis Colon Rectum 2018;61(3):306–13.

46. King BH, Baumgartner JM, Kelly KJ, et al. Preoperative bevacizumab does not increase complications following cytoreductive surgery and hyperthermic intraperitoneal chemotherapy. PLoS One 2020;15(12):e0243252.

47. Shigyo H, Suzuki H, Tanaka T, et al. Safety of early bevacizumab administration after central venous port placement for patients with colorectal cancer. Cancers 2023;15(8):2264.
48. Seishima R, Okabayashi K, Ikeuchi H, et al. Effect of biologics on the risk of advanced-stage inflammatory bowel disease-associated intestinal cancer: a nationwide study. Am J Gastroenterol 2023;118(7):1248–55.
49. Kulaylat AS, Kulaylat AN, Schaefer EW, et al. Association of preoperative anti-tumor necrosis factor therapy with adverse postoperative outcomes in patients undergoing abdominal surgery for ulcerative colitis. JAMA Surg 2017;152(8):e171538.
50. Billioud V, Ford AC, Tedesco ED, et al. Preoperative use of anti-TNF therapy and postoperative complications in inflammatory bowel diseases: a meta-analysis. Journal of Crohn's & Colitis 2013;7(11):853–67.
51. Rempenault C, Lukas C, Combe B, et al. Risk of diverticulitis and gastrointestinal perforation in rheumatoid arthritis treated with tocilizumab compared to rituximab or abatacept. Rheumatology 2022;61(3):953–62.
52. Xie F, Yun H, Bernatsky S, et al. Brief report: risk of gastrointestinal perforation among rheumatoid arthritis patients receiving tofacitinib, tocilizumab, or other biologic treatments. Arthritis Rheumatol 2016;68(11):2612–7.
53. Brahmer JR, Abu-Sbeih H, Ascierto PA, et al. Society for Immunotherapy of Cancer (SITC) clinical practice guideline on immune checkpoint inhibitor-related adverse events. Journal for Immunotherapy of Cancer 2021;9(6):e002435.
54. Eisenberg BL, Harris J, Blanke CD, et al. Phase II trial of neoadjuvant/adjuvant imatinib mesylate (IM) for advanced primary and metastatic/recurrent operable gastrointestinal stromal tumor (GIST): early results of RTOG 0132/ACRIN 6665. J Surg Oncol 2009;99(1):42–7.
55. National Comprehensive Cancer Network (NCCN). Gastrointeoinal Stromal Tumors (Version 1. 2023). 2023; https://www.nccn.org/professionals/physician_gls/pdf/gist.pdf. Accessed August 7, 2023.
56. Moss JG, Wu O, Bodenham AR, et al. Central venous access devices for the delivery of systemic anticancer therapy (CAVA): a randomised controlled trial. Lancet (London, England) 2021;398(10298):403–15.
57. Karanlik H, Odabas H, Yildirim I, et al. Is there any effect of first-day usage of a totally implantable venous access device on complications? Int J Clin Oncol 2015;20(6):1057–62.
58. Narducci F, Jean-Laurent M, Boulanger L, et al. Totally implantable venous access port systems and risk factors for complications: a one-year prospective study in a cancer centre. Eur J Surg Oncol 2011;37(10):913–8.
59. Kakkos A, Bresson L, Hudry D, et al. Complication-related removal of totally implantable venous access port systems: Does the interval between placement and first use and the neutropenia-inducing potential of chemotherapy regimens influence their incidence? A four-year prospective study of 4045 patients. Eur J Surg Oncol 2017;43(4):689–95.
60. Reuss JE, Anagnostou V, Cottrell TR, et al. Neoadjuvant nivolumab plus ipilimumab in resectable non-small cell lung cancer. Journal for immunotherapy of Cancer 2020;8(2):e001282.
61. Wei G, Rafiyath S, Liu D. First-line treatment for chronic myeloid leukemia: dasatinib, nilotinib, or imatinib. J Hematol Oncol 2010;3:47.
62. Mayer RJ, Van Cutsem E, Falcone A, et al. Randomized trial of TAS-102 for refractory metastatic colorectal cancer. N Engl J Med 2015;372(20):1909–19.

63. Fennell DA, King A, Mohammed S, et al. Abemaciclib in patients with p16ink4A-deficient mesothelioma (MiST2): a single-arm, open-label, phase 2 trial. Lancet Oncol 2022;23(3):374–81.
64. Karasic TB, O'Hara MH, Teitelbaum UR, et al. Phase II trial of palbociclib in patients with advanced esophageal or gastric cancer. Oncol 2020;25(12):e1864–8.
65. Liu K, Li YH, Zhang X, et al. Incidence and risk of severe adverse events associated with trastuzumab emtansine (T-DM1) in the treatment of breast cancer: an up-to-date systematic review and meta-analysis of randomized controlled clinical trials. Expert Rev Clin Pharmacol 2022;15(11):1343–50.

Precision Oncology in Breast Cancer Surgery

Ali Benjamin Abbasi, MD[a], Vincent Wu, MD[b], Julie E. Lang, MD[b,*],
Laura J. Esserman, MD, MBA[a]

KEYWORDS

- Precision medicine • Breast surgery • Biomarker • Personalized medicine
- Precision oncology • Precision screening

KEY POINTS

- Breast cancer is a heterogeneous family of diseases that ranges from indolent to aggressive tumor biology.
- Molecular testing biomarkers are useful to rationally select therapies for patients and to identify patients who carry deleterious gene mutations.
- Response predictive subtypes may be used to guide treatment.
- Appropriate de-escalation of cancer treatments based on disease response allows for avoidance of overtreatment.

INTRODUCTION

Despite significant advances in treatment, breast cancer remains the second leading cause of cancer death in women, with more than 40,000 deaths annually in the United States.[1] Although surgical resection remains a cornerstone of therapy, advances in precision oncology have begun to shift the paradigm for treating this disease. Traditionally, breast cancer has been classified according to hormone receptor (HR) status (ie, estrogen receptor [ER] and progesterone receptor [PR]), human epidermal growth factor receptor 2 (HER2) receptor status, and histology (invasive vs carcinoma in situ, and ductal vs lobular, and other rare histologies). In this article, the authors explore the emerging understanding of breast cancer as a very heterogeneous disease, beyond the traditional categorization of receptor status. The authors illustrate how precision approaches to diagnosis, treatment, and screening promise to continue revolutionizing the treatment of breast cancer.

[a] Department of Surgery, San Francisco Breast Care Center, University of California, Box 1710, UCSF, San Francisco, CA 94143, USA; [b] Department of Surgery, Cleveland Clinic Breast Services, 9500 Euclid Avenue, A80, Cleveland Clinic, Cleveland, OH 44195, USA
* Corresponding author. 9500 Euclid Avenue, A80, Cleveland Clinic, Cleveland, OH 44195.
E-mail address: LANGJ2@ccf.org

Surg Oncol Clin N Am 33 (2024) 293–310
https://doi.org/10.1016/j.soc.2023.12.011
1055-3207/24/© 2023 Elsevier Inc. All rights reserved.
surgonc.theclinics.com

The driving force behind precision breast oncology is the recognition that breast cancer is not one disease but includes a heterogeneous family of cancers. Breast cancer biology ranges from ultralow to rapidly metastatic disease. Indolent or ultralow tumors may never or rarely progress to metastatic or life-threatening disease. For these tumors, biology, rather than early detection determines the outcome and only treatments with low risks of adverse events should be given, because the potential for dissemination is quite low.[2,3] Other cancers that are low grade and slow growing have a long tail for recurrence, where rates of recurrence are higher after 5 years, and can recur up to 15 or even 20 years after diagnosis. Still others are fast growing, metastasize early, and warrant prompt and aggressive treatment. The paradigm of precision oncology in breast cancer is to personalize screening based on patients' risk depending on their disease phenotype and to personalize diagnosis and treatment based on the biology of their tumor and their response to treatments (**Fig. 1**).

The movement toward precision oncology in breast cancer has in part been enabled by a shift in the approach to treating the disease. Traditionally, patients with operable breast cancer underwent surgery upfront, followed by adjuvant chemotherapy and hormonal therapy if indicated. However, systemic therapy for faster growing subtypes has increasingly moved to the neoadjuvant setting, which improves rates of breast-conserving therapy and most importantly allows early assessment of response to therapy by evaluating the pathologic response of the tumor specimen.[4,5] Before surgery, the tumor can be evaluated on serial imaging, which enables use of tumor size as a "biomarker" for treatment response, meaning personalized treatments can rapidly be evaluated and adapted. After surgery, pathologic complete response (pCR) is a powerful predictor of Event-free survival (EFS) with a hazard ratio of 0.19[6] across subtypes in the setting of molecularly high-risk disease. This early endpoint enables rapid learning on the impact of personalized therapies and efficient evaluation of drugs.

In this article, the authors focus on precision treatments of operable or potentially operable breast cancer. The authors first discuss the importance of genetic and

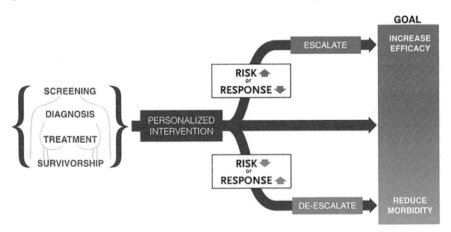

Fig. 1. A new paradigm for precision oncology in breast cancer. Screening should be based on the risk for developing specific breast cancer phenotypes. Diagnosis should establish the molecular subtype of the tumor, which determines personalized treatments based on the predicted risk of the tumor and response to therapy. The aim is to optimize treatment response to escalate in the setting of poor response and de-escalate either in the setting of low risk of developing metastases or in the setting of exceptional response (complete pathologic response) and minimize treatment toxicity for low-risk tumors and great responders.

molecular testing in workup and neoadjuvant treatment of patients with germline mutations and those at average risk. The authors then discuss why treatment response is an important aspect of personalizing therapy and explore future directions in the area of diagnostics and therapeutics. Given the heterogeneous nature of breast cancer, it becomes clear that screening must also take a personalized approach. At the end of this article, the authors therefore focus on precision approaches to screening, based on genetic testing and other factors, as well as discuss ongoing trials addressing this strategy.

PRECISION DIAGNOSIS AND TREATMENT
Genetic Testing in Patients at High-Risk for Breast Cancer

Identification of patients with hereditary cancer syndromes enables surgeons and patients to make informed treatment decisions, allowing for enhanced surveillance, consideration of risk-reducing interventions for patients, and cascade screening in family members. High-penetrance cancer susceptibility genes are associated with 5% to 10% of all breast cancers,[7,8] and although pathogenic germline mutations may occur in one of several different genes, BRCA1 and BRCA2 mutations account for more than 50% of pathogenic germline variants.[9] Current National Comprehensive Cancer Network (NCCN) guidelines for consideration of genetic evaluation and testing incorporate personal and family history. Personal criteria include those ≤50 years of age with breast cancer, triple-negative breast cancer (TNBC), multiple primaries (metachronous or synchronous), and males with breast cancer. In those with breast cancer, criteria for family history include having ≥1 first-, second-, or third-degree relative (same side of family) with breast cancer at age ≤50 year, male breast cancer, ovarian cancer, pancreatic cancer, or prostate cancer (high-risk or very high-risk group, metastatic)[8] (**Table 1**).

Comprehensive, multigene genetic testing has become widely available and incorporated as an integral part of breast cancer evaluation due to advances in next-generation sequencing and regulatory changes leading to lower cost,[10–12] although greater than 99% of all mutations are based on mutations in nine genes. Companies, such as Invitae, Color Genomics, Myriad Genetics, Ambry Genetics, and Natera, provide germline panel testing evaluating 30 to 90 genes associated with hereditary breast cancer or other hereditary cancer risk genotypes. These allow for simultaneous analysis of specific familial cancer predisposition and/or multiple cancer-related genetic mutations (some panels offer testing for up to 500 genes for families with individuals with mixed tumor types).[13] These tests are similar in performance but vary widely in cost. As the turnaround time for these comprehensive panels may take weeks to return and as results may impact decision for breast-conserving therapy (breast-conserving surgery [BCS]) versus mastectomy, unilateral versus bilateral mastectomy, or systemic therapy regimen, breast cancer STAT panels can be used for time-sensitive cases. These panels analyze high-risk genes (such as BRCA1, BRCA2, CDH1, PALB2, PTEN, STK11, and TP53) associated with significantly increased risk of breast cancer in which risk-reducing bilateral mastectomy is strongly considered while providing results in less than 2 weeks.[13] The panels may also detect other moderate-risk genes with an increased risk of breast cancer (such as ATM, BARD1, CHEK2, NF1, and RAD51 C) that have insufficient evidence to recommend risk-reducing mastectomy per National Comprehensive Cancer Center Network (NCCN) guidelines.[8,13]

As the cost of genetic testing has declined substantially, some have called for increased access to genetic testing beyond the criteria supported by the NCCN

Table 1
The National Comprehensive Cancer Network genetic evaluation and hereditary cancer testing guidelines version 4.2023

NCCN Guidelines Version 4.2023	
Personal History of Breast Cancer	
1. ≤50 y of age	
2. Any age	Treatment Indications:
	1. Aid in systemic treatment decisions with PARP inhibitors for breast cancer in metastatic setting
	2. Aid in adjuvant treatment decisions with olaparib for high-risk, HER2-breast cancer
	Pathology or Histology:
	1. Triple-negative breast cancer
	2. Multiple primary breast cancers (synchronous or metachronous)
	3. Lobular breast cancer with a personal or family history of diffuse gastric cancer
	Male breast cancer
	Ashkenazi Jewish Ancestry
	Family History:
	1. ≥1 close blood relative with any of the following: Breast cancer at age ≤50 y; male breast cancer; ovarian cancer; pancreatic cancer; and prostate cancer with metastatic or high- or very-high-risk group
	2. ≥3 diagnoses of breast and/or prostate cancer including patient with breast cancer
Family History of Only Breast, Ovarian, Pancreatic, and/or Prostate Cancer(s)	
1. Affected individual (not meeting criteria above) or unaffected individual with:	1. First- or second-degree blood relative meeting any of the criteria listed above (except unaffected individuals with relatives meeting criteria only for systemic therapy decision-making)
	2. If affected relative has pancreatic cancer or prostate cancer, only first-degree relatives should be offered testing unless indicated based on additional family history
2. Affected or unaffected individual who does not meet criteria above	1. >5% probability of a BRCA1/2 pathogenic variant based on prior probability models (eg, Tyrer-Cuzick, BRCAPro, CanRisk)

guidelines. The American Society of Breast Surgeons consensus guideline states that all women with either newly diagnosed or a personal history of breast cancer should be offered access to genetic testing.[14] The rationale for this stance is that a similar proportion of patients with pathogenic/likely pathogenic mutations may be found in patients meeting the NCCN guidelines versus those not meeting the NCCN guidelines (9.39 vs 7.9%).[15] The approach of testing everyone is controversial since not all mutations are truly actionable, and it is possible that patients might view genetic testing as stressful and added cost. Another study also advocated for expanding the NCCN guidelines to include all patients with breast cancer diagnosed by age 65 years.[16] Direct-to-consumer genetic testing is also available, but there are highly variable levels of evidence to support their claims of accurate detection of genetic variants associated with breast cancer or other diseases.[17]

Tailoring Therapy to Molecular Tumor Types in Patients with Germline Mutations

Tumor and germline genetic testing may provide opportunities for targeted therapy in the neoadjuvant or adjuvant setting. Deleterious mutations in *BRCA1/2* result in deficiency in DNA double-strand break repair and lead to tumor cell dependence on a single-strand break repair pathway regulated by the poly (adenosine diphosphate ribose [ADP-ribose]) poly (ADP-ribose) polymerase (PARP) enzyme. PARP inhibitors (PARPi) have recently emerged as a new therapy in breast cancer gene (BRCA)-related or BRCA-like breast cancers. The Investigation of Serial Studies to Predict Your Therapeutic Response with Imaging and Molecular Analysis 2 (I-SPY2) is an on-going, multicenter, open-label, adaptive phase 2 platform trial designed to assess new agent combinations with standard neoadjuvant therapy in high-risk stage II–III patients with breast cancer.[18] So far, three arms in the trial have included a PARPi. These arms suggest that there is likely to be a 60% to 70% complete response (CR) rate in *BRCA1/2* and *PALB2* mutation carriers. For example, one of these arms included talazoparib (PARPi) with a low dose of irinotecan. Although the arm did not graduate, exploratory analysis revealed that 6 of 10 *BRCA* carriers in the arm attained pCR.[19] Multiple additional ongoing clinical trials, including those by MD Anderson, are assessing PARPi use in the neoadjuvant or adjuvant setting for early-stage HER2-negative breast cancers in those with *BRCA* mutations (NCT05498155, NCT04584255). This is a promising area of development for precision treatments of patients with pathogenic germline mutations.

In patients with metastatic disease and germline *BRCA1/2* pathogenic or likely pathogenic variants, the OlympiA (NCT02032823) trial was conducted as a randomized (1:1), double-blind, placebo-controlled, international study of 1836 patients with HER2-negative high-risk early breast cancer who had received local treatment and neoadjuvant or adjuvant chemotherapy. Patients were randomized to 1 year of oral olaparib (PARPi) or placebo with the primary endpoint of invasive disease-free survival (IDFS). Three-year IDFS was significantly longer in the olaparib group (85.9%) compared with the placebo group (77.1%, Hazard ratio [HR] 0.58; 99.5% CI 0.41–0.82; $P < .001$) and fewer deaths were associated with the olaparib group.[20] Olaparib has since been approved by the Food and Drug Administration (FDA) for adjuvant therapy in this patient population.

Tailoring Therapy to Molecular Tumor Types in Patients Without Germline Mutations

Targeted therapy is also advancing in patients without germline mutations. The goal is to identify which patients are most likely to respond to each drug. This is important for several reasons. First, it allows patients the best opportunity of using the "shots on goal" that have the highest rate of success, thereby increasing the chance of pCR. Second this minimizes the level of toxicity that patients are exposed to. This is important to have the best chance of avoiding cytotoxic chemotherapy altogether and to protect patients from uncommon, but devastating complications of newer treatments like permanent adrenal insufficiency, which can be seen with immune checkpoint inhibitors.[21]

A recent analysis 990 patients treated on nine different arms of the first I-SPY trial illustrates the power of personalized treatments beyond the traditional receptor subtypes.[22] Although the control arm achieved pCR in only 19% of patients, patients on the nine experimental arms achieved pCR at a rate of 35%. With the benefit of hindsight, if all patients had been assigned to the optimal treatment based on their HR and HER2 receptor statuses, the rate of pCR could have been boosted to 51%. By developing new subtypes based on tumor transcriptomics using RNA-sequencing and protein expression using reverse phase protein arrays (RPPA), the response rate could have been boosted even further up to 58% (**Fig. 2**). These tumor subtypes, called response predictive subtypes (RPSs) were developed by clustering mRNA sequencing data and RPPA data into different phenotypes based on tumor biology and treatment response. The final subtyping scheme included immune, DNA repair, HER2-positive basal, and HER2-positive luminal types. This improvement in pCR up to 58% compared with 19% on standard chemotherapy illustrates the promise of precision treatments that go beyond traditional HR/HER2 categorization.

These RPSs are being studied for potential clinical use. For example, the immune phenotype developed in this study was predictive of response to immune oncology (IO) drugs. This was recently developed into a clinical grade assay, called the ImPrint (Agendia), which was evaluated in the immune therapy arms of the I-SPY 2 trial.[23] The ImPrint classifier was most predictive in HR+ disease where 76% of ImPrint+ HR+ tumors achieved pCR, compared with 16% ImPrint-HR+ tumors. In

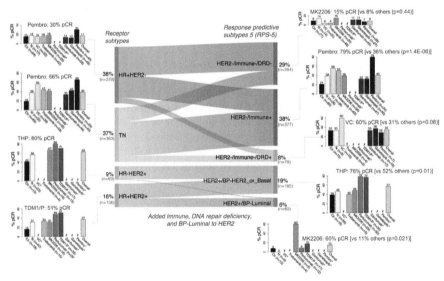

Fig. 2. Response to therapy based on response predictive subtypes (RPS-5) (*right*) as compared with traditional hormone receptor (HR) and HER2 receptor subtypes (*left*). Each bar graph shows the percent of patients achieving pathologic complete response (pCR) in a particular subgroup of patients for each of the nine agents included in I-SPY, as well as the best performing agent in blue above each chart. The middle portion of the figure shows the mapping between the traditional HR and HER2 subtypes versus the RPS-5. If patients had been assigned to optimal therapy based on their HR and HER2 status, pCR could have been achieved in 51% where in patients assigned by RPS-5 directed therapy, pCR could have been achieved 58% of patients. The # denotes subsets with < 5 patients. * denotes arm not open in subtype. BP, blueprint; Ctr, control; DRD, DNA repair deficiency; N, neratinib; P, pertuzumab; TDM1, trastuzumab emtansine; THP, trastuzumab, docetaxel, trastuzumab, and pertuzumab; VC, veliparib carboplatin. (*Adapted from* Wolf DM, Yau C, Wulfkuhle J, Brown-Swigart L, Gallagher RI, Lee PRE, et al. Redefining breast cancer subtypes to guide treatment prioritization and maximize response: Predictive biomarkers across 10 cancer therapies. Cancer Cell. 2022;40(6):609-23 e6.)

TNBC (ie, ER-/PR-/HER-negative), 75% of ImPrint + tumors reached pCR, compared with 37% of ImPrint-tumors. The ImPrint recently received an investigational device exemption by the FDA, which allows its deployment in prospective clinical trials including I-SPY 2.2. The FDA has approved immune checkpoint blockade in combination with a taxane and carboplatin for TNBC patients. The RPS schema shows that about a third of molecularly high-risk HR-positive patients and two-thirds of TNBC patients have the immune signature. This is important because the immune checkpoint inhibitors come with side effects that can be permanent (adrenal insufficiency), so it is best not to expose women with tumor types unlikely to respond. Confirmatory data are emerging that some HR-positive patients indeed respond to the IO agents.

Changing the Surgical Paradigm

The shift to precision neoadjuvant treatments also presents an opportunity for reducing the need for axillary surgery. At the start of the I-SPY trial, patients with clinically positive nodes were required to undergo axillary lymph node dissection (ALND) after completion of neoadjuvant therapy. However, this paradigm has shifted, and the use of ALND has declined dramatically, especially in patients who were node positive before the start of neoadjuvant therapy.[24] Although SLNB alone after neoadjuvant chemotherapy carries a false-positive rate that is too high,[25] removing the clipped node alongside any sentinel nodes has a similar diagnostic accuracy as a full ALND.[26] The ability to reduce the reliance on highly morbid procedures like ALND illustrates the potential benefits of precision neoadjuvant therapy for operable breast cancer.

Precision neoadjuvant therapy also promises to further improve rates of BCS. Although it is accepted that neoadjuvant therapy improves rates of BCS,[27] the previous studies suggested that BCS after neoadjuvant therapy may lead to increased rates of locoregional recurrence (LRR).[28] However, a recent analysis of the I-SPY trial found that therapy followed by BCS does not increase the risk of LRR compared with mastectomy.[29] In fact, the main predictors of locoregional recurrence after BCS in I-SPY were TNBC receptor status and the amount of residual cancer burden on pathology. This suggests that precision neoadjuvant therapy will be able to improve the rates of breast conservation without affecting locoregional disease control.

Evolving Approaches

Predicting pathologic complete response to avoid overtreatment

Despite decades of research, relatively few clinical grade biomarkers exist to predict therapeutic response to chemotherapy, limiting the ability to apply precision oncology to many early-stage breast cancer patients. The American Society of Clinical Oncology (ASCO) Guidelines for adjuvant endocrine and chemotherapy decision-making include ER, PR, HER2, and Ki67 (combined with ER, PR, and HER2 known as IHC4).[30] Genomic classifiers, such as Oncotype DX, MammaPrint, Breast Cancer Index, EndoPredict, and Prosigna assays, may be used for specific indications in patients who are not HER2-positive or TNBC.[30] Research classifiers such as the RPS developed in I-SPY will further push the envelope for personalizing treatment based on predicted pCR rates.

In recent years, several new treatment regimens have been adopted as standard of care in the adjuvant and neoadjuvant setting (eg, combinations including pembrolizumab[31,32] and pertuzumab[33,34]). Patients with cancer with TNBC or HER2-amplified breast cancers are often treated with contemporary guideline-based neoadjuvant therapy and achieve unprecedentedly high pCR rates of 60% to 80%. Breast MRI is often used in patients receiving neoadjuvant chemotherapy to determine treatment response.[35] Although much progress has been made with contrast-enhanced

MRI,[36] radiographic response based on standard breast MRI cannot determine residual cancer burden with 100% accuracy.[37] Thus, surgery is offered despite radiographic CR. However, there exist opportunities to de-escalate surgery, systemic therapy, and radiation to avoid over-treatment of patients with breast cancer who respond favorably to neoadjuvant systemic therapy and achieve a pCR.[38] Several ongoing clinical trials will contribute to provide evidence of whether it is safe to de-escalate various multidisciplinary treatments if pCR occurs.[6,39–41]

Kuerer and colleagues conducted a multicenter, single-arm, Phase II clinical trial enrolling women who had T1-2, N0-1, M0 TNBC, or HER2-amplified breast cancers and who had a residual breast lesion less than 2 cm after neoadjuvant therapy.[40] The goal of the trial was to identify exceptional responders by proving that patients achieved a pCR (or not) with twelve 9-gauge vacuum-assisted core needle biopsies of the tumor bed. Surgery was omitted in 31 patients with no invasive or in situ carcinoma identified. These patients were treated with radiotherapy alone. No ipsilateral local recurrences occurred at a median follow-up of 26.4 months.[40] If these results are maintained on long-term follow-up, this sets the stage for future prospective studies to confirm these results.

Reducing the use of cytotoxic chemotherapy is another promising direction for precision breast oncology. Some oncologists have questioned the overall survival benefit for the addition of anthracyclines to taxane-based chemotherapy in non-metastatic breast cancer.[42] US Oncology Research published a trial comparing adriamycin/cyclophosphamide (AC) to docetaxel/cyclophosphamide (TC) as adjuvant therapy in Stage I–III breast cancer showing better disease-free survival (DFS) for TC versus AC.[43] However, the subsequent ABC trials evaluated six cycles of adjuvant TC (TC6) to taxane+ AC (TaxAC) in a non-inferiority design, but was subsequently halted for futility as TaxAC showed a better DFS rate (90.7% vs 88.2%), particularly in a subset analysis of patients who were N2 or higher.[44] Therefore, it remains controversial what the role of anthracyclines should be in many non-metastatic breast cancer patients. TC6 is an option per the NCCN guidelines, however, anthracycline-based combinations remain an option and are commonly used in both the neoadjuvant and adjuvant setting.

As an evolving platform trial, I-SPY2 evolved into I-SPY2.2, giving patients the potential to avoid standard chemotherapy altogether if they are able to achieve a pCR with new targeted agents such as antibody drug conjugates or bispecific antibodies. Patients are adaptively randomized to Block A, which includes novel targeted treatments tested across tumor RPSs,[22] with the option of early surgery if MRI and biopsy suggest that pCR is not achieved, using a score called the predicted Residual Cancer Burden (preRCB). Patients who do not proceed to surgery move to Block B which is a best-in-class RPS-specific rescue based on the best results from I-SPY2. Block B involves adaptive randomization based on six RPSs with three categories for high-predicted response and three categories for low predicted response. Among the high responders, the goal is to find the least toxic agent, whereas among the low responders the goal is to improve efficacy. This approach allows individual tailoring of therapy to biology based on response despite the use of randomization. There again exists the option of an early surgery based on preRCB or moving on to Block C (AC ± immunotherapy for TNBC). In the most recent analysis, the use of preRCB reduced the use of AC by 22% in the last year of I-SPY 2. Among patients who met preRCB criteria, 95% had a residual cancer burden score on pathology of 0 or 1.[45] This approach allows patients the potential to avoid the short- and long-term toxicities of AC while providing the opportunity to switch therapies (another shot on goal) if the tumor does not respond favorably to the initial neoadjuvant therapy.

Liquid biopsy with next-generation sequencing for precision oncology

The term liquid biopsy includes assays such as circulating tumor cells (CTCs) or circulating tumor DNA (ctDNA). There is considerable interest in the use of liquid biopsies to detect minimal residual disease (MRD) recurrence, as a screening tool, and to predict sensitivity to a specific therapy. The detection of CTCs or ctDNA is associated with worse outcomes in both early and metastatic breast cancer.[46–48] Although the term liquid biopsy is more commonly used to refer to ctDNA testing, our group has shown that CTCs may also be used as a liquid biopsy indicative of tumor biology in both early and advanced breast cancer.[49–51]

There is growing interest in the use of ctDNA assays in non-metastatic breast cancer, but this requires a priori knowledge of specific tumor mutations personalized as a bespoke assay for individual patients for optimal sensitivity.[52,53] Garcia-Murillas and colleagues demonstrated that targeted capture sequencing of ctDNA after completion of neoadjuvant therapy and surgery predicted subsequent metastatic recurrence.[54] Mutation tracking with ctDNA also could predict the genetic events present in distant metastatic biopsies better than sequencing the primary tumor (acquired at an earlier timepoint before metastasis).[54] Several teams published creating patient-specific ctDNA assays to detect MRD. McDonald and colleagues reported that ctDNA concentrations were lower in patients who achieved a pCR.[55] Parsons and colleagues showed that bespoke ctDNA assay sensitivity for detecting MRD is driven by the number of tumor mutations available to track, which varied widely, ranging from $n = 2$ to 346 mutations per tumor.[56] The technologic capabilities of ctDNA assays were refined to allow for detecting very low variant allele fractions to enable use in non-metastatic patients[55] and for following breast cancer survivors for the detection of MRD in advance of subsequent distant metastasis.[57] Coombes and colleagues showed that ctDNA could detect MRD recurrence by as much as 2 years earlier than imaging, providing a window of opportunity for possible therapeutic intervention.[58]

Because the detection of ctDNA after neoadjuvant therapy is associated with early metastatic relapse, the investigators have called for prospective trials testing the utility of ctDNA monitoring for early detection of recurrence.[59] Turner and colleagues conducted the c-TRAK-TN study to prospectively determine if ctDNA can guide clinical management. Patients with early-stage TNBC and residual disease after neoadjuvant chemotherapy underwent ctDNA surveillance with 27.4% of patients testing positive for ctDNA. In turn, the ctDNA-positive patients were randomized 2:1 to receive pembrolizumab, but insufficient numbers of patients were treated to evaluate the potential activity of pembrolizumab, which is now approved for use in TNBC.[60] Careful study design excluding patients who were metastatic at diagnosis, rapidly designing personalized assays, and consideration of best effective treatment available will optimize outcomes of liquid biopsy clinical trials.[60]

Turner and colleagues conducted the plasmaMATCH study as a platform trial assessing the clinical validity of using ctDNA to select targeted therapies in patients with metastatic breast cancer without previous tissue sequencing.[61] This study showed that ctDNA testing for *PIK3CA*, *ESR1*, *HER2*, *AKT1*, *PTEN*, and *TP53* has sufficient accuracy for widespread use without concomitant tumor biopsy testing.[61] The ASCO guidelines recommend testing for *ESR1* and *PIK3CA* mutations, preferably in ctDNA, in metastatic breast cancer at the time of disease progression.[62]

Magbanua and colleagues reported an analysis of the I-SPY2 trial using bespoke tumor-informed assays, which found ctDNA to be present in 73% of patients' plasma specimens before treatment.[63] All patients who achieved pCR were ctDNA negative. The lack of ctDNA clearance predicted for disease recurrence, whereas ctDNA negativity was associated with improved outcomes even in the absence of a pCR.[63] They then performed a second tumor-informed ctDNA study involving a separate cohort of I-SPY2 patients.[64] Early clearance of ctDNA at 3 weeks after initiation of treatment in patients with TNBC was associated with improved outcomes. Again, ctDNA negativity was shown to be associated with improved outcomes even in the absence of a pCR.[64]

Relatively few liquid biopsy assays are FDA-approved for use in breast cancer at this time. The CellSearch assay was the first FDA-approved liquid biopsy test to enumerate CTCs in the peripheral blood.[48] Some liquid biopsy assays have been FDA-approved as companion diagnostic (CDx) ctDNA assays or for use to harvest CTCs for subsequent user-validated downstream analysis, such as the ANGLE Parsortix.[51,65] ctDNA detection of *ESR1* mutation status by the Guardant 360 CDx was FDA-approved as a CDx predicting benefit from elacestrant (an oral ER degrader) in HR-positive, HER2-negative advanced breast cancer.[66] ctDNA detection of *PIK3CA* mutations was FDA-approved as a CDx predicting benefit from alpelisib in HR-positive, HER2-negative advanced breast cancer.[67]

The Qiagen therascreen PIK3CA RGQ polymerase chain reaction kit and also the FoundationOne CDx are FDA-approved as companion diagnostic tests for detecting PIK3CA mutations for candidacy for alpelisib treatment.[67,68] The Natera Signatera received FDA Breakthrough Device Designation for the detection of MRD.[58] Although screening patients with a liquid biopsy to enhance population-based mammographic screening is an appealing concept, this remains an unmet need in breast cancer research. The heterogeneity of breast cancer and the rarity of ctDNA transcripts in the very early stages of breast cancer create challenges for ctDNA testing in screening; therefore, there are no current FDA-approved liquid biopsy assays for screening for breast cancer.

PRECISION SCREENING
Precision Screening in Average-Risk Individuals

The recommended approach to screening for breast cancer has been a highly controversial topic, with a range of recommendations from different guideline bodies.[69] In part, the controversy surrounding screening reflects the fact that there likely should not be a one size fits all approach. Given the heterogeneous nature of breast cancer that we have described above, screening decisions should be made based on each patient's individual risk.[70] The goal of screening should not be to maximize the number of breast cancers detected, but rather to minimize the number of cancers that are detected in advanced stages of disease. Over-detection of early-stage cancers is a problem, because it can expose patients to the risks of procedures or drugs, despite that fact that some early-stage tumors are unlikely to progress to life-threatening disease.[71]

Precision screening should depend on a patient's individual risk for fast or slow-growing tumors and our understanding of the genetics that underpin breast cancer risk. Although the notion that clinical risk factors and germline mutations in genes like *BRCA1/2* increase the risk of breast cancer is well established, we are beginning to uncover single nucleotide polymorphisms (SNPs) that also result in increases in breast cancer risk. Although each SNP alone results only in a small increase in risk, taken together they are thought to explain 15% to 20% of the variance in breast cancer risk.[72,73] Several ongoing trials are evaluating precision screening using genetic information.

The Women Informed to Screen Depending on Measures of risk (WISDOM) study (NCT02620852) is a large, randomized trial that evaluates a personalized approach to screening, compared with standard screening.[74,75] In WISDOM, patients are randomized to annual screening or risk-based screening. The trial uses a preference sensitive design in which women who do not wish to randomize can opt to be in the observational arm of the study where they can choose which arm they join. Sixty-five percent of all women have chosen to randomize. In WISDOM, risk is estimated using the Breast Cancer Surveillance Consortium (BCSC) breast density model,[76] modified by testing for pathogenic germline mutations in *BRCA1, BRCA2, TP53, STK11, PTEN, CDH1, ATM, PALB2,* and *CHEK2*, as well as a polygenic risk score (PRS) from SNP testing. Screening recommendations are determined based on 5-year risk of cancer, with options ranging from no recommended screening before age 50 years and biennial screening thereafter for the lowest risk women to annual mammography alternating with annual MRI for the highest risk, including carriers of germline mutations. The primary endpoint is the number of late-stage cancers diagnosed (>IIB) and rates of recall and breast biopsy.

Another study testing personalized approaches to screening, the European My Personalized Breast Screening (MyPEBS) study (NCT03672331) is currently enrolling, randomizing women to screening according to their national guidelines, or risk-based screening every 1 to 4 years, based on their 5-year cancer risk.[77] In MyPEBS, women with low family risk are screened using the MammoRisk test, which incorporates a proprietary PRS but not germline testing. Women with high family risk are stratified using the Tyrer-Cuzick risk score. The primary outcome of this trial is incidence of stage 2+ breast cancer in a non-inferiority design. Both WISDOM and MyPEBS are expected to result in 2025 and have committed to pooling their data.

Better Tools for High-Risk Individuals

Although screening mammography has contributed to reducing breast cancer mortality, up to 10% of breast cancers potentially are not detected by mammogram. A blood test to detect cancer using liquid biopsy technology could add value to conventional breast cancer screening by detecting abnormal DNA or proteins in the blood of patients at elevated risk for breast cancer. Lennon and colleagues studied the concept of detecting malignancies with a blood test for cancer in combination with PET-CT scans for those patients testing positive by liquid biopsy.[78] Of 10,006 women with no history of cancer studied, 26 cancers were detected by blood testing and 9 were surgically excised. The assay detected only one out of 20 (5%) breast cancers present in the cohort, highlighting the problem that this expensive test is neither sufficiently sensitive nor specific for breast cancer and shows the problem of establishing an accurate blood test strategy suitable for screening for breast cancer, especially without enriching for risk.[78]

Artificial intelligence (AI) with radiomics and computational pathology may help address challenges in the detection and treatment of breast cancer.[79] Deep-learning methodology may be applied to address challenges in breast cancer detection, treatment, monitoring, and prognosis.[79–81] Recently, AI was found to outperform the BCSC model at predicting risk of breast cancer from 0 to 5 years after a negative screening mammogram.[82]

Ductal Carcinoma in Situ Is an Opportunity for Personalized Risk Assessment

Ductal carcinoma in situ (DCIS) is a premalignant breast lesion that is often captured on screening mammography. The incidence of DCIS has increased by 500% since the advent of widespread screening in the 1980s.[83] Although it is not life-threatening in itself, DCIS has traditionally been treated similarly to stage I breast cancer, following a series of trials that optimized the risk of local recurrence.[84] However, we are beginning to realize that much like invasive breast cancer, DCIS is a very heterogeneous disease, and many cases may never progress to invasive disease. The ongoing COMET trial is reevaluating this approach by randomizing patients with screen-detected DCIS to routine management with excision (with or without radiotherapy and/or endocrine therapy) versus active surveillance and is expected to result within the next year.[85] New active surveillance trials (RECAST DCIS) are on the horizon using MR markers to assess suitability for surveillance and risk reduction.[86] Several personalized approaches to treating DCIS are also being developed. For example, about 20% of DCIS are HR-negative or HER2-positive and are associated with immune infiltrates and there are early phase studies evaluating the role of immunotherapy in treating these lesions.[87] However, much remains to be discovered about precision treatments for DCIS, and we would argue that there is an urgent need for changing the treatment paradigm.[88]

SUMMARY

Treatment of localized breast cancer has long been informed by immunohistochemical diagnostics, such as the HR and HER2 receptor status. Recent advances in genomic analysis in the setting of response to therapy in early-stage high-risk breast cancer have begun to unlock personalized therapies beyond these biomarkers. The shift toward neoadjuvant chemotherapy has enabled personalized evaluation of response on serial imaging, enabling rapid evaluation, and individualization of therapies. Early endpoints like pCR have enabled more rapid evaluation of novel therapies in women with molecularly high-risk disease at risk for early recurrence, where pCR predicts EFS and distant recurrence free at 3 to 5 years. Liquid biopsies are also under investigation and have the potential to become another important early endpoint to predict recurrence, as well as guide the length of both neoadjuvant and adjuvant therapies. Neoadjuvant treatment approaches also can be applied to the precancerous setting to test strategies to reverse DCIS and avoid traditional local and regional treatments. It may also serve as a window to test preventive interventions. Furthermore, better understanding the individualized risk factors that predispose to both fast-growing and slow-growing tumors will enable us to transform the way we screen and prevent breast cancer by personalized approaches starting first with risk assessment. In summary, personalized approaches promise to revolutionize all aspects of care for patients with localized breast cancer.

CLINICS CARE POINTS

- Precision screening for breast cancer should be based on the risk for developing fast- versus slow-growing cancers, as well as informing when to start/stop and how often and with what modality to inform interventions to reduce the lifetime risk for breast cancer.
- Precision diagnosis should include the molecular profiling of a patient's tumor, as well as the individual predisposition (eg, germline risk), which should guide personalized treatments based on predicted risk, the timing of risk, and the likely response to various therapeutic interventions.
- Precision treatments can be optimized based on response, with the goal of de-escalating treatments in the setting of low-risk disease and/or complete and rapid response to minimize toxicity while escalating therapy in the setting of poor response to prevent progression to metastatic disease.

REFERENCES

1. Division of Cancer Prevention and Control CfDCaP. An Update on Cancer Deaths in the United States. Available at: https://www.cdc.gov/cancer/dcpc/research/update-on-cancer-deaths/index.htm. Accessed December 1, 2023.

2. van 't Veer LJ, Dai H, van de Vijver MJ, et al. Gene expression profiling predicts clinical outcome of breast cancer. Nature 2002;415(6871):530–6.
3. Esserman LJ, Yau C, Thompson CK, et al. Use of molecular tools to identify patients with indolent breast cancers with ultralow risk over 2 decades. JAMA Oncol 2017;3(11):1503–10.
4. Fisher B, Bryant J, Wolmark N, et al. Effect of preoperative chemotherapy on the outcome of women with operable breast cancer. J Clin Oncol 1998;16(8): 2672–85.
5. Bear HD, Anderson S, Smith RE, et al. Sequential preoperative or postoperative docetaxel added to preoperative doxorubicin plus cyclophosphamide for operable breast cancer:National Surgical Adjuvant Breast and Bowel Project Protocol B-27. J Clin Oncol 2006;24(13):2019–27.
6. Consortium IST, Yee D, DeMichele AM, et al. Association of event-free and distant recurrence-free survival with individual-level pathologic complete response in neoadjuvant treatment of stages 2 and 3 breast cancer: three-year follow-up analysis for the I-SPY2 adaptively randomized clinical trial. JAMA Oncol 2020; 6(9):1355–62.
7. Wooster R, Weber BL. Breast and ovarian cancer. N Engl J Med 2003;348(23): 2339–47.
8. NCCN Clinical Practice Guidelines in Oncology (NCCN Guidelines®) Genetic/Familial High-Risk Assessment: Breast, Ovarian, and Pancreatic. Version 4.2023 National Comprehensive Cancer Network2023 Available at: www.NCCN.org. Accessed December 1, 2023.
9. Cancer Genome Atlas N. Comprehensive molecular portraits of human breast tumours. Nature 2012;490(7418):61–70.
10. Domchek SM, Bradbury A, Garber JE, et al. Multiplex genetic testing for cancer susceptibility: out on the high wire without a net? J Clin Oncol 2013;31(10): 1267–70.
11. Kurian AW, Ford JM. Multigene panel testing in oncology practice: how should we respond? JAMA Oncol 2015;1(3):277–8.
12. Offit K, Bradbury A, Storm C, et al. Gene patents and personalized cancer care: impact of the Myriad case on clinical oncology. J Clin Oncol 2013;31(21):2743–8.
13. NCCN Clinical Guidelines in Oncology (NCCN Guidelines) Breast Cancer Risk Reduction. Version 1.2023 2023. Available at: www.NCCN.org. Accessed December 1, 2023.
14. Available at: https://www.breastsurgeons.org/docs/statements/Consensus-Guideline-on-Genetic-Testing-for-Hereditary-Breast-Cancer.pdf. Accessed December 1, 2023.
15. Beitsch PD, Whitworth PW, Hughes K, et al. underdiagnosis of hereditary breast cancer: are genetic testing guidelines a tool or an obstacle? J Clin Oncol 2019; 37(6):453–60.
16. Yadav S, Hu C, Hart SN, et al. Evaluation of germline genetic testing criteria in a hospital-based series of women with breast cancer. J Clin Oncol 2020;38(13): 1409–18.
17. Available at: https://www.fda.gov/medical-devices/in-vitro-diagnostics/direct-consumer-tests. Accessed December 1, 2023.
18. Wang H, Yee D. I-SPY 2: a neoadjuvant adaptive clinical trial designed to improve outcomes in high-risk breast cancer. Curr Breast Cancer Rep 2019;11(4):303–10.
19. Schwab R. Abstract CT136: evaluation of talazoparib in combination with irinotecan in early stage, high-risk HER2 negative breast cancer: results from the I-SPY2 trial. Atlanta, GA: American Association for Cancer Research; 2019.

20. Tutt ANJ, Garber JE, Kaufman B, et al, OlympiA Clinical Trial Steering Committee and Investigators. Adjuvant Olaparib for Patients with BRCA1- or BRCA2-Mutated Breast Cancer. N Engl J Med 2021;384(25):2394–405.
21. Cui K, Wang Z, Zhang Q, et al. Immune checkpoint inhibitors and adrenal insufficiency: a large-sample case series study. Ann Transl Med 2022;10(5):251.
22. Wolf DM, Yau C, Wulfkuhle J, et al. Redefining breast cancer subtypes to guide treatment prioritization and maximize response: Predictive biomarkers across 10 cancer therapies. Cancer Cell 2022;40(6):609–623 e6.
23. Wolf D, Yau C, Campbell MJ, et al. Biomarkers predicting response to 5 immunotherapy arms in the neoadjuvant I-SPY2 trial for early-stage breast cancer (BC): Evaluation of immune subtyping in the response predictive subtypes (RPS). J Clin Oncol 2023;41(16_suppl):102.
24. Boughey JC, Yu H, Dugan CL, et al. Changes in surgical management of the axilla over 11 years - report on more than 1500 breast cancer patients treated with neoadjuvant chemotherapy on the prospective I-SPY2 trial. Ann Surg Oncol 2023;30(11):6401–10.
25. Tee SR, Devane LA, Evoy D, et al. Meta-analysis of sentinel lymph node biopsy after neoadjuvant chemotherapy in patients with initial biopsy-proven node-positive breast cancer. Br J Surg 2018;105(12):1541–52.
26. Caudle AS, Yang WT, Krishnamurthy S, et al. Improved axillary evaluation following neoadjuvant therapy for patients with node-positive breast cancer using selective evaluation of clipped nodes: implementation of targeted axillary dissection. J Clin Oncol 2016;34(10):1072–8.
27. Golshan M, Loibl S, Wong SM, et al. Breast conservation after neoadjuvant chemotherapy for triple-negative breast cancer: surgical results from the brightness randomized clinical trial. JAMA Surg 2020;155(3):e195410.
28. Early Breast Cancer Trialists' Collaborative G. Long-term outcomes for neoadjuvant versus adjuvant chemotherapy in early breast cancer: meta-analysis of individual patient data from ten randomised trials. Lancet Oncol 2018;19(1):27–39.
29. Mukhtar RA, Chau H, Woriax H, et al, ISPY-2 Locoregional Working Group. Breast conservation surgery and mastectomy have similar locoregional recurrence following neoadjuvant chemotherapy: results from 1,462 patients on the prospective, randomized I-SPY2 trial. Ann Surg 2023;278(3):320–7.
30. Andre F, Ismaila N, Allison KH, et al. Biomarkers for adjuvant endocrine and chemotherapy in early-stage breast cancer: ASCO guideline update. J Clin Oncol 2022;40(16):1816–37.
31. Schmid P, Cortes J, Dent R, et al, KEYNOTE-522 Investigators. Event-free survival with pembrolizumab in early triple-negative breast cancer. N Engl J Med 2022;386(6):556–67.
32. Nanda R, Liu MC, Yau C, et al. Effect of pembrolizumab plus neoadjuvant chemotherapy on pathologic complete response in women with early-stage breast cancer: an analysis of the ongoing phase 2 adaptively randomized I-SPY2 trial. JAMA Oncol 2020;6(5):676–84.
33. Hurvitz SA, Martin M, Symmans WF, et al. Neoadjuvant trastuzumab, pertuzumab, and chemotherapy versus trastuzumab emtansine plus pertuzumab in patients with HER2-positive breast cancer (KRISTINE): a randomised, open-label, multicentre, phase 3 trial. Lancet Oncol 2018;19(1):115–26.
34. Schneeweiss A, Chia S, Hickish T, et al. Pertuzumab plus trastuzumab in combination with standard neoadjuvant anthracycline-containing and anthracycline-free chemotherapy regimens in patients with HER2-positive early breast cancer:

a randomized phase II cardiac safety study (TRYPHAENA). Ann Oncol 2013; 24(9):2278–84.

35. Partridge SC, Gibbs JE, Lu Y, et al. MRI measurements of breast tumor volume predict response to neoadjuvant chemotherapy and recurrence-free survival. AJR Am J Roentgenol 2005;184(6):1774–81.

36. Partridge SC, Zhang Z, Newitt DC, et al, ACRIN 6698 Trial Team and I-SPY 2 Trial Investigators. Diffusion-weighted MRI findings predict pathologic response in neoadjuvant treatment of breast cancer: the ACRIN 6698 multicenter trial. Radiology 2018;289(3):618–27.

37. Sener SF, Sargent RE, Lee C, et al. MRI does not predict pathologic complete response after neoadjuvant chemotherapy for breast cancer. J Surg Oncol 2019;120(6):903–10.

38. Mandish SF, Gaskins JT, Yusuf MB, et al. The effect of omission of adjuvant radiotherapy after neoadjuvant chemotherapy and breast conserving surgery with a pathologic complete response. Acta Oncol 2020;59(10):1210–7.

39. Morrow M, Khan AJ. Locoregional management after neoadjuvant chemotherapy. J Clin Oncol 2020;38(20):2281–9.

40. Kuerer HM, Smith BD, Krishnamurthy S, et al, Exceptional Responders Clinical Trials Group. Eliminating breast surgery for invasive breast cancer in exceptional responders to neoadjuvant systemic therapy: a multicentre, single-arm, phase 2 trial. Lancet Oncol 2022;23(12):1517–24.

41. van Hemert AKE, van Olmen JP, Boersma LJ, et al. De-ESCAlating RadioTherapy in breast cancer patients with pathologic complete response to neoadjuvant systemic therapy: DESCARTES study. Breast Cancer Res Treat 2023;199(1):81–9.

42. Hurvitz SA, McAndrew NP, Bardia A, et al. A careful reassessment of anthracycline use in curable breast cancer. NPJ Breast Cancer 2021;7(1):134.

43. Jones SE, Savin MA, Holmes FA, et al. Phase III trial comparing doxorubicin plus cyclophosphamide with docetaxel plus cyclophosphamide as adjuvant therapy for operable breast cancer. J Clin Oncol 2006;24(34):5381–7.

44. Blum JL, Flynn PJ, Yothers G, et al. Anthracyclines in early breast cancer: the ABC trials-USOR 06-090, NSABP B-46-I/USOR 07132, and NSABP B-49 (NRG Oncology). J Clin Oncol 2017;35(23):2647–55.

45. DeMichele A, Price E, Venters S, et al. PreRCB in ISPY 2.0. Madrid, Spain: ESMO; 2023.

46. Radovich M, Jiang G, Hancock BA, et al. Association of circulating tumor DNA and circulating tumor cells after neoadjuvant chemotherapy with disease recurrence in patients with triple-negative breast cancer: preplanned secondary analysis of the BRE12-158 randomized clinical trial. JAMA Oncol 2020;6(9):1410–5.

47. Lucci A, Hall CS, Lodhi AK, et al. Circulating tumour cells in non-metastatic breast cancer: a prospective study. Lancet Oncol 2012;13(7):688–95.

48. Cristofanilli M, Budd GT, Ellis MJ, et al. Circulating tumor cells, disease progression, and survival in metastatic breast cancer. N Engl J Med 2004;351(8):781–91.

49. Lang JE, Ring A, Porras T, et al. RNA-seq of circulating tumor cells in stage II-III breast cancer. Ann Surg Oncol 2018;25(8):2261–70.

50. Ring A, Campo D, Porras TB, et al. Circulating tumor cell transcriptomics as biopsy surrogates in metastatic breast cancer. Ann Surg Oncol 2022;29(5): 2882–94.

51. Cohen EN, Jayachandran G, Moore RG, et al. A multi-center clinical study to harvest and characterize circulating tumor cells from patients with metastatic breast cancer using the parsortix((R)) PC1 system. Cancers 2022;14(21):5238.

52. Dawson SJ, Tsui DW, Murtaza M, et al. Analysis of circulating tumor DNA to monitor metastatic breast cancer. N Engl J Med 2013;368(13):1199–209.

53. Murtaza M, Dawson SJ, Pogrebniak K, et al. Multifocal clonal evolution characterized using circulating tumour DNA in a case of metastatic breast cancer. Nat Commun 2015;6:8760.

54. Garcia-Murillas I, Schiavon G, Weigelt B, et al. Mutation tracking in circulating tumor DNA predicts relapse in early breast cancer. Sci Transl Med 2015;7(302): 302ra133.

55. McDonald BR, Contente-Cuomo T, Sammut SJ, et al. Personalized circulating tumor DNA analysis to detect residual disease after neoadjuvant therapy in breast cancer. Sci Transl Med 2019;11(504):eaax7392.

56. Parsons HA, Rhoades J, Reed SC, et al. Sensitive detection of minimal residual disease in patients treated for early-stage breast cancer. Clin Cancer Res 2020;26(11):2556–64.

57. Lipsyc-Sharf M, de Bruin EC, Santos K, et al. Circulating tumor DNA and late recurrence in high-risk hormone receptor-positive, human epidermal growth factor receptor 2-negative breast cancer. J Clin Oncol 2022;40(22):2408–19.

58. Coombes RC, Page K, Salari R, et al. Personalized detection of circulating tumor DNA antedates breast cancer metastatic recurrence. Clin Cancer Res 2019; 25(14):4255–63.

59. Cailleux F, Agostinetto E, Lambertini M, et al. Circulating tumor DNA after neoadjuvant chemotherapy in breast cancer is associated with disease relapse. JCO Precis Oncol 2022;6:e2200148.

60. Turner NC, Swift C, Jenkins B, et al, c-TRAK TN investigators. Results of the c-TRAK TN trial: a clinical trial utilising ctDNA mutation tracking to detect molecular residual disease and trigger intervention in patients with moderate- and high-risk early-stage triple-negative breast cancer. Ann Oncol 2023;34(2):200–11.

61. Turner NC, Kingston B, Kilburn LS, et al. Circulating tumour DNA analysis to direct therapy in advanced breast cancer (plasmaMATCH): a multicentre, multi-cohort, phase 2a, platform trial. Lancet Oncol 2020;21(10):1296–308.

62. Burstein HJ, DeMichele A, Somerfield MR, et al. Testing for ESR1 mutations to guide therapy for hormone receptor-positive, human epidermal growth factor receptor 2-negative metastatic breast cancer: ASCO guideline rapid recommendation update. J Clin Oncol 2023;41(18):3423–5.

63. Magbanua MJM, Swigart LB, Wu HT, et al. Circulating tumor DNA in neoadjuvant-treated breast cancer reflects response and survival. Ann Oncol 2021;32(2): 229–39.

64. Magbanua MJM, Brown Swigart L, Ahmed Z, et al. Clinical significance and biology of circulating tumor DNA in high-risk early-stage HER2-negative breast cancer receiving neoadjuvant chemotherapy. Cancer Cell 2023;41(6): 1091–10102 e4.

65. Snow A, Chen D, Lang JE. The current status of the clinical utility of liquid biopsies in cancer. Expert Rev Mol Diagn 2019;19(11):1031–41.

66. Bidard FC, Kaklamani VG, Neven P, et al. Elacestrant (oral selective estrogen receptor degrader) Versus Standard Endocrine Therapy for Estrogen Receptor-Positive, Human Epidermal Growth Factor Receptor 2-Negative Advanced Breast Cancer: Results From the Randomized Phase III EMERALD Trial. J Clin Oncol 2022;40(28):3246–56.

67. Andre F, Ciruelos EM, Juric D, et al. Alpelisib plus fulvestrant for PIK3CA-mutated, hormone receptor-positive, human epidermal growth factor receptor-2-negative

advanced breast cancer: final overall survival results from SOLAR-1. Ann Oncol 2021;32(2):208–17.

68. Juric D, Rugo HS, A R, et al. Alpelisib (ALP) + fulvestrant (FUL) in patients (pts) with hormone receptor–positive (HR+), human epidermal growth factor receptor 2–negative (HER2–) advanced breast cancer (ABC): biomarker (BM) analyses by next-generation sequencing (NGS) from the SOLAR-1 study. J Clin Oncol 2022;40(suppl 16):1006.

69. Ren W, Chen M, Qiao Y, et al. Global guidelines for breast cancer screening: A systematic review. Breast 2022;64:85–99.

70. Esserman LJ, Thompson IM, Reid B, et al. Addressing overdiagnosis and over-treatment in cancer: a prescription for change. Lancet Oncol 2014;15(6): e234–42.

71. Houssami N. Overdiagnosis of breast cancer in population screening: does it make breast screening worthless? Cancer Biol Med 2017;14(1):1–8.

72. Michailidou K, Beesley J, Lindstrom S, et al. Genome-wide association analysis of more than 120,000 individuals identifies 15 new susceptibility loci for breast cancer. Nat Genet 2015;47(4):373–80.

73. Michailidou K, Hall P, Gonzalez-Neira A, et al. Large-scale genotyping identifies 41 new loci associated with breast cancer risk. Nat Genet 2013;45(4):353–61, 61e1-361.

74. Shieh Y, Eklund M, Madlensky L, et al, Athena Breast Health Network Investigators. Breast Cancer Screening in the Precision Medicine Era: Risk-Based Screening in a Population-Based Trial. J Natl Cancer Inst 2017;109(5).

75. Esserman LJ, Study W, Athena I. The WISDOM Study: breaking the deadlock in the breast cancer screening debate. NPJ Breast Cancer 2017;3:34.

76. Tice JA, Cummings SR, Smith-Bindman R, et al. Using clinical factors and mammographic breast density to estimate breast cancer risk: development and validation of a new predictive model. Ann Intern Med 2008;148(5):337–47.

77. Available at: https://www.mypebs.eu/the-project/. Accessed December 1, 2023.

78. Lennon AM, Buchanan AH, Kinde I, et al. Feasibility of blood testing combined with PET-CT to screen for cancer and guide intervention. Science 2020; 369(6499).

79. Corredor G, Bharadwaj S, Pathak T, et al. A review of AI-based radiomics and computational pathology approaches in triple-negative breast cancer: current applications and perspectives. Clin Breast Cancer 2023;23(8):800–12.

80. Ris F, Hellan M, Douissard J, et al. Blood-based multi-cancer detection using a novel variant calling assay (DEEPGEN(TM)): early clinical results. Cancers 2021;13(16):4104.

81. Hermann BT, Pfeil S, Groenke N, et al. DEEPGEN(TM)-a novel variant calling assay for low frequency variants. Genes 2021;12(4):507.

82. Arasu VA, Habel LA, Achacoso NS, et al. Comparison of Mammography AI Algorithms with a Clinical Risk Model for 5-year Breast Cancer Risk Prediction: An Observational Study. Radiology 2023;307(5):e222733.

83. Kerlikowske K. Epidemiology of ductal carcinoma in situ. J Natl Cancer Inst Monogr 2010;2010(41):139–41.

84. Wapnir IL, Dignam JJ, Fisher B, et al. Long-term outcomes of invasive ipsilateral breast tumor recurrences after lumpectomy in NSABP B-17 and B-24 randomized clinical trials for DCIS. J Natl Cancer Inst 2011;103(6):478–88.

85. Hwang ES, Hyslop T, Lynch T, et al. The COMET (Comparison of Operative versus Monitoring and Endocrine Therapy) trial: a phase III randomised controlled

clinical trial for low-risk ductal carcinoma in situ (DCIS). BMJ Open 2019;9(3): e026797.

86. Glencer AC, Miller PN, Greenwood H, et al. Identifying Good Candidates for Active Surveillance of Ductal Carcinoma In Situ: Insights from a Large Neoadjuvant Endocrine Therapy Cohort. Cancer Res Commun 2022;2(12):1579–89.

87. Glencer AC, Wong JM, Hylton NM, et al. Modulation of the immune microenvironment of high-risk ductal carcinoma in situ by intralesional pembrolizumab injection. NPJ Breast Cancer 2021;7(1):59.

88. Esserman L, Shieh Y, Thompson I. Rethinking screening for breast cancer and prostate cancer. JAMA 2009;302(15):1685–92.

Precision Oncology in Lung Cancer Surgery

Patrick Bou-Samra, MD[a], Sunil Singhal, MD[b],*

KEYWORDS

- Precision surgery • Neoadjuvant and adjuvant therapy
- Minimally invasive thoracic surgery • Intraoperative molecular imaging
- Sublobar resection

KEY POINTS

- Precision surgery involves patient- and tumor-specific perioperative medical treatment, refining operative techniques, and using innovative tumor visualization methods to enhance detection of previously occult disease.
- The latest guidelines recommend evaluating all patients before surgery to assess the need for neoadjuvant therapy, considering factors such as resectability criteria and molecular analysis for personalized treatment.
- Video-assisted thoracoscopic surgery and robot-assisted thoracoscopic surgery offer benefits over traditional thoracotomy, including reduced morbidity, shorter hospital stays, improved disease-free survival, and better postoperative outcomes.
- Sublobar resection, compared with lobectomy, can achieve similar overall and disease-free survival rates for early-stage non-small cell lung cancer.
- Intraoperative molecular imaging using fluorescent probes and near-infrared imaging can assist in tumor localization and guide the preservation of healthy parenchymal tissue during surgery for occult lesions.

BACKGROUND

In 1912, Dr Hugh Morriston Davies first introduced the concept of an oncologic lung resection by individual ligation of hilar vessels and suture closure of the bronchus. His patient unfortunately died because of the poor understanding of management of the pleural spaces postoperatively.[1] Since then, the role of surgery in the management of thoracic tumors has incrementally increased, most recently in the management of early-stage non-small cell lung cancer (NSCLC).[2] Meanwhile, our understanding of the biology of tumors has evolved over time as well. Lung cancers fall into different

---

[a] The University of Pennsylvania - Stemmler Hall, 3450 Hamilton Walk, Philadelphia, PA 19104, USA; [b] Department of Thoracic Surgery, Perelman School of Medicine, University of Pennsylvania, 14th Floor PCAM South Tower, 3400 Civic Center Boulevard, Philadelphia, PA 19104, USA
* Corresponding author.
E-mail address: sunil.singhal@pennmedicine.upenn.edu

Surg Oncol Clin N Am 33 (2024) 311–320
https://doi.org/10.1016/j.soc.2023.12.003
1055-3207/24/© 2023 Elsevier Inc. All rights reserved.

histologic subtypes that are not only morphologically different but also molecularly distinct. In the realm of precision medicine, tumor microenvironment and genomic sequencing has allowed us to tailor treatments to specific tumors.[3] Tyrosine kinase inhibitors (TKIs) in lung adenocarcinoma patients with EGFR mutations and ALK-rearrangement have led to remarkable responses that are superior to traditional cytotoxic chemotherapy.[4,5] Newer drugs, such as immune checkpoint inhibitors, have revolutionized lung cancer care and have shown durable responses in a subset of lung cancer patients with programmed death-1 (PD-1) expression. Albeit a relatively new concept, this has allowed us to treat patients who are at high risk of a recurrence with PD-1 inhibitors before embarking on a resection.[6] Meanwhile, in the general surgery world, an analogous concept was introduced: precision surgery. It was first applied in colorectal surgery and identifying the different prognosis of colorectal cancer related to different genetic mutations. Given the recent advances in understanding the role of molecular alterations in pharmaceutical therapy in thoracic malignancies, we describe the different considerations of precision surgery in lung cancer.

Precision in Perioperative Treatment Course

One aspect of surgical oncology is deciding on neoadjuvant therapy (NAT) or adjuvant therapy (AT). Surgical resection with curative intent is indicated for patients with early stages of NSCLC: stage I, stage II, and some patients with stage IIIA. There is evidence that in early-stage NSCLC, AT improved survival by 4% at 5 years compared with surgery alone.[7] However, in stages II–IIIA, the relapse rate remained high with a relative high toxicity.[8] Also in stage IIIA NSCLC, randomized trials have been unable to show a clear advantage of NAT compared with definitive chemoradiation.[9] Unfortunately, most of the patients with stage III NSCLC are nonsurgical candidates and will benefit most from chemotherapy followed by immunotherapy.[10]

The most recent NCCN guidelines recommend that all patients should be evaluated preoperatively for NAT. Patients with resectable tumors ($\geq$4 cm) or node positive disease that have no contraindications for immune checkpoint inhibitors should be strongly considered for nivolumab and chemotherapy.[11] However, NAT should not be used in an attempt to make a tumor resectable if the patients do not meet resectability criteria to start with.

In addition, the NCCN guidelines recommend molecular testing for ALK, EGFR, BRAF, METex14, NTRK1/2/3, RET, and ROS1.[12] This additional phenotypic stratification of tumors allows for administration of targeted therapies. Patients with EGFR and ALK arrangements may benefit from TKIs. In an open-label phase 3 clinical trial, crizotinib, a TKI, was shown to be superior to standard first-line pemetrexed-plus-platinum patients with previously untreated ALK-positive NSCLC.[13] Likewise, patients with the EGFR mutation had a superior response with using gefitinib, a TKI, compared with standard chemotherapy.[4] In terms of timing of administration, there has been increasing appeal to administering it as NAT, but the data on this are not fully mature yet and remain restricted to clinical trials.[14]

Although there is a role for targeted therapies in patients with a targetable mutation, most patients do not have one. These patients, without these driver mutations, may benefit from immunotherapy with programmed death-ligand 1 (PD-L1) inhibitors. In fact, PD-L1 testing is a standard recommendation for all patients with a newly diagnosed lung cancer, particularly those with advanced NSCLC.[15] Initially reserved for patients with advanced stage NSCLC or metastatic disease, several trials have shown a role of PD-L1 inhibitors in early-stage disease as well. The extent of PD-L1 expression also predicts treatment response as those with a PD-L1 expression greater than or equal to 50% are offered a checkpoint inhibitor, such as pembrolizumab, either as monotherapy or in combination with platinum-based chemotherapy.[16] If PD-L1 expression is less than 50%, patients are offered a combination of chemotherapy and the checkpoint inhibitor. When deciding on timing, immunotherapy in the NAT setting is thought to create an "auto-vaccine" that targets micro-metastases throughout the body thus reducing the chances of relapse.[17] In the AT, the rational for its use is to eradicate residual disease and prevent recurrence. There are currently several studies investigating the administration of NAT versus AT and the data are patient and stage-dependent.[18] For instance, the FDA approved the use of pembrolizumab for resectable NSCLC cancer as NAT or AT, depending on patient stage and disease presentation.

This addition of molecular and biochemical analysis has introduced a paradigm shift in lung cancer care. The personalization of treatment in the modern era is not just stage reliant but also tumor biology-dependent.

Precision in Operative Technique

Thoracotomies were introduced in the nineteenth century by Professor Moitz Schiff and Ludqig Rehn where it was first performed in the setting of repair of a cardiac wound and open cardiac message. The techniques from these procedures, when combined, formed the basis of the modern procedure known as resuscitative thoracotomy, which is a fundamental damage control intervention.[19,20] Although lifesaving and still indicated in particular situations, traditional thoracotomy may be a traumatic approach. As such, much effort was invested in developing less invasive techniques that allow similar visibility and outcomes. In 1910, Professor Hans Christian Jacobaeus performed thoracic pneumolysis in Stockholm and published on the use of thoracoscopy in staging tuberculous pleurisy, malignant pleural effusion, and rheumatoid disease. Starting in the early 1990s, several researchers reintroduced the concept of thoracoscopy, taking advantage of the scopes, cameras, and instruments that had become available due to the advancements in laparoscopic surgery. Initially, the term "video-assisted thoracic surgery" (VATS) was broadly used to describe any procedure that involved port placement, a utility incision, and some form of endoscopic visualization. Over time, VATS became more precisely defined as a minimally invasive procedure characterized by an access incision of less than 8 cm, one or more port incisions, reliance on thoracoscopic visualization alone, and the complete avoidance of rib-spreading or cutting.[21]

There were a few concerns with relying on VATS as opposed to traditional open techniques. The first was the increased cost associated with VATS. A retrospective review involving 123,498 patients showed that VATS was associated with a decreased length of stay and overall morbidity that offsets the initial added cost of purchasing minimally invasive surgery equipment.[22] The second concern was its ability to have analogous oncologic outcomes to open surgery. A study involving 546 patients comparing open and thoracoscopic approaches showed similar oncologic outcomes between the two subgroups and a superior disease-free survival (DFS) in the thoracoscopic approach.[23] Another propensity matched analysis comparing VATS and open lobectomy following induction therapy for stage III NSCLC showed equivalent postoperative and oncologic outcome without an increased risk of procedure-related locoregional recurrence.[24] VATS was also associated with decreased gastrointestinal and respiratory complications, a better quality of life, and less postoperative pain than open thoracotomy at least for the first year postoperatively.[25]

Robot-assisted thoracic surgery (RATS) has also made its way into thoracic oncology. It does not seem to be a significant advantage for an established VATS lobectomy surgeon based on clinical outcomes despite the improved visibility and range of motion on the robot.[26] However, in the realm of precision surgery and the overall direction of the field to a more targeted sublobar dissection, RATS can provide a valuable tool that allows the dexterity to more easily preform these sub-anatomical dissections.[27] The RATS technique is advantageous in allowing full-wristed dexterity, in having a tremor filter, and in visualization of the lesion with up to 10x magnification.[28] There has also been report of improved mediastinal lymph node (LN) dissection using RATS over VATS without any reported change in postoperative complications.[29] Meanwhile, some of the critiques include being distant from the patient while manipulating the robot at the console, where it would be more challenging to respond expeditiously to emergent situations. However, over time, as the era of robotics has become mainstream with both VATS and RATS providing significant improvements in postoperative morbidity.

Precision in Extent of Dissection

When deciding on more conservative approaches, there are three main issues that need to be addressed. First, do sublobar resections compromise oncologic outcomes such as survival and recurrence? Second, what is the ideal LN yield? Last, do sublobar resections that improve postoperative pulmonary function tests (PFTs) when compared with lobectomies? Several studies have attempted to address these questions.

When it comes to oncologic outcomes, a study from the Mayo Clinic has shown that the overall survival and DFS of patients with T1a NSCLC undergoing segmentectomy was similar to those undergoing lobectomy.[30] Furthermore, a recent multicenter non-inferiority trial (CALGB 140503) showed that patients diagnosed with early-stage NSCLC who had tumors measuring 2 cm or smaller and no presence of cancer in the LNs near the lungs and chest, achieved similar DFS outcomes whether they underwent sublobar resection or lobectomy.[31] This was also echoed in a Japanese phase III, randomized, controlled non-inferiority trial involving 1106 patients.[32] Patients in that trial with NSCLC who were clinical stage IA were randomly assigned to lobectomy or segmentectomy. There was improved overall survival in the segmentectomy subgroup.

One of the major concerns of sublobar resection is the concern for local recurrence. In fact, in the phase III Japanese study, the proportions of patients with stage IA NSLC with local relapse were 10.5% for segmentectomy and 5.4% for lobectomy ($P = .0018$).[32] Local recurrence can be attributed to three potential scenarios. First, the surgeon may fail to completely resect the primary tumor and leave behind residual microscopic disease. Second, the cancer might have already spread to the nodes and that has been undetected or not surgically removed. Last, the cancer might have satellite synchronous lesions either ipsilaterally or contralaterally that are missed.

When it comes to LN yield, a study by Yendumari and colleagues showed that many patients having sublobar resection for early NSCLC in the United States do not have a single LN removed. The same study showed that the association between survival and LN yield is greater than that with the extent of resection.[33] The optimal number of harvested LNs to ensure accurate staging of cancer is still uncertain. Different studies have suggested varying ranges, from 10 to 16 LNs. In 2015, the American College of Surgeons Commission on Cancer (COC) used these studies to recommend the sampling of 10 or more LNs during surgery as a quality measure.[34,35] However, the adherence to this guideline has consistently been low which prompted the COC to update them in 2020.[36] The updated guidelines now require the resection of LNs from one or more specific hilar station and three or more distinct mediastinal stations.[37]

When it comes to PFTs, a Japanese study showed no functional advantage for segmentectomy compared with lobectomy likely due to the compensatory lung regrowth after lobectomy.[38] Meanwhile, a study involving 159 patients showed that parenchymal-sparing resections resulted in a better preservation of pulmonary function at a median of 1 year.[39] This heterogeneity in the result might be due to several reasons such as different types of a segmentectomy which could include wedge resections and the heterogeneity of the patients. Regardless, it advocates for the potential benefits of segmentectomy in select subgroups.

Precision in Tumor Visualization

Lung parenchymal diseases have often no clear visual cues to identify specific areas of lung involvement. Tactile sensation emerges as a potential solution; however, two challenges hinder its effectiveness. First, certain lesions may be imperceptible to touch. Second, when using the more commonly used minimally invasive procedures, tactile feedback cannot be used as a diagnostic tool. As a result, the surgeon resorts to a more extensive resection that has a higher likelihood of yielding an R0 resection at the expense of removal of more normal parenchyma than potentially needed.

One solution is the implementation of intraoperative molecular imaging (IMI) as a tool to identify disease and guide surgical resection. There are multiple facets of IMI all of which use either inherent or induced tools to help the surgeon localize the area of concern and perform the most parenchymal-sparing dissection. One technique of IMI uses fluorescent probes.[40]

IMI-probe-guided surgery requires three essential components: a targeted fluorophore that can be injected throughout the body and reach a tumor, a laser that can emit a specific wavelength, and a camera capable of detecting the near-infrared (NIR) fluorescence emitted by the cancer. These components have been developed over the past 2 decades to identify different targets and have been increasingly used in clinical settings. Unlike traditional imaging, IMI relies on NIR wavelengths because they can penetrate deeper into tissues and reduce background fluorescence. The cameras used are designed to detect the emitted wavelength from the fluorophore and are commonly available in most medical institutions for measuring perfusion (Fig. 1). The delivery of fluorescent dyes can be achieved through three main strategies. The first strategy is passive targeting, which takes advantage of the tumor's leaky blood vessels and allows the dye to accumulate preferentially in the tumor tissue (enhanced permeability and retention [EPR]). Another approach involves targeting specific receptors or enzymes that are overexpressed in tumors, providing a more precise tumor targeting. The third strategy involves "activatable" dyes that can be activated by tumor-specific microenvironments or enzymes.[40,41]

Typically, regardless of the type of probe, patients receive a tumor-specific fluorescent probe the day of or the day before surgery. Intraoperatively, the NIR camera is used to detect fluorescence emitted by the probe and direct the surgeon to the area of interest. Then, depending on the location of the lesion, nodal status, and the surgeon's judgment, they decide whether to proceed with a sublobar resection or a lobar resection. Assuming the surgeon proceeds with a sublobar resection, the lesion can be analyzed on the back table using an exoscope to determine its proximity to the margin. The surgeon can then decide whether they are comfortable with the resected lesion or more needs to be done. IMI can also be used to assess for nodal involvement and for any residual disease once the specimen has been removed from the body.

There are several types of probes. First, there are non-targeted passive probes. These include indocyanine green (ICG), which is in cancer tissue due to the EPR around tumor tissue.[42,43] ICG has shown to detect residual disease in mesothelioma patients during cytoreductive surgical procedures.[44] It has also helped identify known and occult sarcomatous lesions and served as a useful intraoperative adjunct to

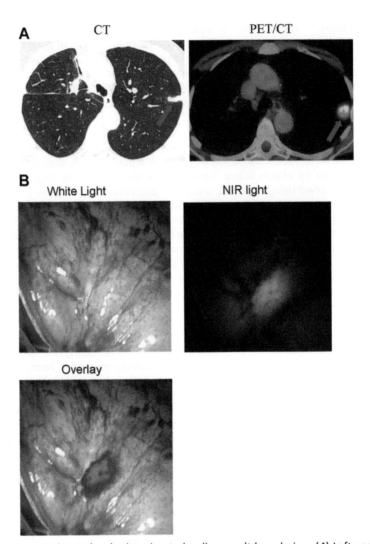

Fig. 1. Intraoperative molecular imaging to localize occult lung lesion. (*A*) Left upper lobe lesion seen on computed tomography (CT) and PET/CT. (*B*) Video-assisted thoracoscopy view of lesion in question on left with near infra-red light imaging on the right showing the location of the lesion. An overlay image overlaps white light and near-infrared light. The *red arrow* is pointing at the lesion in question.

improve metastasectomy.[45] Another separate class is targeted probes. Those include fluorescent probes that target receptors overexpressed on cancer cells such as folate receptor. A recent phase III, 12-center trial to study the utility of pafolacianine, a folate receptor agonist fluorescent probe, in lung cancer showed that IMI helped locating primary nodules that the surgeon could not locate with white light or palpation, identify close margins, and identify synchronous occult disease culminating in its Food and Drug Administration approval for lung cancer.[46] Another class of contrast agents, pegsitacianine is activatable. A phase 2 clinical study is currently underway to evaluate the effectiveness and safety of pegsitacianine, a fluorescent dye, in patients undergoing surgery for suspected lung cancer. It is activated in the tumor acidic microenvironment and is otherwise non-fluorescent. At this time, patients are being recruited for the phase II study (NCT05048082). Another example of "smart" contrast agents is VGT-309, a quenched activity-based probe. The probe has a fluorochrome, a linker, and a quencher. The presence of a quencher prevents the probe from emitting fluorescence until it encounters a specific class of enzymes, cysteine cathepsins, which is selectively upregulated in tumor cells.[47] When the enzyme cleaves the quencher, the fluorochrome is released and becomes visible. It has shown very promising results and the phase 2 clinical trial was just concluded (NCT05400226).

Other forms of IMI use the inherent autofluorescent properties of proteins without the need for a contrast agent.[48] In addition, there are techniques being developed that rely on photoacoustics and do not require a contrast agent. However, these methods are still in the early stages of development.[49]

SUMMARY

Overall, precision in surgical oncology encompasses decision-making for perioperative therapy, refined operative techniques, optimal extent of dissection, and innovative tumor visualization methods. These advancements aim to improve patient outcomes, minimize complications, and provide personalized care in the modern era of lung cancer treatment.

First, in terms of the perioperative treatment course, the decision between NAT and adjuvant AT is crucial. AT has shown improved survival in early-stage NSCLC compared with surgery alone. However, for stages II-IIIA, NAT has not demonstrated clear advantages over definitive chemoradiation. The latest guidelines suggest evaluating all patients preoperatively for NAT, considering resectability criteria and molecular analysis for personalized treatment. Second, precision in operative technique has evolved to minimize the site of entry and improve outcomes. VATS has been associated with decreased morbidity, shorter hospital stays, improved DFS, and better postoperative outcomes compared with traditional thoracotomy. Third, precision in the extent of dissection involves addressing concerns about sublobar resections. Studies have shown that a sublobar resection can achieve similar overall survival and DFS compared with lobectomy for early-stage NSCLC. The optimal LN yield for accurate staging remains uncertain, but recent updates require resection from specific hilar and mediastinal stations. Last, precision in tumor visualization has been aided by IMI techniques. IMI-probe-guided surgery uses fluorescent probes and NIR imaging to localize tumors and guide parenchymal-sparing dissection. This approach has shown promise in improving surgical precision.

CLINICS CARE POINTS

- Precision in surgical oncology encompasses decision-making for perioperative therapy, refined operative techniques, optimal extent of dissection, and innovative tumor visualization methods. These advancements aim to improve patient outcomes, minimize complications, and provide personalized care in the modern era of lung cancer treatment.

- The latest guidelines suggest evaluating all patients preoperatively for neoadjuvant therapy, considering resectability criteria and molecular analysis for personalized treatment.

- Video-assisted thoracoscopic surgery and robot-assisted thoracoscopic surgery have been associated with decreased morbidity, shorter hospital stays, and better postoperative outcomes compared with traditional thoracotomy.

- A sublobar resection can achieve similar overall and disease-free survival compared with lobectomy for early-stage non-small cell lung cancer.
- Optimal lymph node yield for accurate staging remains uncertain, but recent updates require resection from specific hilar and mediastinal stations.
- Intraoperative molecular imaging using fluorescent probes and near-infrared imaging can help localize tumors and guide parenchymal-sparing dissection in occult lesions.

DISCLOSURE

The authors have nothing to disclose.

REFERENCES

1. Meyer JA. Hugh Morriston Davies and lobectomy for cancer, 1912. Ann Thorac Surg 1988;46(4):472–4.
2. Montagne F, Guisier F, Venissac N, et al. The Role of Surgery in Lung Cancer Treatment: Present Indications and Future Perspectives-State of the Art. Cancers 2021;13(15). https://doi.org/10.3390/cancers13153711.
3. Cannone G, Comacchio GM, Pasello G, et al. Precision Surgery in NSCLC. Cancers 2023;15(5). https://doi.org/10.3390/cancers15051571.
4. Mok TS, Wu YL, Thongprasert S, et al. Gefitinib or carboplatin-paclitaxel in pulmonary adenocarcinoma. N Engl J Med 2009;361(10):947–57.
5. Shaw AT, Kim DW, Nakagawa K, et al. Crizotinib versus chemotherapy in advanced ALK-positive lung cancer. N Engl J Med 2013;368(25):2385–94.
6. Onoi K, Chihara Y, Uchino J, et al. Immune checkpoint inhibitors for lung cancer treatment: a review. J Clin Med 2020;9(5):1362.
7. Burdett S, Pignon JP, Tierney J, et al. Adjuvant chemotherapy for resected early-stage non-small cell lung cancer. Cochrane Database Syst Rev 2015;3: Cd011430.
8. Pignon JP, Tribodet H, Scagliotti GV, et al. Lung adjuvant cisplatin evaluation: a pooled analysis by the LACE Collaborative Group. J Clin Oncol 2008;26(21): 3552–9.
9. Preoperative chemotherapy for non-small-cell lung cancer: a systematic review and meta-analysis of individual participant data. Lancet (London, England) 2014;383(9928):1561–71.
10. Alexander M, Kim SY, Cheng H. Update 2020: Management of Non-Small Cell Lung Cancer. Lung 2020;198(6):897–907.
11. Liang W, Cai K, Cao Q, et al. International expert consensus on immunotherapy for early-stage non-small cell lung cancer. Transl Lung Cancer Res 2022;11(9): 1742–62.
12. Ettinger DS, Wood DE, Aisner DL, et al. NCCN Guidelines Insights: Non-Small Cell Lung Cancer, Version 2.2021. J Natl Compr Canc Netw 2021;19(3):254–66.
13. Solomon BJ, Mok T, Kim DW, et al. First-line crizotinib versus chemotherapy in ALK-positive lung cancer. N Engl J Med 2014;371(23):2167–77.
14. Huang Q, Li J, Sun Y, et al. Efficacy of EGFR tyrosine kinase inhibitors in the adjuvant treatment for operable non-small cell lung cancer by a meta-analysis. Chest 2016;149(6):1384–92.
15. Brahmer JR, Govindan R, Anders RA, et al. The Society for Immunotherapy of Cancer consensus statement on immunotherapy for the treatment of non-small cell lung cancer (NSCLC). J Immunother Cancer 2018;6(1):75.

16. Kim H, Chung JH. PD-L1 testing in non-small cell lung cancer: past, present, and future. J Pathol Transl Med 2019;53(4):199–206.

17. Mamdani H, Matosevic S, Khalid AB, et al. Immunotherapy in Lung Cancer: Current Landscape and Future Directions. Front Immunol 2022;13:823618.

18. Indini A, Rijavec E, Bareggi C, et al. Novel treatment strategies for early-stage lung cancer: the oncologist's perspective. J Thorac Dis 2020;12(6):3390–8.

19. Vallejo-Manzur F, Varon J, Fromm R Jr, et al. Schiff and the history of open-chest cardiac massage. Resuscitation 2002;53(1):3–5.

20. Blatchford JW 3rd. Ludwig Rehn: the first successful cardiorrhaphy. Ann Thorac Surg 1985;39(5):492–5.

21. Swanson SJ, Herndon JE, D'Amico TA, D'Amico TA, et al. Video-assisted thoracic surgery lobectomy: report of CALGB 39802–a prospective, multi-institution feasibility study. J Clin Oncol 2007;25(31):4993–7.

22. Jawitz OK, Wang Z, Boffa DJ, et al. The differential impact of preoperative comorbidity on perioperative outcomes following thoracoscopic and open lobectomies. Eur J Cardio Thorac Surg 2017;51(1):169–74.

23. Yamashita SI, Tokuishi K, Moroga T, et al. Long-term survival of thoracoscopic surgery compared with open surgery for clinical N0 adenocarcinoma. J Thorac Dis 2020;12(11):6523–32.

24. Hireche K, Lounes Y, Bacri C, et al. VATS versus Open Lobectomy following Induction Therapy for Stage III NSCLC: A Propensity Score-Matched Analysis. Cancers 2023;15(2). https://doi.org/10.3390/cancers15020414.

25. Bendixen M, Jørgensen OD, Kronborg C, et al. Postoperative pain and quality of life after lobectomy via video-assisted thoracoscopic surgery or anterolateral thoracotomy for early stage lung cancer: a randomised controlled trial. Lancet Oncol 2016;17(6):836–44.

26. Guo F, Ma D, Li S. Compare the prognosis of Da Vinci robot-assisted thoracic surgery (RATS) with video-assisted thoracic surgery (VATS) for non-small cell lung cancer: A Meta-analysis. Medicine (Baltim) 2019;98(39):e17089.

27. Eguchi T, Miura K, Hamanaka K, et al. Adoption of Robotic Core Technology in Minimally Invasive Lung Segmentectomy: Review. J Pers Med 2022;12(9). https://doi.org/10.3390/jpm12091417.

28. Bedetti B, Zalepugas D, Arensmeyer JC, et al. [Robotics in thoracic surgery]. Pneumologie 2023;77(6):374–85. Robotik in der Thoraxchirurgie.

29. Ureña A, Moreno C, Macia I, et al. A Comparison of Total Thoracoscopic and Robotic Surgery for Lung Cancer Lymphadenectomy. Cancers 2023;15(13). https://doi.org/10.3390/cancers15133442.

30. Deng B, Cassivi SD, de Andrade M, et al. Clinical outcomes and changes in lung function after segmentectomy versus lobectomy for lung cancer cases. J Thorac Cardiovasc Surg 2014;148(4):1186–92.e3.

31. Altorki N, Wang X, Kozono D, et al. Lobar or Sublobar Resection for Peripheral Stage IA Non-Small-Cell Lung Cancer. N Engl J Med 2023;388(6):489–98.

32. Saji H, Okada M, Tsuboi M, et al. Segmentectomy versus lobectomy in small-sized peripheral non-small-cell lung cancer (JCOG0802/WJOG4607L): a multicentre, open-label, phase 3, randomised, controlled, non-inferiority trial. Lancet (London, England) 2022;399(10335):1607–17.

33. Yendamuri S, Dhillon SS, Groman A, et al. Effect of the number of lymph nodes examined on the survival of patients with stage I non-small cell lung cancer who undergo sublobar resection. J Thorac Cardiovasc Surg 2018;156(1):394–402.

34. Boffa DJ, Kosinski AS, Paul S, et al. Lymph node evaluation by open or video-assisted approaches in 11,500 anatomic lung cancer resections. Ann Thorac Surg 2012;94(2):347–53, discussion 353.
35. Bott MJ, Patel AP, Crabtree TD, et al. Pathologic Upstaging in Patients Undergoing Resection for Stage I Non-Small Cell Lung Cancer: Are There Modifiable Predictors? Ann Thorac Surg 2015;100(6):2048–53.
36. Odell DD, Feinglass J, Engelhardt K, et al. Evaluation of adherence to the Commission on Cancer lung cancer quality measures. J Thorac Cardiovasc Surg 2019;157(3):1219–35.
37. Nissen AP, Vreeland TJ, Teshome M, et al. American College of Surgeons Commission on Cancer Standard for Curative-intent Pulmonary Resection. Ann Thorac Surg 2022;113(1):5–8.
38. Suzuki H, Morimoto J, Mizobuchi T, et al. Does segmentectomy really preserve the pulmonary function better than lobectomy for patients with early-stage lung cancer? Surg Today 2017;47(4):463–9.
39. Macke RA, Schuchert MJ, Odell DD, et al. Parenchymal preserving anatomic resections result in less pulmonary function loss in patients with Stage I non-small cell lung cancer. J Cardiothorac Surg 2015;10:49.
40. Bou-Samra P, Muhammad N, Chang A, et al. Intraoperative molecular imaging: 3rd biennial clinical trials update. J Biomed Opt 2023;28(5):050901.
41. Azari F, Kennedy GT, Bou-Samra P, et al. Intraoperative molecular imaging in thoracic oncology: pushing the boundaries of precision resection for occult non-small cell lung cancer in the era of minimally invasive surgery. J Thorac Dis 2022;14(10):3688–91.
42. Jiang JX, Keating JJ, Jesus EM, et al. Optimization of the enhanced permeability and retention effect for near-infrared imaging of solid tumors with indocyanine green. Am J Nucl Med Mol Imaging 2015;5(4):390–400.
43. Keating J, Newton A, Venegas O, et al. Near-Infrared Intraoperative Molecular Imaging Can Locate Metastases to the Lung. Ann Thorac Surg 2017;103(2):390–8.
44. Predina JD, Newton AD, Corbett C, et al. A Clinical Trial of TumorGlow to Identify Residual Disease During Pleurectomy and Decortication. Ann Thorac Surg 2019; 107(1):224–32.
45. Predina JD, Newton AD, Corbett C, et al. Near-infrared intraoperative imaging for minimally invasive pulmonary metastasectomy for sarcomas. J Thorac Cardiovasc Surg 2019;157(5):2061–9.
46. Sarkaria IS, Martin LW, Rice DC, et al, ELUCIDATE Study Group. Pafolacianine for intraoperative molecular imaging of cancer in the lung: The ELUCIDATE trial. J Thorac Cardiovasc Surg 2023. https://doi.org/10.1016/j.jtcvs.2023.02.025.
47. Kennedy GT, Holt DE, Azari FS, et al. A Cathepsin-Targeted Quenched Activity-Based Probe Facilitates Enhanced Detection of Human Tumors during Resection. Clin Cancer Res 2022;28(17):3729–41.
48. Alfonso-Garcia A, Bec J, Sridharan Weaver S, et al. Real-time augmented reality for delineation of surgical margins during neurosurgery using autofluorescence lifetime contrast. J Biophotonics 2020;13(1):e201900108.
49. Hu P, Li L, Wang LV. Location-Dependent Spatiotemporal Antialiasing in Photoacoustic Computed Tomography. IEEE Trans Med Imaging 2023;42(4):1210–24.

Precision Oncology in Gastrointestinal and Colorectal Cancer Surgery

Hannah G. McDonald, MD[a], Daniel M. Kerekes, MD, MHS[b],
Joseph Kim, MD, FSSO[a], Sajid A. Khan, MD, FSSO[c],*

KEYWORDS

- Precision oncology • GI malignancies • Molecular medicine • Targeted therapies
- Multiomics

KEY POINTS

- Precision medicine individualizes care of patients with gastrointestinal (GI) tract cancers.
- Molecular biomarkers enhance multimodality cancer care including surgery.
- Colorectal cancer is the subject of many cutting-edge molecular assays, which may supplant historically used clinical criteria.
- Multiomic studies will dictate future trends and guidelines for management of GI cancers.

PRECISION MEDICINE

Precision medicine in oncology is treatment tailored toward patient-specific histopathologic and molecular tumor biology. The treatment of patients with gastrointestinal (GI) cancers has been transformed by highly sensitive diagnostic assays, advances in molecular methodologies, risk-stratification modalities, and novel therapies. This includes classification of molecular subtypes with different prognostic implications, identification of biomarkers for targeted systemic, immune checkpoint inhibitors (ICIs) and surgical therapies, and molecularly guided therapeutic regimens to maximize benefit while minimizing toxicity. In this article, the authors discuss the molecular underpinnings and precision treatment of colorectal, esophageal, gastric, and small bowel cancers with cutting-edge modalities for diagnosis, prognosis, and beyond.

[a] Department of General Surgery, Division of Surgical Oncology, The University of Kentucky, 800 Rose Street, Lexington, KY 40508, USA; [b] Department of General Surgery, Division of Surgical Oncology, Yale University, 15 York Street, New Haven, CT 06510, USA; [c] Department of Surgery, Yale University, 15 York Street, New Haven, CT 06510, USA
* Corresponding author.
E-mail address: Sajid.Khan@yale.edu

Surg Oncol Clin N Am 33 (2024) 321–341
https://doi.org/10.1016/j.soc.2023.12.007
1055-3207/24/© 2023 Elsevier Inc. All rights reserved.

COLORECTAL CANCER

Colorectal cancer (CRC) continues to rank third in cancer incidence and mortality in the United States, but second in mortality worldwide. The overall incidence of CRC is on the decline and is diagnosed equally in men and women. Five year overall survival (OS) varies for localized (91%); locoregional (73%), and metastatic disease (16%). Factors associated with late-stage diagnosis include socioeconomic status, race, and younger age. Additional factors that impact survival include comorbidities and male sex.

Molecular Tumorigenesis

The development of CRC occurs via one of three major genetic pathways: chromosomal instability (CIN), microsatellite instability (MSI), and cytosine phosphoguanine (CpG) island methylation phenotype (CIMP).

CIN accounts for 60% of CRC and refers to a high rate of gains or losses of large portions of chromosomes leading to aneuploidy, chromosome amplification, chromosomal rearrangement, accumulation of oncogenic mutations, and loss of heterozygosity of tumor suppressor genes. This pathway is classically secondary to a biallelic mutation in *APC*, rendering the Wnt/β-catenin pathway constitutively active. This can also occur via *POLE/POLD1* (<1%) or *MutY-Homolog* (*MYH* or *MUTYH*; 1%–2%) mutations.[1]

MSI occurs in ∼15% of sporadic CRC and greater than 95% of hereditary nonpolyposis colorectal cancers. It is characterized by DNA sequences consisting of tandem repeats and a high frequency of replication errors in this region, primarily due to the slippage of DNA polymerase. MSI is due to DNA mismatch repair (MMR) deficiency, primarily of MLH1 and MSH2. MMR gene impairment is secondary to mutational or epigenetic inactivation through CpG island methylation of the promoter regions of the genes. For *sporadic* MSI-high (MSI-H) CRCs, a *BRAF* mutation is responsible for inhibition of apoptosis leading to polyps with gene silencing secondary to CpG island promoter methylation. This occurs upstream of MMR genes, causing dysfunctional DNA repair and subsequent MSI.[2]

The CIMP subtype accounts for ∼15% of CRC with similar clinical features as MSI-CRC and is secondary to inactivation by DNA hypermethylation at promoter CpG islands of tumor-suppressor genes, causing gene silencing. It is considered an early event and is characteristic for the serrated pathway of CRC tumorigenesis.[3]

Consensus Molecular Subtypes

Although certain mutations (such as Kirsten rat sarcoma virus or *KRAS*) may be present across all subtypes, the mechanism for mutation, downstream pathway activation, and cellular composition vary widely. Consensus molecular subtypes (CMSs) were developed in 2015 by the CRC Subtyping Consortium.[4] International data identified differential transcriptomic and immune landscapes to guide precision treatment of CRC. From this effort, four molecular subtypes were identified: CMS1–4 (**Table 1**). CMS1 (MSI immune subtype, 14%) is characterized by MSI-H with hypermutation and strong immune activation. Associated mutations include *MSH5, NRF43, ATM, TGRBR2, BRAF*, and *PTEN*. CMS2–4 tumors develop via the CIN pathway. CMS2 (canonical subtype, 37%) has *APC* mutations leading to Wnt and MYC activation with an epithelial phenotype. CMS3 (metabolic subtype, 13%) has *KRAS* mutation-mediated metabolic deregulation and an epithelial phenotype. CMS4 (mesenchymal subtype, 23%) has prominent TGF-β activation, mesenchymal phenotype, stromal invasion, and angiogenesis.[2,4,5]

> **Table 1**
> Consensus molecular subtypes including prevalence, pathway for development, immune cell involvement, and mutations/downstream effectors[2,4,5]
>
> | CMS Group | Subtype | Percentage (%) | Pathway | Immune Infiltration | Mutations/ Downstream Effectors |
> |---|---|---|---|---|---|
> | CMS1 | MSI immune | 14 | Hypermethylation | Yes (activating) | MSH5, ATM, BRAF, PTEN |
> | CMS2 | Canonical | 37 | CIN | No | APC |
> | CMS3 | Metabolic | 13 | CIN | No | KRAS |
> | CMS4 | Mesenchymal | 23 | CIN | Yes (suppressive) | TGF-β |

The CMS groups are centered on differential transcriptomic and immune landscapes to guide precision treatment of CRC. Subtypes may be differentiated based on mutation profile, pathway activation, and cellular composition. For example, CMS2 and CMS4 have overlapping mutation profiles. However, pathway activation between the two is distinct. Similarly, CMS1 and CMS4 show immune cell infiltration. However, CMS1 has an immunogenic phenotype with abundant cytotoxic T cells and expression of immune checkpoints such as PDL1, whereas CMS4 has an immune suppressive phenotype. Poorly immunogenic subtypes CMS2 and CMS3 are microsatellite stable (MSS), non-hypermutated, lack T-cells, and PDL1. These differences have clinical implications for therapy choice and disease progression.[5]

Special Populations

Young patients

Despite an overall decline in the last 20 years, the incidence of CRC has been on the rise in young patients. Early-onset CRC (EO-CRC) is diagnosed before the age of 50 years and accounts for approximately 13% of new cases. EO-CRC ranks 1st versus 3rd (all CRC) in cancer incidence, as well as 1st for men versus 2nd for women less than 50 years in mortality. For this reason, in 2021, the recommended age to initiate screening colonoscopy decreased from 50 to 45 year old. EO-CRC is a biologically distinct entity and requires an individualized approach to diagnosis and treatment.

There seems to be a strong birth-cohort effect, with elevated generational risk leading to higher incidence of EO-CRC. Many modifiable risk factors have been linked to EO-CRC, including obesity and sedentary lifestyle, tobacco exposure, heavy alcohol use, type 2 diabetes, and diet high in processed/red meats or high-fructose corn syrup. Many studies over the past 20 years have shown a proportional increase of CRC risk (HR 1.03 per 1 kg/m^2) with increasing body mass index (BMI). Risk for developing CRC is 20% to 40% higher in obese individuals (RR 1.54) and 50% to 70% higher in obese men, specifically.[6,7]

Family history also remains the most important risk factor, as $\geq$ 40% of EO-CRC patients have family history of CRC and 16% of these are related to a hereditary syndrome.[8,9] The US Preventative Task Force recommends screening at age 40 years for those with a family history of CRC *or* advanced polyps.[10] Studies have shown that young CRC patients are more likely to be MSI-H tumor and/or have Lynch syndrome (LS), and less likely to have tumors harboring $BRAF^{V600E}$ mutations.[11] A large database review showed improved OS for EO-CRC, however, when adjusted for markers such as $BRAF^{V600E}$, this survival benefit disappeared.[12] This reinforces the importance of tumor biology for treatment decisions and for determining prognosis.

Hereditary Cancer Syndromes

Inherited CRC syndromes begin with a "first hit" germline mutation in a tumor suppressor gene, for example, *APC* or DNA repair gene(s). A somatic "second hit" mutation subsequently leads to the development of cancer.[2] Prominent hereditary cancer syndromes associated with CRC include familial adenomatous polyposis (FAP), mutY Homolog-associated polyposis (MAP), LS, Peutz–Jeghers syndrome (PJS), and juvenile polyposis syndrome (JPS). Each of these syndromes has unique implications and recommendations for CRC and extraintestinal cancers (**Table 2**).[10,13,14]

FAP (1:10,000) is caused by a germline mutation in tumor suppressor gene *APC*, which regulates cell proliferation, differentiation, and adhesion. Classically, patients with FAP develop between 100 and 1000 colorectal adenomas; however, greater than 1000 are observed in severe cases, and less than 100 may be seen in attenuated FAP (AFAP). Seventy-five percent of cases are inherited, and 25% are *de novo* with germline *APC* mutation occurring in the absence of family history. Polyp formation occurs at average age of 13 to 14 years, and CRC will develop by around age 39 years without preventative measures.[15] Screening flexible proctosigmoidoscopy is recommended. However, if polyps are found on proctosigmoidoscopy, full colonoscopy is required. Surgery is warranted in patients with symptoms, large polyps or polyps with high-grade dysplasia not amenable to endoscopic mucosal resection, and family history of severe disease.[2,16] Planned surgery is recommended by the age of 20 years in patients who are asymptomatic with mild disease. Exceptions to this include patients with AFAP (may wait until 25 years) or women who wish to bear children (with strict screening). Surgical options for patients with FAP include total abdominal colectomy (TAC) with ileorectal anastomosis (IRA) or proctocolectomy with either ileal pouch-anal anastomosis (IPAA) or permanent end ileostomy. However, patients who undergo TAC with IRA may not have greater than 20 rectal adenomas, adenomas greater than 3 cm in diameter, anal sphincter dysfunction, or adenomas with severe dysplasia/cancer. Of note, female patients, patients with history of abdominal surgery, family history of desmoid tumors, or those with *APC* mutations at the 3′ region of codon 1399 have elevated risk of developing (mesenteric) desmoid tumors. Therefore, surgery may be delayed on a case-by-case basis.[16] Gardner syndrome and Turcot syndrome are subsets characterized by FAP with inclusion cysts, osteomas, and desmoid tumors, or with malignant central nervous system (CNS) tumors, respectively. Additional screening includes annual thyroid ultrasound and esophagogastroduodenoscopy based on the Spigelman criteria.[17]

MAP is caused by a biallelic germline mutation in *MUTYH*. MAP is phenotypically similar to AFAP; those affected typically have less than 100 adenomas and may be distinguished by driver mutation (*MUTYH* vs *APC*). Unlike AFAP, patients with MAP may develop CRC in the absence of adenomatous polyps (serrated, hyperplastic, or no precursor).[18,19] About 20% of patients with MAP will have duodenal polyposis as well. Screening and surgical recommendations are similar to FAP.

LS is the most common cause of hereditary CRC making up 3% to 5% of all CRC cases and up to 20% of cases less than 50 year old.[2,17] Germline mutations in MMR genes including *MLH1/MSH2* (up to 90%), *MSH6*, *PMS2*, and *EpCAM* lead to the development of MSI-H tumors.[20] Patients with LS carry a lifetime cancer risk up to 78%, characterized by an accelerated adenoma-to-carcinoma pathway of as little as 3 years.[17,21] Of note, the presence of a *BRAF* mutation with MSI-H is classic for sporadic tumors (15%) and is not observed in LS.[2] CRCs in this population show a predilection for the proximal colon, and surgery for LS is indicated when CRC is diagnosed. The choice of surgery should weigh recurrence risk with postoperative quality

Table 2
Inherited syndromes with clinical, molecular, screening, and treatment recommendations

Inherited	Mutation Type Mutated Gene	Lifetime Risk of CRC	Age of Onset (Average Years)	Colonoscopy Onset (Years)/Interval	Surgery Recommendations	Extraintestinal Mmanifestations	Extraintestinal Surveillance
FAP	AD APC[5q21–22]	100%	39	12/flexible sigmoidoscopy q1y	TAC/IRA, PC/EI, PC/IPAA	Gastric (0%, 1%–7.1%), duodenal (<1%–10%), small bowel (<1%), CNS (I%), and thyroid (1.2%–12%) cancers, intra-abdominal desmoid tumors (10%–24%), hepatoblastoma (0.4%–2.5%), CHRPE	Upper endoscopy (age 20–25 y, interval guided by Spigelman score), thyroid ultrasound (late teens) q2-5 y
AFAP	AD APC[5q21–22]	70%	56	Late teens/q1-2 y[a]	TAC/IRA[d]	Same as above	Upper endoscopy (age 20–25 y, interval guided by Spigelman score), thyroid ultrasound (late teens) q2-5 y
MAP	AR MUTYH 1p32.1–34.3	80%–90%	47	25–35/q1-2 y[a]	TAC/IRA[d]	Duodenal polyps (20%) and cancer (<5%)	Upper endoscopy (age 30–35 y, interval guided by Spigelman score)
Lynch	AD MLH1	46%–61%	44	20–25/q1-2 y[a]	Segmental resection vs TAC/IRA	Endometrial (34%–54%), ovarian (4%–20%), urothelial (0.2%–7%), gastric (5%–7%), small bowel (0.4%–11%), pancreatic (6.2%), biliary (1.9%–3.7%), prostate (4.4%–13.8%), and brain (0.7%–1.7%) cancers	Upper endoscopy with antral biopsy (age 30–40 y) q2-4 y, may consider, endometrial and ovarian screening and surgery on a case-by-case basis, annual urinalysis (age 30–35 y), and annual pancreas EUS or magnetic resonance cholangiopancreatograohy (MRCP; age 50 y)

(continued on next page)

Table 2
(continued)

Inherited	Mutation Type Mutated Gene	Lifetime Risk of CRC	Age of Onset (Average Years)	Colonoscopy Onset (Years)/ Interval	Surgery Recommendations	Extraintestinal Mmanifestations	Extraintestinal Surveillance
	AD MSH2	33%–52%	44	20–25/q1-2 y[a]	Segmental resection vs TAC/IRA	Endometrial (21%–57%), ovarian (8%–38%), urothelial (2.2%–28%), gastric (0.2%–9%), small bowel (1.1%–10%), pancreatic (0.5%–1.6%), biliary (0.02%–1.7%), prostate (3.9%–23.8%), and brain (2.5%–7.7%) cancers	Upper endoscopy with antral biopsy (age 30–40 y) q2-4 y, may consider, endometrial and ovarian screening and surgery on a case-by-case basis, annual urinalysis (age 30–35 y), and annual pancreas EUS or MRCP (age 50 y)
	AD MSH6	10%–44%	42–69	30–35/q1-3 y[b]	Segmental resection vs TAC/IRA	Endometrial (16%–49%), ovarian (1%–13%), urothelial (0.7%–8.2%), gastric (<1–7.9%), small bowel (<1–4%), pancreatic (1.4%–1.6%), biliary (0.2%–1%), prostate (2.5%–11.6%), and brain (0.8%–1.8%) cancers	Upper endoscopy with antral biopsy (age 30–40 y) q2-4 y, may consider, endometrial and ovarian screening and surgery on a case-by-case basis, annual urinalysis (age 30–35 y), and annual pancreas EUS or MRCP (age 50 y)
	AD PMS2	8.7%–20%	61–66	30–35/q1-3 y[b]	Segmental resection vs TAC/IRA	Endometrial (13%–26%), ovarian (1.3%–3%), urothelial (<1–3.7%), prostate (4.6%–11.6%), brain (0.6%–1%) cancers	May consider: upper endoscopy (age 30–40 y) q2-4 y; endometrial and ovarian screening and surgery on a case-by-case basis; annual urinalysis (age 30–35 y)

PJS	AD STK11(19p)	39%	46	8–10/q2-3 y[c]	Segmental resection vs TAC/IRA	Breast (32%–54%), gastric (29%), small intestine (13%), pancreatic (11%–36%), cervical (10%+) ovarian (20%+), lung (7%–17%), and testicular (9%), cancers	Mammogram/breast MRI annually (age 30), upper endoscopy and capsule endoscopy vs CT/MR enterography (18yrs) q2-3yrs, annual pancreas EUS or MRCP (30-35yrs), annual pelvic exam and ultrasound with biopsy if bleeding (18-20yrs)
JPS	AD SMAD4(18p) or BMPR1A[10q]	≤50%	34	30–35/q1-3 y[b]	Segmental resection vs TAC/IRA	Gastric (up to 21%), hereditary hemorrhagic telangiectasia (HHT: 22%)	Upper endoscopy (age 18 y) q1-3 y (5 y if no polyps)

Abbreviations: AD, autosomal dominant; AFAP, attenuated familial adenomatous polyposis; AR, autosomanal recessive; CHRPE, congenital hypertrophy of the retinal pigment epithelium; FAP, familial adenomatous polyposis; JPS, juvenile polyposis syndrome; MAP, MUTYH-associated polyposis; PC/EI, proctocolectomy with end-ileostomy; PC/IPA, proctocolectomy with end-ileostomy; PC/IPAA, proctocolectomy with ileal pouch-anal anastomosis; PJS, Peutz-Jeghers syndrome; TAC/IRA, total abdominal colectomy with ileorectal anastomosis (if rectal polyps are amendable to endoscopic surveillance and resection).

[a] Or 2 to 5 y before earliest CRC diagnosis if before age 25 y.
[b] Or 2 to 5 y before earliest CRC diagnosis if before age 30 y.
[c] If no polyps at age 8 to 10 y, resume age 18 q2-3 y.
[d] If adenoma burden is not amendable to endoscopic resection, TAC/IRA is preferred unless dense rectal polyposis not amendable to endoscopic resection.

of life. Segmental colectomy is acceptable in this population and is associated with improved quality of life without a survival disadvantage.[22] For young patients with intact sphincter function, TAC with IRA may be considered as the risk for developing metachronous CRC increases each decade after surgery (16% at 10 years, 41% at 20 years, and 62% at 30 years).[23] In contrast, patients with LS-associated rectal cancer should be treated as sporadic. Extensive surgery such as pancreaticoduodenectomy has been described for colon cancer invading into the duodenum.[24] In addition, the frequency of extraintestinal malignant manifestations vary based on gene mutation and include endometrial, breast, ovarian, urinary, and pancreatic cancers; gastric and small bowel cancers occur more frequently in men.[17,25]

PJS is inherited in 50% of cases and is characterized by benign hamartomatous GI polyps, mucocutaneous pigmentation, and both intestinal and extraintestinal cancers. The lifetime risk of cancer is 90%, with 39% risk of CRC. Surgery for PJS is reserved for obstruction or malignancy. Extracolonic malignant manifestations include small bowel, gastric, pancreatic, esophageal, ovarian, lung, uterine, breast, and testicular cancers. Screening for these patients is imperative and extensive (see **Table 2**).

JPS is localized to the GI tract and, like PJS, is characterized by hamartomatous polyps. The clinical diagnosis of PJS requires ≥ 5 hamartomatous polyps in the colon or rectum, multiple polyps within the GI tract, or any number of polyps with a family history of JPS.

Inflammatory Bowel Disease

CRC develops in up to 5.7% of patients with inflammatory bowel disease (IBD).[26] Patients with CRC in the setting of ulcerative colitis and Crohn's disease (CD) tend to be younger, develop multifocal tumors at an accelerated rate, and have higher mortality (5-year OS 50%) compared with those without IBD.[27] This is thought to be due to chronic inflammation leading to dysplasia followed by malignancy. Inflammation-induced oxidative stress and DNA damage lead to activating (oncogene) and inactivating (tumor suppressor gene) mutations within diseased mucosa. Tumors develop via the same pathways as previously described; however, mutations may be present within inflamed mucosa before development of dysplasia or malignancy. This phenomenon is known as "field cancerization," which has been described in CD ileocolitis, and involves in the presence of genomic alterations in segments adjacent to but spared from cancer. In patients with colonic IBD, colonoscopy should be performed every 1 to 3 years, starting 8 to 10 years after IBD diagnosis. Patients diagnosed with CRC in the setting of IBD should undergo total colectomy.

MOLECULAR ASSAYS IN COLORECTAL CANCER
Introduction

The ability to detect CRC development, recurrence, and progression has been rapidly improving with the emergence of new technologies. Multiple DNA and antigen-based molecular assays have been developed to this end, some of which are approved for routine use and others which are currently undergoing clinical validation.

Diagnostic Assays

Although colonoscopy remains the gold standard for screening, several molecular-based diagnostic tests are available for noninvasive detection of occult CRC (or precursor lesions). Commonly used stool-based assays include fecal immunochemical (FIT) and multitarget stool DNA (mt-sDNA) tests. FIT is an antibody-based assay, which detects hemoglobin subunits with high sensitivity and specificity. The mt-sDNA test (Cologuard) detects DNA methylation and *KRAS* mutations, as well as fecal hemoglobin.[28] When detecting (pre)cancerous lesions ≥10 mm, Cologuard has sensitivity and specificity comparable to colonoscopy and has shown superiority to FIT.[29,30] As such, annual FIT or mt-sDNA assay every 3 years may be considered alternative to colonoscopy. Epi proColon, a blood-based assay which detects mutated methylated septin9 DNA, is FDA-approved for those who refuse all other screening modalities.[10,31] Any abnormal noninvasive study should trigger invasive evaluation. Importantly, none of these assays are approved for those at *greater than average* risk. This includes patients with history of precancerous lesion, inherited syndrome, IBD, cystic fibrosis, childhood cancer, or family history of advanced polyps or CRC.[10]

Prognostic and Predictive Assays

In addition to molecular modalities for *screening*, multiple assays have proven efficacious to predict treatment response and prognosis. Currently, determining the need for adjuvant treatment of stage II CRC is based on predicted risk of recurrence. Patients are categorized as "high-risk" based on lymphovascular invasion or perineural invasion, high-grade, obstructing tumors, localized perforation, insufficient nodal examination, or narrow/positive margins. Many gene-based scoring systems have shown heterogeneity in recurrence risk that is not captured by clinical scoring systems. ColoPrint is an 18-gene assay developed to predict response to therapy in stage II (and III) patients being considered for adjuvant therapy.[32] A validation study of greater than 400 patients showed effective risk stratification by 5-year recurrence rate (RR, without adjuvant therapy) into low risk (10% RR) and high risk (21% RR), in both MSS and MSI-H. ColoPrint can also predict development of distant metastasis.[33] Importantly, the National Comprehensive Cancer Network and the American Society of Clinical Oncology clinical risk factors were not predictive of RR or metastasis, respectively, in this population.[34] The hazard ratio (HR) associated with ColoPrint (high risk) was 4.28 for stage II disease, showing great promise to guide the use of adjuvant therapy. ColDx, a 634-probe DNA microarray, has also shown efficacy in predicting recurrence in patients with stage II colon cancer (HR 2.21).[35] OncotypeDx is a 12-gene panel which can predict recurrence in stage II/III colon cancer (HR 2.05) and shows correlation with oxaliplatin benefit.[36,37] Unlike gene-based assays, immunoscore characterizes immune cell distribution within the tumor. This assay follows decades of research showing heterogeneity of tumor progression and therapy response related to the immune microenvironment. Immunoscore quantifies cytotoxic and memory T cells to stratify by predicted tumor immune reactivity.[38] Immunoscore has prognostic value in stage I/II CRC, predicting disease-free survival (DFS) and OS (HR 23.08 and 11.53, respectively).

Circulating Tumor DNA and Circulating Tumor Cells

Tumor-specific genetic information found in the bloodstream may come in the form of circulating tumor DNA (ctDNA) or circulating tumor cells (CTCs). ctDNA or cell-free DNA is found outside of the cell, whereas CTCs remain intact, both have utility in diagnosis, prognosis, treatment, and surveillance. ctDNA assays can detect tumor mutational burden (TMB), specific mutations, and MSI. ctDNA is a promising modality for detecting minimal residual disease after surgery, response to therapy, and recurrence with sensitivity and convenience superior to standard of care (SOC) imaging. Many clinical trials are investigating the efficacy of ctDNA in these contexts. The GALAXY trial found that detection of 4-week postoperative ctDNA in patients with stage II/III colon cancer correlated with DFS. This trial demonstrated that patients with positive postoperative ctDNA had a significantly higher rate of disease clearance if treated with adjuvant chemotherapy (HR 17.1, $P < .001$). This group also showed that patients with undetectable ctDNA following adjuvant therapy had higher DFS (HR 52.3, $P < .001$).[39] ctDNA has the potential to predict who may benefit from chemotherapy in a shorter time frame and with higher sensitivity than standard imaging. Thus, ctDNA is a promising clinical trial endpoint, allowing dissemination of results before long-term survival endpoints. Multiple trials are now underway assessing the use of ctDNA to predict benefit from adjuvant therapy in patients with low-risk stage II colon cancer. Other trials are investigating whether (undetectable) ctDNA may be used to de-escalate treatment and minimize chemotherapy-related toxicity.[40] Importantly, ctDNA does not offer the same sensitivity for every patient. For example, patients with liver metastases have a higher likelihood of ctDNA detection (and correlation with tissue sequencing) than those with peritoneal or lung metastases.[41] CTCs have been used for cell surface biomarker recognition, single-cell analysis, and expansion in vitro. The presence of CTCs has been associated with worse PFS and OS in multiple CRC studies. Targeted analysis of programmed death-ligand 1 (PD-L1) expression in CTCs has been used to guide therapy and predict survival.[42]

TREATMENT OF COLORECTAL CANCER
Treatment of Colon Cancer

Genomic and molecular characterization of tumor tissue is achieved via next-generation sequencing (NGS), which can detect mutations, methylation, and even transcriptional changes. NGS, however, is a time-consuming and costly tool that may become less prevalent in the wake of newer blood-based assays. Those with metastatic CRC (mCRC) should undergo NGS to assess for MSI-H or rat sarcoma virus (RAS)/BRAF mutations, as this will guide the choice of treatment. Treatment is based on stage and molecular characteristics. Neoadjuvant therapy should be considered for bulky nodal disease or clinical T4b (cT4b) tumors.[43] For those with MSS tumors, FOLFOX (or CAPEOX) is SOC. The randomized control trial (RCT), FOxTROT, showed patients with cT3-4 colon tumors had a 28% decrease in recurrence and higher rate of complete resection when treated with neoadjuvant therapy.[44] This trial also showed decreased efficacy of FOLFOX or CAPEOX in patients with MSI-H tumors. In those with MSI-H tumors, ICI therapy is SOC. NICHE and NICHE-2 trials demonstrated efficacy of neoadjuvant (anti-CTLA-4) ipilimumab and (anti-PD1) nivolumab for MSI-H cT3-T4 tumors.[45] Amenable tumors without evidence of metastasis should undergo oncologic resection with ($\geq$12 nodes) lymphadenectomy. If pathologic examination shows pT3-4 or any "high-risk" factors, adjuvant therapy should be discussed. Patients with stage III disease may receive 3 months of CAPEOX versus 6 months of FOLFOX (low risk), or 6 months of either regimen (high risk).[46] Despite cutting-edge molecular assays with promising results, data are insufficient to direct adjuvant therapy.

Treatment of Rectal Cancer

Transabdominal resection is indicated for those with cT1-2N0 rectal cancer, whereas transanal excision is considered for amenable cT1N0 tumors. Patients with cT3-4 tumors or nodal disease should undergo chemotherapy with radiation (CRT); however, upfront resection may be considered for those with low-risk proximal cT3N0 tumors. Patients with MSS tumors should receive either neoadjuvant induction (first) or consolidation (second) chemotherapy with FOLFOX or CAPEOX preceded/followed by CRT (capecitabine vs 5-fluorouracil and RT); those with MSI-H should receive (anti-PD1) ICI therapy with nivolumab, pembrolizumab, or dostarlimab-gxly. Following therapy and restaging CT and MRI, patients may undergo resection versus further therapy (if unresectable), or total neoadjuvant therapy (TNT) if complete clinical response is confirmed with flexible endoscopy, digital rectal examination and MRI pelvis. Biopsy is not needed and has a high false-negative rate in posttreatment patients with rectal cancer.[47] TNT includes a long course of CRT followed by consolidation chemotherapy (CC). A meta-analysis of eight RCTs including RAPIDO, STELLAR, POLISH II, and PRODIGE 23, showed a higher rate of pathologic complete response (pCR) with TNT with an odds ratio (OR) of 1.77 when compared with standard CRT followed by surgery.[48] Importantly, higher pCR is associated with CRT before CC compared with the inverse (OR 1.59). Additional benefits of TNT include compliance with therapy and organ preservation.[48]

Treatment of Metastatic Colorectal Cancer

Patients with mCRC follow the same algorithm for diagnosis with divergence in targeted treatment strategies. Although the prevalence of *BRAF, KRAS*, and *NRAS* mutations does not differ between metastatic and localized disease, MSI-H occurs at a lower frequency (4%–5%).[49,50] Despite the lower rate of MSI-H in mCRC, these patients benefit from ICI therapy. KEYNOTE-177 Phase III RCT demonstrated superior PFS in MSI-H mCRC when treated with pembrolizumab versus chemotherapy.[51] This led to the establishment of pembrolizumab as SOC in patients with MSI-H mCRC in 2020.[40] In addition, Phase II trial Checkmate 142 demonstrated enhanced efficacy of anti-PD1 (nivolumab) combined with anti-CTLA-4 (ipilimumab) therapy in patients with recurrent micrometastatic CRC. These findings led to approval of this combination in patients with disease progression after first-line therapy.[52] Treatment with targeted therapy for mCRC will be discussed in detail in the following section.

GENOMIC ALTERATIONS AND TARGETED THERAPY IN COLORECTAL CANCER
Molecular Markers for Management

Patients with mCRC should undergo molecular testing for (MSI and) *BRAF/KRAS/NRAS* mutations and human epidermal growth factor receptor 2 (HER2) amplification/NTRK fusion. These genomic alterations serve as biomarkers of heterogenous treatment response and thoughtful consideration is required when selecting therapy for metastatic disease. Those with mCRC should be treated with systemic therapy including FOLFIRI, FOLFOX, CAPEOX, or FOLFIRINOX with anti-VEGF therapy (bevacizumab) for tumors throughout the colon. Anti-epidermal growth factor receptor (EGFR) therapy such as panitumumab and cetuximab (if WT for *BRAF/KRAS/NRAS*) may be used in (left-sided) colon and rectal tumors.[43]

KRAS and BRAF
The adenoma to carcinoma pathway begins with *APC* mutations, leading to subsequent mutations in *KRAS, BRAF*, and others. EGFR activation stimulates downstream effectors such as KRAS, BRAF, and mitogen-activated kinase (MAPK). *KRAS* and *BRAF* mutations are mutually exclusive, suggesting one mutation is sufficient for tumorigenesis. Furthermore, in the absence of targeted inhibitors, *KRAS* and *BRAF* mutations render EGFR-inhibitors ineffective due to autonomous downstream pathway activation. *KRAS* is the most commonly mutated oncogene (40%) in CRC, associated with poor prognosis and metastasis.[53] *KRAS* mutations are typically activating mutations of codons 12 and 13; *KRAS* (or *NRAS*) mutations in exons 2 to 4 should not be treated with EGFR inhibitors.[54,55] KRAS^{G12C} inhibitors (eg, sotorasib and adagrasib) are under investigation for use in this population which typically does not benefit from anti-EGFR therapy.[40,56,57] *BRAF* mutations occur in 5% to

16% of patients with CRC and are associated with poor prognosis. *BRAF* encodes a protein kinase downstream of RAS; therefore, *BRAF* mutations lead to constitutive activation of the RAS/Raf/MAPK pathway with dysregulated colonocyte growth and proliferation. Most *BRAF* mutations involve a codon 600 glutamic acid for valine substitution (BRAF[V600E]); however, those with BRAF[V600E] require BRAF inhibitor treatment to benefit from EGFR-inhibitors.[58–60] After the BEACON trial showed enhanced OS, BRAF-inhibitor encorafenib and anti-EGFR antibody cetuximab gained FDA-approval as second-line therapy in *BRAF*-mutated mCRC.[61] Ongoing trials may lead to approval of the combination as first-line therapy in this subset of patients. Minimization of toxicity is important to consider in those who require long-term chemotherapy. Maintenance with cetuximab has been associated with a 5.3 month PFS, superior to observation alone, providing opportunity for a chemotherapy holiday in those on maintenance chemotherapy for mCRC.[62]

Other targets

HER2 amplification (HER2+) is found in 3% to 5% of colon cancers.[63] Targeted therapy (eg, trastuzumab) should be considered in HER2+ patients (WT for *KRAS, NRAS,* and *BRAF*). NTRK fusions are rare (~0.35%) but when present should be considered for treatment with an NTRK inhibitor (eg, entrectinib or larotrectinib). POLE and POLD1 encode for proofreading DNA polymerases. Alterations in the exonuclease domain lead to accumulation of mutations, high TMB, and neoantigen generation, making patients with these alterations potential candidates for treatment with ICIs. Another common mutation includes *PIK3CA* (10%–20%), a downstream effector of EGFR associated with poor prognosis.[64] Certain targeted and non-targeted therapies have shown efficacy in patients with this mutation including alpelisib and aspirin, respectively, among others.[65,66]

Microsatellite Instability

MSI-H, present in up to 15% of CRCs, is caused by mutations in MMR genes such as *MLH1, MLH3, MSH2, MSH3, MSH6,* or *PMS2*. Defects in these genes lead to the accumulation of mutations within microsatellite regions, generating high TMB.[2,17] High TMB leads to translocation of mutated protein fragments to the cell surface to be recognized by the immune system as "neoantigens." Not all pathways leading to MSI-H are equal. For example, those with mutations in *MSH2* and *MSH6* show higher TMB than those with mutations in *MLH1* and *PMS2*.[67] MSI-H is associated with early-stage tumors in the proximal colon, lower rate of metastasis, and improved response to immunotherapy. MSI-H is more commonly found in the elderly, however, when found in younger patients should raise suspicion for LS. ICI therapy has higher efficacy and should be considered in this patient population; however, studies have shown lack of efficacy with cytotoxic chemotherapeutics such as 5-fluorouracil (5-FU; in stage II).[68] Other studies have shown benefit from irinotecan (over oxaliplatin)-based therapies as well as (anti-VEGF) bevacizumab.[69]

It is important to evaluate for associated mutations in MSI-H patients. These patients should be tested for BRAF[V600E] mutation, which indicates sporadic cancer rather than LS (99%).[70] Mutations associated with favorable prognosis in MSI-H CRC include beta-2-microglobulin (B2M) and heat shock protein 110 (HSP110).[50,71] B2M is found in approximately 30% of MSI-H CRC and is associated with resistance to ICI therapy. However, those with this mutation have a greater OS and lower rate of metastasis.[71] Silencing mutations of HSP110 result in infiltration of tumor-suppressive macrophages, leading to increased efficacy of cytotoxic chemotherapy, and provides a promising target to improve efficacy of ICIs.[72] Mutations associated with poor prognosis include *SMAD4* (associated with juvenile polyposis) shown to decrease survival in patients with MSI-H CRC.[73]

ESOPHAGEAL CANCER

Esophageal cancer (EC) ranks eighth in incidence and sixth in mortality worldwide and can be divided into esophageal adenocarcinoma (EAC) and squamous cell carcinoma (ESCC) histologic subtypes. Risk factors for development of EAC include gastro-esophageal reflux disease and resultant metaplasia (Barrett's esophagus) and for ESCC include consumption of alcohol, nitrosamines, and hot beverages. Tobacco is a risk factor for both subtypes. The two subtypes have distinct molecular features, wherein EAC resembles gastric cancer and ESCC is closely related to head and neck cancers. Although both subtypes are treated with neoadjuvant chemoradiation for $\geq$ cT2 tumors, options for targeted therapy vary widely based on molecular characteristics. NGS is warranted for patients with locally advanced or distant disease, assessing for HER2, PD-L1, and MSI-H status. The backbone for chemotherapy in EC includes a fluoropyrimidine (5-FU or capecitabine) and platinum agent (oxaliplatin or cisplatin). For those with HER2 overexpression, trastuzumab should be added. Similarly, for those with PD-L1 expression (combined positive score [CPS] $\geq$10, defined as number of PD-L1 positive cells divided by viable cells multiplied by 100), the addition of anti-PD1 nivolumab (or pembrolizumab) is recommended, after increased OS and PFS in multiple RCTs.[74,75] Adjuvant chemotherapy with nivolumab is given to those with evidence of residual disease on pathology following resection. This recommendation stems from 2021 RCT CHECKMATE-577, which showed significantly increased DFS in those given adjuvant nivolumab following chemoradiation and surgery.[76] Efforts to better target ESCC-related pathways such as Ras/Raf/MEK/ERK and PI3K/AKT/mTOR are underway.[77]

GASTRIC CANCER

Gastric cancer (GC) ranks fifth in incidence and third in mortality worldwide. In the Lauren classification system, GC is classified into diffuse- or intestinal-type (or indeterminate) based on histopathology, with intestinal-type associated with a better prognosis. In 2010, the World Health Organization (WHO) recognized four major histopathologic types of GC: tubular, papillary, mucinous, and poorly cohesive, along with 20 subtypes. More recently, the WHO has recommended HER2+, MSI-H, and Epstein–Barr virus (EBV) as markers of prognosis and/or response to therapies.[78] Despite recent advances in precision oncology for GC, the backbone of therapy for GC remains resection with adjuvant or neoadjuvant cytotoxic chemotherapy and radiation with/without immunotherapy.

Classifying Gastric Cancer

High intra-tumor and inter-tumor heterogeneity has been a barrier to developing targeted therapy and identifying clinically meaningful biomarkers in GC. As a consequence, many groups have developed molecular classification systems for GC. The most comprehensive and widely adopted of these are the Cancer Genome Atlas (TCGA)[79] and the Asian Cancer Research Group (ACRG)[80] systems.

The TCGA classification system was developed using a biobank of 295 GC specimens and includes four classes: EBV-associated, genomically stable (GS), MSI-H, and chromosomal unstable.[79] Each class is associated with distinct characteristics. EBV-associated tumors carry *PIK3CA* mutations, extreme DNA hypermethylation, and amplification of *JAK2*, *PD-L1*, and *PD-L2* (also known as *PDCD1LG2*). GS tumors have *RHOA* mutations or fusions involving Rho-family GTPase-activating proteins. MSI-H tumors display elevated mutation rates, often of oncogenic proteins, which may serve as targets for intervention. Chromosomal unstable tumors display aneuploidy and receptor tyrosine kinase amplification. Subtype analysis demonstrated that EBV had the best prognosis, and CIN had the best response to chemotherapy and GS, the worst prognosis with least benefit from chemotherapy.[81]

ACRG used a biobank of 300 GC tumors to define four classes: MSI-H, MSS with active TP53 (MSS/TP53+), MSS with inactive TP53 (MSS/TP53−), and MSS with epithelial-mesenchymal transition (MSS/EMT).[80] An important difference between ACRG and TCGA cohorts is that the ACRG had a higher proportion of diffuse-type GC (45% vs 24%). ACRG subtypes are associated with a wide range of unique somatic alterations, with the MSS/EMT subtype bearing the worst prognosis and highest recurrence risk.

Treatment of Gastric Cancer

Currently, four molecular characteristics have therapeutic relevance in GC: HER2+, PD-L1+, MSI-H, and TMB. HER2 expression guides the use of trastuzumab, whereas the latter three predict efficacy of immunotherapy. In patients with advanced HER2+ tumors, trastuzumab added to SOC chemotherapy offers advantages in overall response rate (ORR), PFS, and OS.[82] Significant intra-tumor heterogeneity led to a consensus statement from two expert consortia recommending initial evaluation of a ≥5 biopsy specimens using immunohistochemistry (IHC), with fluorescence in situ hybridization techniques for equivocal HER2 expression on IHC.[83] The benefit of immunotherapy can also be guided by molecular characteristics of the tumor. Patients with advanced GC and PD-L1+, MSI-H, or high TMB should be considered for first-line treatment with immunotherapy with or without cytotoxic chemotherapy. The KEYNOTE-062 trial found pembrolizumab monotherapy to be non-inferior to chemotherapy for OS in patients with PD-L1 CPS ≥1 with a more favorable side effect profile; for patients with CPS ≥10, treatment with pembrolizumab was associated with a significant improvement in OS compared with chemotherapy alone.[84] The CheckMate 649 trial, which compared chemotherapy alone to chemotherapy with nivolumab, found patients with CPS ≥5 to have significantly improved OS with the addition of nivolumab.[85] The benefit of using immunotherapy for patients with MSI-H tumors primarily stems from post hoc analyses of existing RCTs.[85,86] Several studies have found an association between high TMB and improved response to immunotherapy.[87,88]

SMALL BOWEL ADENOCARCINOMA

Small bowel cancer is diagnosed in 2.5 per 100,000 people each year, with nearly half (30%–40%) adenocarcinoma primarily (60%) located within the duodenum.[89] Duodenal adenocarcinoma develops de novo, in the setting of polyps (eg, FAP, MAP, LS, and PJS), or chronic inflammation such as with CD. In those who have resectable disease, pancreaticoduodenectomy is often required due to anatomic location. Adjuvant treatment for (≥pT3) MSS tumors with high-risk features includes fluoropyrimidine chemotherapy ± oxaliplatin. For MSS advanced or metastatic disease, treatment includes a fluoropyrimidine with bevacizumab and either oxaliplatin, irinotecan, or both. For MSI-H advanced or metastatic disease, treatment includes nivolumab ± ipilimumab or pembrolizumab.[90] Common mutations in small bowel adenocarcinoma include TP53, KRAS, APC, SMAD4, and PIK3CA, with ERBB2 (HER2) being more common in duodenal adenocarcinoma. In addition, rates of MSI-H have been reported between 14.2% and 21.6%.[91,92] Some studies have assessed molecular subtypes, identifying an "immunologic," "DNA Damage Repair Like," and "Colon-like" subtype to guide therapy.[93]

EMERGING AREAS OF RESEARCH IN GASTROINTESTINAL CANCERS

Big data and high-throughput techniques have ushered in an era of "omics," in which a large-scale study is performed to characterize the molecular biology or pathology of an entity. After the first human genome was sequenced in 2003, technological advances allowed for rapid, affordable sequencing of tissues. "Omics" techniques advanced to transcriptomics, followed by proteomics. Downstream, fields such as metabolomics and study of the microbiome are emerging as promising pathways for development of targeted and complementary therapies.

Metabolomics

Metabolomics focuses on small molecule intermediates and end products of different cellular pathways. Disruption of cellular metabolism is a major mechanism by which tumors support nutrient consumption resulting in proliferation. Studies of metabolomics in GI cancers are based on analysis of wide-ranging specimen types such as tumor, urine, stool, plasma, and serum. Mass spectrometry is by far the most popular method of analysis. Metabolic differences between cancerous and noncancerous tissue may be exploited to identify novel biomarkers for targeted therapy and provide insight into pathway derangements leading to cancer development and progression. Promising application of metabolomics in GI cancer has enabled for a higher level of understanding of sex differences and environmental exposures precipitating cancer development.[94,95] There is significant therapeutic potential in targeting metabolic processes in GI cancers that is yet to be maximized.

Microbiome

An area of great interest in metabolomics is the interplay between a host's microbiome and colon cancer. Many studies have linked gut microbiota and their metabolites to CRC development.[96] Different aspects of the microbiome have been associated with the development of CRC: bacterial diversity,[97] species, and release of oncogenic metabolites impacting immune response and inflammation.[98] The most heavily implicated species in CRC is *Fusobacterium nucleatum*,[99] associated with both tumor progression and resistance to therapy.[100] The microbiome impacts other GI malignancies such as GC, most prominently via *Helicobacter pylori*. As with *H pylori*, the use of antibiotics and/or probiotics may be used to prevent or treat GI malignancies.

SUMMARY

Exponential advances by the scientific community have improved the clinical understanding of GI cancers. Cutting edge diagnostic and prognostic tools have enabled cancer surgeons to provide personalized care to patients based on tumor biology. We expect precision oncology to become paramount in clinical care as "omics" research continues to uncover key regulatory mechanisms in the development and progression of GI cancers.

CLINICS CARE POINTS

- Management of gastrointestinal cancers must account for inherited risk and molecular features to determine optimal treatment strategies.

- Diagnostic and prognostic assays should be thoughtfully employed to ensure expeditious treatment of GI malignancies.
- Investigation of multiomic pathways such as metabolomics and the microbiome will continue to uncover opportunities for multimodal targeting of GI malignancies

DISCLOSURES

H.G. McDonald was supported by NIH T32CA60003.

REFERENCES

1. Church JM. Molecular Genetics of Colorectal Cancer. Current Therapy in Colon and Rectal Surgery. Third edition, 2017:273-274.
2. Susan Galandiuk UN, Morpurgo Emilio, Tosato Sara Maria, et al. Sabiston Textbook of Surgery. In: Townsend CM, editor. Sabiston textbook of surgery. 21 edition. Elsevier Inc; 2022. p. 1320–400.e1.
3. Weisenberger DJ, Siegmund KD, Campan M, et al. CpG island methylator phenotype underlies sporadic microsatellite instability and is tightly associated with BRAF mutation in colorectal cancer. Nat Genet 2006;38:787–93.
4. Guinney J, Dienstmann R, Wang X, et al. The consensus molecular subtypes of colorectal cancer. Nat Med 2015;21:1350–6.
5. Dienstmann R, Vermeulen L, Guinney J, et al. Consensus molecular subtypes and the evolution of precision medicine in colorectal cancer. Nat Rev Cancer 2017;17:79–92.
6. O'Sullivan DE, Sutherland RL, Town S, et al. Risk Factors for Early-Onset Colorectal Cancer: A Systematic Review and Meta-analysis. Clin Gastroenterol Hepatol 2022;20:1229–40.e5.
7. Jochem C, Leitzmann M. Obesity and Colorectal Cancer. Recent Results Cancer Res 2016;208:17–41.
8. Chen FW, Sundaram V, Chew TA, et al. Low Prevalence of Criteria for Early Screening in Young-Onset Colorectal Cancer. Am J Prev Med 2017;53:933–4.
9. Pearlman R, Frankel WL, Swanson B, et al. Prevalence and Spectrum of Germline Cancer Susceptibility Gene Mutations Among Patients With Early-Onset Colorectal Cancer. JAMA Oncol 2017;3:464–71.
10. NCCN Colorectal Cancer Screening v 1.2023.
11. Willauer AN, Liu Y, Pereira AAL, et al. Clinical and molecular characterization of early-onset colorectal cancer. Cancer 2019;125:2002–10.
12. Jin Z, Dixon JG, Fiskum JM, et al. Clinicopathological and Molecular Characteristics of Early-Onset Stage III Colon Adenocarcinoma: An Analysis of the ACCENT Database. J Natl Cancer 2021;113:1693–704.
13. Weiss JM, Gupta S, Burke CA, et al. NCCN Guidelines® Insights: Genetic/Familial High-Risk Assessment: Colorectal, Version 1.2021. J Natl Compr Cancer Netw 2021;19:1122–32.
14. Giardiello FM, Brensinger JD, Tersmette AC, et al. Very high risk of cancer in familial Peutz–Jeghers syndrome. Gastroenterology 2000;119:1447–53.
15. Kennedy RD, Potter DD, Moir CR, et al. The natural history of familial adenomatous polyposis syndrome: A 24 year review of a single center experience in screening, diagnosis, and outcomes. J Pediatr Surg 2014;49:82–6.
16. Campos FG. Surgical treatment of familial adenomatous polyposis: dilemmas and current recommendations. World J Gastroenterol 2014;20:16620–9.

17. Stoffel EM, Mangu PB, Gruber SB, et al. Hereditary colorectal cancer syndromes: American Society of Clinical Oncology Clinical Practice Guideline endorsement of the familial risk-colorectal cancer: European Society for Medical Oncology Clinical Practice Guidelines. J Clin Oncol 2015;33:209–17.

18. Boparai KS, Dekker E, van Eeden S, et al. Hyperplastic Polyps and Sessile Serrated Adenomas as a Phenotypic Expression of MYH-Associated Polyposis. Gastroenterology 2008;135:2014–8.

19. Wang L, Baudhuin LM, Boardman LA, et al. MYH mutations in patients with attenuated and classic polyposis and with young-onset colorectal cancer without polyps. Gastroenterology 2004;127:9–16.

20. Peltomäki P. Deficient DNA mismatch repair: a common etiologic factor for colon cancer. Hum Mol Genet 2001;10:735–40.

21. Aarnio M, Mecklin JP, Aaltonen LA, et al. Life-time risk of different cancers in hereditary non-polyposis colorectal cancer (HNPCC) syndrome. Int J Cancer 1995;64:430–3.

22. You YN, Chua HK, Nelson H, et al. Segmental vs. extended colectomy: measurable differences in morbidity, function, and quality of life. Dis Colon Rectum 2008;51:1036–43.

23. Parry S, Win AK, Parry B, et al. Metachronous colorectal cancer risk for mismatch repair gene mutation carriers: the advantage of more extensive colon surgery. Gut 2011;60:950–7.

24. Zhu R, Grisotti G, Salem RR, et al. Pancreaticoduodenectomy for locally advanced colon cancer in hereditary nonpolyposis colorectal cancer. World J Surg Oncol 2016;14:12.

25. Engel C, Loeffler M, Steinke V, et al. Risks of Less Common Cancers in Proven Mutation Carriers With Lynch Syndrome. J Clin Oncol 2012;30:4409–15.

26. Faye AS, Holmer AK, Axelrad JE. Cancer in Inflammatory Bowel Disease. Gastroenterol Clin N Am 2022;51:649–66.

27. Keller DS, Windsor A, Cohen R, et al. Colorectal cancer in inflammatory bowel disease: review of the evidence. Tech Coloproctol 2019;23:3–13.

28. Young GP, Symonds EL, Allison JE, et al. Advances in Fecal Occult Blood Tests: the FIT revolution. Dig Dis Sci 2015;60:609–22.

29. Rex DK, Rahmani EY, Haseman JH, et al. Relative sensitivity of colonoscopy and barium enema for detection of colorectal cancer in clinical practice. Gastroenterology 1997;112:17–23.

30. Imperiale TF, Ransohoff DF, Itzkowitz SH. Multitarget stool DNA testing for colorectal-cancer screening. N Engl J Med 2014;371:187–8.

31. Issa IA, Noureddine M. Colorectal cancer screening: An updated review of the available options. World J Gastroenterol 2017;23:5086–96.

32. Salazar R, Roepman P, Capella G, et al. Gene expression signature to improve prognosis prediction of stage II and III colorectal cancer. J Clin Oncol 2011;29:17–24.

33. Maak M, Simon I, Nitsche U, et al. Independent Validation of a Prognostic Genomic Signature (ColoPrint) for Patients With Stage II Colon Cancer. Ann Surg 2013;257:1053–8.

34. Kopetz S, Tabernero J, Rosenberg R, et al. Genomic classifier ColoPrint predicts recurrence in stage II colorectal cancer patients more accurately than clinical factors. Oncol 2015;20:127–33.

35. Kennedy RD, Bylesjo M, Kerr P, et al. Development and independent validation of a prognostic assay for stage II colon cancer using formalin-fixed paraffin-embedded tissue. J Clin Oncol 2011;29:4620–6.

36. Yamanaka M, Hayashi M, Yamada S, et al. A Possible Definition of Oligometa-stasis in Pancreatic Cancer and Associated Survival Outcomes. Anticancer Res 2021;41:3933–40.

37. Yothers G, O'Connell MJ, Lee M, et al. Validation of the 12-gene colon cancer recurrence score in NSABP C-07 as a predictor of recurrence in patients with stage II and III colon cancer treated with fluorouracil and leucovorin (FU/LV) and FU/LV plus oxaliplatin. J Clin Oncol 2013;31:4512–9.

38. Pagès F, Kirilovsky A, Mlecnik B, et al. In Situ Cytotoxic and Memory T Cells Pre-dict Outcome in Patients With Early-Stage Colorectal Cancer. J Clin Oncol 2009; 27:5944–51.

39. Kotaka M, Shirasu H, Watanabe J, et al. Association of circulating tumor DNA dynamics with clinical outcomes in the adjuvant setting for patients with colo-rectal cancer from an observational GALAXY study in CIRCULATE-Japan. J Clin Oncol 2022;40:9.

40. Fabregas JC, Ramnaraign B, George TJ. Clinical Updates for Colon Cancer Care in 2022. Clin Colorectal Cancer 2022;21:198–203.

41. Kagawa Y, Elez E, García-Foncillas J, et al. Combined Analysis of Concordance between Liquid and Tumor Tissue Biopsies for RAS Mutations in Colorectal Can-cer with a Single Metastasis Site: The METABEAM Study. Clin Cancer Res 2021; 27:2515–22.

42. Satelli A, Batth IS, Brownlee Z, et al. Potential role of nuclear PD-L1 expression in cell-surface vimentin positive circulating tumor cells as a prognostic marker in cancer patients. Sci Rep 2016;6:28910.

43. NCCN Guidelines Version 2.2023 Colon Cancer. .

44. Foxtrot Collaborative G. Feasibility of preoperative chemotherapy for locally advanced, operable colon cancer: the pilot phase of a randomised controlled trial. Lancet Oncol 2012;13:1152–60.

45. Morton D, Seymour M, Magill L, et al. Preoperative Chemotherapy for Operable Colon Cancer: Mature Results of an International Randomized Controlled Trial. J Clin Oncol 2023;41:1541–52.

46. Grothey A, Sobrero AF, Shields AF, et al. Duration of Adjuvant Chemotherapy for Stage III Colon Cancer. N Engl J Med 2018;378:1177–88.

47. NCCN Guidelines Version 3.2023 Rectal Cancer.

48. Liu S, Jiang T, Xiao L, et al. Total Neoadjuvant Therapy (TNT) versus Standard Neoadjuvant Chemoradiotherapy for Locally Advanced Rectal Cancer: A Sys-tematic Review and Meta-Analysis. Oncol 2021;26:e1555–66.

49. Etienne-Grimaldi MC, Formento JL, Francoual M, et al. K-Ras mutations and treatment outcome in colorectal cancer patients receiving exclusive fluoropyri-midine therapy. Clin Cancer Res 2008;14:4830–5.

50. Battaglin F, Naseem M, Lenz HJ, et al. Microsatellite instability in colorectal can-cer: overview of its clinical significance and novel perspectives. Clin Adv Hem-atol Oncol 2018;16:735–45.

51. André T, Shiu K, Kim T, et al. O-8 Final overall survival for the phase 3 KN177 study: Pembrolizumab versus chemotherapy in microsatellite instability-high/ mismatch repair deficient metastatic colorectal cancer. Ann Oncol 2021;32: S220–1.

52. Overman MJ, McDermott R, Leach JL, et al. Nivolumab in patients with metasta-tic DNA mismatch repair-deficient or microsatellite instability-high colorectal cancer (CheckMate 142): an open-label, multicentre, phase 2 study. Lancet On-col 2017;18:1182–91.

53. Zhu G, Pei L, Xia H, et al. Role of oncogenic KRAS in the prognosis, diagnosis and treatment of colorectal cancer. Mol Cancer 2021;20:143.

54. Lièvre A, Bachet JB, Boige V, et al. KRAS mutations as an independent prognostic factor in patients with advanced colorectal cancer treated with cetuximab. J Clin Oncol 2008;26:374–9.

55. Amado RG, Wolf M, Peeters M, et al. Wild-type KRAS is required for panitumumab efficacy in patients with metastatic colorectal cancer. J Clin Oncol 2008;26:1626–34.

56. Fakih MG, Kopetz S, Kuboki Y, et al. Sotorasib for previously treated colorectal cancers with KRAS(G12C) mutation (CodeBreaK100): a prespecified analysis of a single-arm, phase 2 trial. Lancet Oncol 2022;23:115–24.

57. Ou SI, Jänne PA, Leal TA, et al. First-in-Human Phase I/IB Dose-Finding Study of Adagrasib (MRTX849) in Patients With Advanced KRAS(G12C) Solid Tumors (KRYSTAL-1). J Clin Oncol 2022;40:2530–8.

58. Di Nicolantonio F, Martini M, Molinari F, et al. Wild-type BRAF is required for response to panitumumab or cetuximab in metastatic colorectal cancer. J Clin Oncol 2008;26:5705–12.

59. Bokemeyer C, Van Cutsem E, Rougier P, et al. Addition of cetuximab to chemotherapy as first-line treatment for KRAS wild-type metastatic colorectal cancer: pooled analysis of the CRYSTAL and OPUS randomised clinical trials. Eur J Cancer 2012;48:1466–75.

60. Pietrantonio F, Petrelli F, Coinu A, et al. Predictive role of BRAF mutations in patients with advanced colorectal cancer receiving cetuximab and panitumumab: a meta-analysis. Eur J Cancer 2015;51:587–94.

61. Tabernero J, Grothey A, Van Cutsem E, et al. Encorafenib Plus Cetuximab as a New Standard of Care for Previously Treated BRAF V600E-Mutant Metastatic Colorectal Cancer: Updated Survival Results and Subgroup Analyses from the BEACON Study. J Clin Oncol 2021;39:273–84.

62. Boige V, Francois E, Ben Abdelghani M, et al. Maintenance treatment with cetuximab versus observation in RAS wild-type metastatic colorectal cancer: Results of the randomized phase II PRODIGE 28-time UNICANCER study. J Clin Oncol 2021;39:15.

63. Siena S, Sartore-Bianchi A, Marsoni S, et al. Targeting the human epidermal growth factor receptor 2 (HER2) oncogene in colorectal cancer. Ann Oncol 2018;29:1108–19.

64. Lech G, Słotwiński R, Słodkowski M, et al. Colorectal cancer tumour markers and biomarkers: Recent therapeutic advances. World J Gastroenterol 2016;22:1745–55.

65. Gu M, Nishihara R, Chen Y, et al. Aspirin exerts high anti-cancer activity in PIK3CA-mutant colon cancer cells. Oncotarget 2017;8:87379–89.

66. Juric D, Rodon J, Tabernero J, et al. Phosphatidylinositol 3-Kinase α-Selective Inhibition With Alpelisib (BYL719) in PIK3CA-Altered Solid Tumors: Results From the First-in-Human Study. J Clin Oncol 2018;36:1291–9.

67. Salem ME, Grothey A, Kim ES, et al. Impact of MLH1, PMS2, MSH2, and MSH6 alterations on tumor mutation burden (TMB) and PD-L1 expression in 1,057 microsatellite instability-high (MSI-H) tumors. J Clin Oncol 2018;36:3572.

68. Sargent DJ, Marsoni S, Monges G, et al. Defective mismatch repair as a predictive marker for lack of efficacy of fluorouracil-based adjuvant therapy in colon cancer. J Clin Oncol 2010;28:3219–26.

69. Tougeron D, Sueur B, Sefrioui D, et al. A large multicenter study evaluating prognosis and chemosensitivity of metastatic colorectal cancers with microsatellite instability. J Clin Oncol 2017;35:3536.

70. Parsons MT, Buchanan DD, Thompson B, et al. Correlation of tumour BRAF mutations and MLH1 methylation with germline mismatch repair (MMR) gene mutation status: a literature review assessing utility of tumour features for MMR variant classification. J Med Genet 2012;49:151–7.

71. Janikovits J, Müller M, Krzykalla J, et al. High numbers of PDCD1 (PD-1)-positive T cells and B2M mutations in microsatellite-unstable colorectal cancer. Oncolmmunology 2018;7. e1390640.

72. Dorard C, de Thonel A, Collura A, et al. Expression of a mutant HSP110 sensitizes colorectal cancer cells to chemotherapy and improves disease prognosis. Nat Med 2011;17:1283–9.

73. Isaksson-Mettävainio M, Palmqvist R, Dahlin AM, et al. High SMAD4 levels appear in microsatellite instability and hypermethylated colon cancers, and indicate a better prognosis. Int J Cancer 2012;131:779–88.

74. Sun JM, Shen L, Shah MA, et al. Pembrolizumab plus chemotherapy versus chemotherapy alone for first-line treatment of advanced oesophageal cancer (KEYNOTE-590): a randomised, placebo-controlled, phase 3 study. Lancet 2021;398:759–71.

75. Janjigian YY, Shitara K, Moehler M, et al. First-line nivolumab plus chemotherapy versus chemotherapy alone for advanced gastric, gastro-oesophageal junction, and oesophageal adenocarcinoma (CheckMate 649): a randomised, open-label, phase 3 trial. Lancet 2021;398:27–40.

76. Kelly RJ, Ajani JA, Kuzdzal J, et al. Adjuvant Nivolumab in Resected Esophageal or Gastroesophageal Junction Cancer. N Engl J Med 2021;384:1191–203.

77. Yang Y-M, Hong P, Xu WW, et al. Advances in targeted therapy for esophageal cancer. Signal Transduct Targeted Ther 2020;5:229.

78. Nagtegaal ID, Odze RD, Klimstra D, et al. The 2019 WHO classification of tumours of the digestive system. Histopathology 2020;76:182–8.

79. Cancer Genome Atlas Research N. Comprehensive molecular characterization of gastric adenocarcinoma. Nature 2014;513:202–9.

80. Cristescu R, Lee J, Nebozhyn M, et al. Molecular analysis of gastric cancer identifies subtypes associated with distinct clinical outcomes. Nat Med 2015; 21:449–56.

81. Sohn BH, Hwang J-E, Jang H-J, et al. Clinical significance of four molecular subtypes of gastric cancer identified by The Cancer Genome Atlas project. Clin Cancer Res 2017;23:4441–9.

82. Bang Y-J, Van Cutsem E, Feyereislova A, et al. Trastuzumab in combination with chemotherapy versus chemotherapy alone for treatment of HER2-positive advanced gastric or gastro-oesophageal junction cancer (ToGA): a phase 3, open-label, randomised controlled trial. Lancet (London, England) 2010;376: 687–97.

83. Bartley AN, Washington MK, Ventura CB, et al. HER2 Testing and Clinical Decision Making in Gastroesophageal Adenocarcinoma: Guideline From the College of American Pathologists, American Society for Clinical Pathology, and American Society of Clinical Oncology. Arch Pathol Lab Med 2016;140:1345–63.

84. Shitara K, Van Cutsem E, Bang Y-J, et al. Efficacy and Safety of Pembrolizumab or Pembrolizumab Plus Chemotherapy vs Chemotherapy Alone for Patients With First-line, Advanced Gastric Cancer: The KEYNOTE-062 Phase 3 Randomized Clinical Trial. JAMA Oncol 2020;6:1571–80.

85. Shitara K, Ajani JA, Moehler M, et al. Nivolumab plus chemotherapy or ipilimumab in gastro-oesophageal cancer. Nature 2022;603:942–8.
86. Chao J, Fuchs CS, Shitara K, et al. Assessment of Pembrolizumab Therapy for the Treatment of Microsatellite Instability-High Gastric or Gastroesophageal Junction Cancer Among Patients in the KEYNOTE-059, KEYNOTE-061, and KEYNOTE-062 Clinical Trials. JAMA Oncol 2021;7:895–902.
87. Jang JY, Jeong SY, Kim ST. Tumor mutational burden as a potential predictive marker for the efficacy of immunotherapy in advanced gastric cancer. J Clin Oncol 2023;41:324.
88. Lee K-W, Van Cutsem E, Bang Y-J, et al. Association of Tumor Mutational Burden with Efficacy of Pembrolizumab±Chemotherapy as First-Line Therapy for Gastric Cancer in the Phase III KEYNOTE-062 Study. Clin Cancer Res 2022; 28:3489–98.
89. Pedersen KS, Raghav K, Overman MJ. Small Bowel Adenocarcinoma: Etiology, Presentation, and Molecular Alterations. J Natl Compr Cancer Netw 2019;17: 1135–41.
90. NCCN. NCCN Clinical Practice Guidelines in Oncology - Small Bowel Adenocarcinoma Version 1.2023, 2023.
91. Laforest A, Aparicio T, Zaanan A, et al. ERBB2 gene as a potential therapeutic target in small bowel adenocarcinoma. Eur J Cancer 2014;50:1740–6.
92. Hänninen UA, Katainen R, Tanskanen T, et al. Exome-wide somatic mutation characterization of small bowel adenocarcinoma. PLoS Genet 2018;14: e1007200.
93. Casadei-Gardini A, Lonardi S, Smiroldo V, et al. Extensive molecular reclassification: new perspectives in small bowel adenocarcinoma? Med Oncol 2021; 38:17.
94. Shen X, Cai Y, Lu L, et al. Asparagine Metabolism in Tumors Is Linked to Poor Survival in Females with Colorectal Cancer: A Cohort Study. Metabolites 2022;12.
95. Kerekes DM, Khan SA. Lipid Metabolism in Biliary Tract Cancer: A New Therapeutic Target? Ann Surg Oncol 2022;29:2750–1.
96. Louis P, Hold GL, Flint HJ. The gut microbiota, bacterial metabolites and colorectal cancer. Nat Rev Microbiol 2014;12:661–72.
97. Chen W, Liu F, Ling Z, et al. Human intestinal lumen and mucosa-associated microbiota in patients with colorectal cancer. PLoS One 2012;7:e39743.
98. Brennan CA, Garrett WS. Gut Microbiota, Inflammation, and Colorectal Cancer. Annu Rev Microbiol 2016;70:395–411.
99. Kostic AD, Chun E, Robertson L, et al. Fusobacterium nucleatum potentiates intestinal tumorigenesis and modulates the tumor-immune microenvironment. Cell Host Microbe 2013;14:207–15.
100. Yu T, Guo F, Yu Y, et al. Fusobacterium nucleatum Promotes Chemoresistance to Colorectal Cancer by Modulating Autophagy. Cell 2017;170:548–63.e16.

Precision Oncology in Hepatopancreatobiliary Cancer Surgery

Timothy E. Newhook, MD[a], Susan Tsai, MD, MHS[b],
Funda Meric-Bernstam, MD[c],*

KEYWORDS

- Genomics • Pancreatic cancer • Cholangiocarcinoma • Liver cancer
- Targeted therapy

KEY POINTS

- Although hepatocellular carcinoma, cholangiocarcinoma, and pancreatic ductal adenocarcinoma (PDAC) arise from sites in close proximity, these tumors differ significantly in the molecular drivers.
- Several genomic alterations are proven therapeutic targets in advanced biliary tract cancers including *FGFR2* fusions, *IDH* mutations and BRAF V600 E mutations, and *HER2* amplifications/overexpression, and several are emerging in the management of PDAC.
- Molecular profiling including assessment of mutations, copy number changes, and fusions should be included for patients with advanced/metastatic hepatopancreatobiliary cancer.
- Further work is needed to optimize precision oncology including immunotherapy for operable hepatopancreatobiliary cancer.

INTRODUCTION

Advances in technology have allowed for the characterization of tumors at the genomic, transcriptomic, and proteomic levels. Coincidentally, with the rapid advances in

Funding: This work was supported in part by the Clinical and Translational Sciences Award (F. Meric-Bernstam, UL1TR003167) and the MD Anderson Cancer Support Grant (F. Meric-Bernstam, P30CA016672). Funded by: NIHHYB. Grant number(s): UL1TR00316.
[a] Department of Surgical Oncology, Division of Surgery, University of Texas MD Anderson Cancer Center, 1515 Holcombe Boulevard, Houston, TX 77030, USA; [b] Division of Surgical Oncology, Department of Surgery, Ohio State University Comprehensive Cancer Center, N924 Doan Hall, 410 West 10th Avenue, Columbus, OH 43210, USA; [c] Department of Investigational Cancer Therapeutics, Division of Cancer Medicine, University of Texas MD Anderson Cancer Center, 1400 Holcombe Boulevard, FC8.3044, Houston, TX 77030, USA
* Corresponding author.
E-mail address: fmeric@mdanderson.org

Surg Oncol Clin N Am 33 (2024) 343–367
https://doi.org/10.1016/j.soc.2023.12.016
1055-3207/24/© 2023 Elsevier Inc. All rights reserved.

genomic sequencing technology, significant gains have been achieved in the development of available molecularly matched therapeutics across oncology, which may be disease-specific, such as the classic example of imatinib for KIT tyrosine kinase–mutated gastrointestinal stromal tumors, or disease agnostic, such as pembrolizumab for tumor mutation burden–high tumors.[1,2] Increasingly, molecular profiling is being performed on not only tumor samples (somatic testing for alterations in the tumor) but also normal tissue (germline testing) and blood (circulating biomarkers). Germline testing has been recommended by practice guidelines for the majority of hepatopancreatobiliary (HPB) cancers.[3] However, alterations identified in tumor-only testing or matched tumor-normal testing to identify somatic alterations may identify pathogenic germline mutations or may trigger germline-specific testing. Knowledge of germline alterations in the absence of targeted therapies may be valuable, as standard chemotherapeutic options may be tailored based on susceptibilities in homologous recombination repair and mismatch repair pathways. Increasingly, the interpretation of both somatic and germline data can be complicated. Information about paired tumor and germline analysis, knowledge of co-occurring alterations, mutational heterogeneity, and subclonal mutations are important aspects to consider. In this article, the authors touch on recent developments in the understanding of the pathogenesis of HPB cancers and review potential therapeutic targets for patients with HPB cancers.

PANCREATIC DUCTAL ADENOCARCINOMA
Overview of the Genomic Landscape and Molecular Subtypes

Over the last 10 years, important advances in large sequencing efforts have culminated in the report of a series of comprehensive integrated genomic analyses summarized in **Table 1**.[4–7] For several decades, it has been well established that pancreatic cancer was the product of the accumulation of successive genetic mutations. The progression from dysplasia to invasive carcinoma is paralleled by a series of genetic mutations that include the activation of the KRAS oncogene and the inactivation of the tumor suppressor genes, CDKN2A, TP53, and SMAD4.[4,8] These 4 genomic alterations were confirmed in the seminal report of genomic sequencing for pancreatic cancer by Jones and colleagues[4] in 2008, which sequenced a total of 114 metastatic pancreatic cancers. In addition, the sequencing revealed a diverse heterogeneity of genetic mutations. Given that most cellular pathways and processes involve multiple proteins that function in a concerted manner, the investigators identified 12 core signaling pathways which were altered in most pancreatic cancer specimens. Unfortunately, many of the pathways were not targetable, and interestingly, no tumors carried mutations in homologous recombination deficiency (HRD). However, this study laid the framework for future studies categorizing pancreatic cancer into subtypes and ignited the search for new therapeutic options for pancreatic cancer.

Subsequent large-scale transcriptomic analysis of pancreatic ductal adenocarcinoma (PDAC) has allowed several groups to describe transcriptomic subtypes in pancreatic cancer, with mostly consistent findings concerning 2 major lineages: a basallike subtype with aggressive tumor biology and worse prognosis and a more favorable differentiated classical subtype. The COMPASS trial was the first trial to utilize molecular profiling in patients with metastatic pancreatic cancer. The trial utilized a modified Moffitt classifier and observed a significantly worse overall survival (OS) in the basallike versus classical subtypes (5.9 vs 9.3 months, $P=.0001$).[9] Furthermore, the investigators identified a transcription factor, GATA6, as a potential biomarker of classical subtype with loss of GATA6 expression associated with basallike subtypes. Retrospective analysis of prospectively collected clinical trial specimens demonstrated

Table 1
Comparison of recent large-scale next-generation sequencing studies in pancreatic cancer

Study	Type of Tissue Utilized	Methodology	Classification
Jones et al,[4] 2008	114 pancreatic cancers—metastatic patients	Sequencing of protein coding exons with PCR	Identification of 12 core signaling pathways
Collison et al,[5] 2011	27 microdissected tumors from surgical specimens + human and murine pancreatic cancer cell lines	Gene expression microarrays	3 Subtypes identified: Classical: associated with adhesion and epithelial genes Quasi-mesenchymal: mesenchyme-associated genes Exocrinelike: associated with digestive enzyme genes
Moffitt et al,[6] 2015	357 primary and metastatic pancreatic cancers, normal tissue, pancreatic cancer cell lines.	Virtual microdissection with microarrays and RNA sequencing	2 Subtypes of tumors: Classical: high-adhesion associated, ribosomal, and epithelial gene expression, elevated GATA-6 Basallike: laminin and keratins 2 Subtypes of stroma: Normal: markers for pancreatic stellate cells Activated: genes associated with macrophages and tumor promotion.
Bailey et al,[7] 2016	456 primary resected pancreatic cancers	Integrated genomic analysis	4 subtypes: Squamous: enriched for integrin signaling and activated EGF signaling. Aberrantly differentiated endocrine-exocrine: Transcriptional networks in later stages of pancreatic development and differentiation. Genes associated with endocrine differentiation Pancreatic progenitor: Genes regulated pancreatic development, fatty acid oxidation, steroid hormone biosynthesis, pancreatitis, and regeneration. Immunogenic: immune infiltrate. B cell signaling pathways, antigen presentation, T cell and toll-like receptor signaling pathways.

Abbreviations: PCR, polymerase chain reaction; RNA, ribonucleic acid.

classical subtype tumors to have superior response to the multiagent regiment of fluo-rouracil, oxaliplatin, and irinotecan (FOLFIRINOX) as compared to basallike tumors.[10] This was further corroborated in organoid-derived signatures of chemotherapeutic response, with oxaliplatin-sensitive signatures being enriched in classical subtype tu-mors.[11] The predictive ability of ribonucleic acid subtypes is currently under investiga-tion in multiple clinical trials (NCT 04469556, NCT 04683315) in both patients with metastatic disease in the first-line setting and in patients with localized pancreatic can-cer in the neoadjuvant setting.

Targeted Approaches

The advantage of molecular subtyping is only realized if the information provided sub-stantially impacts the selection of treatments for the disease. Although the ability to characterize pancreatic cancers into molecular subtypes has evolved substantially over the past decade, its translation into clinical practice has been markedly slower. One of the first reported precision medicine trials for patients with pancreatic cancer was the IMPaCT trial.[12] This was a pilot study of 76 patients with metastatic or recur-rent pancreatic cancer who underwent targeted sequencing of BRCA1, BRCA2, PALB2, ATM, or KRAS genes as well as an assessment of HER2 amplification from formalin-fixed paraffin-embedded samples. Patients were then randomized to single-agent gemcitabine or target-specific therapy (deficient in the homologous re-combinant deoxyribonucleic acid [DNA] repair pathway received 5-fluorouracil and mitomycin C, HER2 amplification received gemcitabine and trastuzumab, KRAS wild-type received gemcitabine and erlotinib). A genomic target was identified in 22 (28%) patients (14 KRAS wild type, 5 HER2 amplification, 2 BRCA2, and 1 ATM). The median time from enrollment to relay of test results was 21.5 days, but no patient was suc-cessfully treated on trial. The investigators recognized that the rapid disease progres-sion made the return of genomic results in a meaningful timeframe challenging.

The Know Your Tumor Initiative was an observational study developed as a joint collaboration between PanCAN and Perthera with the goal of offering patients with pancreatic cancer multi-omic molecular profiling and was recently reported.[13] The study recruited patients from 44 states, including academic and community practices. Next-generation sequencing and immunohistochemical profiling was performed in commercial laboratories (Foundation Medicine, PGDx, Caris Life Sciences, or Neo-Geonomics). A virtual tumor board reviewed the molecular profile and a report with treatment options was created for the treating oncologists. In total, 640 tumor spec-imens were sent for next-generation sequencing and immunohistochemistry (IHC), 591 of which were pancreatic adenocarcinoma. After obtaining tissue from the local pathologist, the median time to report delivery was 30 days. Of 640 patients, 458 (72%) had metastatic disease, 137 (21%) had locally advanced disease, and 45 (7%) had resectable or borderline resectable disease. Of 640 patients, at least 1 mu-tation was identified in 616 samples (median 4 mutations per sample). The tumor board identified actionable genomic alterations in 50% of patients (with 27% highly actionable) and actionable proteomic alterations (excluding chemopredictive markers) in 5%. Highly actionable alterations were identified as those in the homolo-gous recombinant DNA repair pathway (15%), cell cycle genes (11%), and AKT/mTOR (19%) pathways. As a result of the molecular profiling, 156 (24%) of 640 patients were transitioned to a new treatment regimen, 173 (27%) remained on their treatment started prior to sequencing, 111 (17%) passed away prior to transitioning to a new treatment based on tumor sequencing, and 200 (31%) patients were lost to follow-up. A subset analysis of patients with highly actionable biomarkers who received profile-directed therapy (n = 17) demonstrated a significantly longer median progression-free survival (PFS) than those with unmatched therapy (n = 18) (Hazard ratio [HR]: 0.47, P=.003).

Kirsten Rat Sarcoma Virus (KRAS) Inhibitors

KRAS mutations occur in over 90% of pancreatic cancers, with single point mutations at codon G12 representing the vast majority of KRAS mutations, with the most common mutations being G12D, G12V, and G12R.[14] KRAS is a small GTPase that functions as a binary on-off molecular switch, cycling between an active guanosine triphosphate (GTP)–bound and inactive guanosine diphosphate (GDP)–bound state.[15] In normal cells, RAS is predominantly GDP bound and inactive. Cancer-associated RAS mutations result in a persistently GTP bound and constitutively active state and result in downstream activation of effector signaling pathways that drive cancer growth. In recent years, intrinsic biochemical and downstream biologic functions have been identified between different mutant alleles which have greatly informed the complexity of developing effective mutant-specific inhibitors and combination strategies. Currently there are 2 approaches to target RAS activation, either with direct inhibitors or by targeting downstream of RAS. Unfortunately, targeting downstream KRAS signaling has been unsuccessful to date.[16,17]

One of the most exciting developments in recent years is the ability to target KRAS mutations. KRAS G12C mutations occur in 1% to 3% of PDACs. Sotorasib is the first Food and Drug Administration (FDA)–approved KRAS inhibitor for patients with non–small-cell lung cancer harboring a KRAS G12C mutation. In a phase IB expansion cohort, 12 patients with PDAC were enrolled and the disease control rate was 75% with 1 patient achieving a partial response (PR). More recently, the KRYSTAL-1 trial updated the outcome of 12 patients with advanced pancreatic adenocarcinoma. PRs were seen in 50% of patients with evaluable disease and the disease control rate was 100% with median PFS of 6.6 months.[18] There is significant ongoing development of mutation-specific drugs for more common KRAS mutant alleles as well as pan-RAS inhibitors, many of which are currently being testing in clinical trials.

Wild-Type RAS

Up to 10% of PDACs occur in the absence of a KRAS mutation. In this small proportion of patients, there is an enrichment of kinase fusion genes, which occur in 20% to 30% of KRAS wildtype cases.[19] The fusion genes are mutually exclusive and occur most frequently in NRG1, ALK, NTRK, and ROS1. Successful therapeutic targeting of kinase fusion genes have been reported for PDAC. Zenocutuzumab, a bispecific antibody against HER2 and HER3 demonstrated a 42% response rate in 12 patients with advanced NRG1 fusion-positive PDAC.[20] Entrectinib, a pan-NTRK, ROS1, and ALK inhibitor demonstrated a 57% objective response rate (ORR) and median duration of response of 10 months in patients with NTRK fusion-positive tumors.[21] Approximately 25% of KRAS wild-type cases have downstream activation of the MAP kinase pathway, including B-type Raf oncogene (BRAF). Case series have indicated response to crizotinib in ALK fusion-positive tumors and the BRAF plus MEK/ERK inhibitors in BRAF-altered tumors.[22] The diversity of potential therapeutic targeted therapies emphasizes the importance of transcriptomic sequencing to identify potential actionable fusion proteins which may otherwise be missed with targeted genomic sequencing.

Targeting Homologous Recombination Deficiency

Over the last decade, the chemotherapeutic options for patients with PDAC have evolved from single-agent gemcitabine to multiagent regimens, such as FOLFIRINOX or gemcitabine/nab-paclitaxel, which have produced significant gains in OS.[23,24] In addition, with the multiagent regimens, exceptional responders have been reported, most notably among patients with genetic defects in the homologous recombination DNA repair pathway.[25] The molecular basis for these exceptional responders was uncovered when these patients received poly(adenosine diphosphate [ADP]-ribose) polymerase (PARP) inhibitor-based and/or platinum-based therapies. Platinum-based agents cause DNA cross-linking and induce DNA strand breaks which are unable to be repaired in cells with deficient DNA repair mechanisms, such as *BRCA1* and *BRCA2*. In addition to platinum-based therapy, tumors with deficient DNA repair mechanisms also have increased sensitivity to PARP inhibitors. PARP is involved in ribosylation of ADP necessary for DNA repair pathways and apoptosis. In a study by O'Reilly and colleagues, 9 patients with *BRCA* mutations received PARP inhibitor in combination with gemcitabine and cisplatin.[26] Five of 9 (55.6%) patients demonstrated a PR and the remaining 4 patients (44.4%) demonstrated stable disease. Olaparib was evaluated in a phase III trial which enrolled 154 patients with confirmed germline *BRCA1/2* mutation and advanced PDAC.[27] Patients had to have demonstrated disease control for at least 16 weeks with a platinum-based therapy prior. The study demonstrated an improvement in PFS (median 7.4 months vs 3.8 months; $P=.004$) but did not demonstrate an improvement in OS. In 2019, the FDA approved Olaparib as maintenance therapy for patients with germline *BRCA1/2* mutant advanced PDAC. This was the first approval of a molecularly targeted agent in a genetically selected population with PDAC. Currently, the only clinically validated HRD biomarkers in PDAC are *BRCA1/2* and *PALB2*.

The lack of an OS advantage in the POLO trial as well as prior unsuccessful trials utilizing PARP inhibitors in the first-line setting for patients with advanced PDAC suggests that additional challenges in identifying modifiers of the HRD phenotype which may be associated with therapeutic resistance.[28] Currently, somatic and germline mutational profiling of candidate HRD-associated genes includes next-generation sequencing techniques to identify mutational and transcriptomic signatures characteristic of HRD (including telomeric allelic imbalance, loss of heterozygosity, and large scale transitions). Computational scores have been developed to identify HRD in the absence of gene mutations but have yet to be prospectively validated.[29,30] A recent meta-analysis of documented HRD prevalence suggests that up to 16.5% of PDACs may have an HRD phenotype, suggesting that this may be another important underappreciated therapeutic target.[31]

On the Horizon

An abundance of tumor stroma is a defining characteristic of PDACs and a potential therapeutic target, as the dense extracellular compartment has been shown to create a uniquely hypoxic and immunodeficient microenvironment. Prior attempts to target the tumor stroma have been unsuccessful, such as treatment with hyaluronidase, focal adhesion kinase inhibitors, and hedgehog inhibitors.[32–34] Molecular profiling has often utilized microdissection of the epithelial compartment, and identifying molecular targets in the stroma compartment has lagged behind. Transcriptomic data have identified 2 distinct stromal-specific gene expression signatures: normal, dominated by pancreatic stellate cells, and activated stroma, which is characterized by inflammatory signatures. Future characterization of PDAC may need to include considerations for stroma profiling, and improved understanding of the interaction between tumor cells and the stromal components is urgently needed to understand if the stromal subtypes demonstrate cellular plasticity and can evolve in response to therapeutic pressures.

The challenge for precision medicine for pancreatic cancer will continue to be limitations regarding tissue acquisition, not only in addressing the low cellularity of tumor epithelium in biopsy samples but also in tissue acquisition, especially in patients with localized disease. In this regard, characterization of somatic alterations using liquid biopsy would be a significant advancement. Novel blood-based biomarkers, including cell-free DNA, circulating tumor cells, and tumor-derived exosomes, that allow for somatic tumor profiling and quantification would be revolutionary diagnostic adjuncts for this disease.

HEPATOCELLULAR CARCINOMA
Background

Hepatocellular carcinoma (HCC) is the most common liver cancer globally with a rising incidence due in part to aging populations and nonalcoholic steatohepatitis (NASH) associated with obesity and metabolic syndrome.[35–37] Associated with hepatitis B (HBV) and C (HCV) viruses, the increase in sustained virological response to antiviral drugs has decreased the risk for HCC attributable to HCV.[38] Chronic liver disease is the most common cause of HCC, including factors that lead to chronic liver inflammation or scarring, such as cirrhosis. Most patients with HCC are diagnosed at advanced stages of disease or may have poor liver function, which limits treatment opportunities. The foundation of treatment for HCC remains hepatectomy or liver transplantation, and continued improvements in patient selection, surgical technique, and perioperative management have led to significant improvements in outcomes for patients with disease amenable to surgery.[39,40] However, there has been recent advancements in systemic therapies, particularly with immunotherapy and targeted therapies, which have had significant impact on treatment opportunities for patients with both resectable or unresectable HCC. Overall, many of these systemic therapy options are relegated to more advanced stages of the disease not commonly treated by surgeons. However, a fundamental knowledge of the molecular underpinnings of HCC is important as novel therapies and trials emerge in the perioperative setting.

Molecular Pathogenesis and Key Signaling Pathways

The development of HCC is complex and heterogeneous owing to the multiple underlying risk factors that may lead to the disease. The majority of patients with HCC (70%–80%) have underlying cirrhosis commonly associated with alcohol or HCV infection, and the development of HCC in this setting may follow a more classical pathway from dysplastic or regenerative nodule to carcinoma sequence.[41,42] However, HCC may develop in the absence of overt cirrhosis in patients with HBV or NASH, which is increasingly associated with the development of HCC at an alarming rate. The foundation of HCC, regardless of etiology, is a background inflammation that promotes the malignant transformation of mature hepatocytes or liver stem cells with the sequential accumulation of detrimental somatic mutations over time being critical to the development of the disease.

Genomic analysis is critical to understand the underlying biology and prognosis for patients with HCC and hopefully identify actionable targets that may improve patient outcomes. Exome sequencing of tumors have identified genomic alterations associated with HCC and on average 40 to 70 somatic mutations can be found in coding regions of the genome.[42,43] However, few of these mutations are driver mutations and even fewer are "actionable." Genes commonly altered have been identified across cell signaling pathways involved in growth and differentiation (ie, receptor tyrosine kinase, MAPK pathways), Wnt-β-catenin signaling, telomere maintenance, cell cycle, chromatin modification, and oxidative stress.[44] The most commonly identified mutations occur in telomerase reverse transcriptase (*TERT*) (54%), *CTNNB1* (29%), *TP53* (28%), and *ARID1A* (8%).[44] Mutations in *TERT* impact the promoter region of this gene and activate this regulator of telomere length, and 20% of dysplastic nodules harbor this mutation.[43,45] Unfortunately, most of these mutations are not actionable currently with the minority of tumors having mutations that have targeted agents.

Molecular Subtypes

HCC is seemingly a heterogeneous disease, developing in both damaged and at times, undamaged liver. A significant effort has been made to understand the molecular underpinnings of this tumor diversity via deep genomic sequencing and epigenomic profiling across tumors arising from various liver backgrounds and global regions. The ability to combine datasets from prior gene expression studies have allowed the investigation into shared patterns of expression between tumors. This has led to the description of molecular HCC subtypes, which offer insight into patient prognostication and potential treatment strategies.

As work continues, the complexity of molecular classifications increases for HCC and there are seemingly multiple proposed classification schemes. However, these classifications have yet to be fully integrated into clinical decision-making. In a study from investigators from the National Cancer Institute (NCI), Lee and colleagues described 2 major molecular subtypes of HCC associated with survival using gene expression profiling from 91 tumors from patients with predominantly HBV-associated HCC.[46] They described 2 subtypes of HCC based upon signatures associated with survival termed the NCI proliferation (NCIP) signature: HCC cluster A (poor-prognosis) and HCC cluster B (good prognosis). Characterization of gene expression patterns revealed that tumors within the poor-prognosis cluster A had higher expression of genes involved in cell growth and maintenance, anti-apoptosis, ubiquitination, and histone modification.[46] Specifically, the authors found increased expression of *HIF1a* in cluster A with concomitant downregulation of genes involved in regulation of *HIF1a* indicating this hypoxia-related gene's impact on survival of patients with HCC. Kim and colleagues[47] further evaluated the NCIP signature to develop a recurrence risk score (from 0–100) associated with recurrence-free survival (RFS) and OS. Interestingly, mutations in β-catenin were associated with lower risk scores whereas AKT and IGF1R were associated with higher risk scores.

Hoshida and colleagues[48] analyzed gene expression data from 603 patients with HCC across 8 previously published studies and described 3 distinct cohorts (S1, S2, and S3) associated with common clinical factors. Further dissection of these signatures revealed individual genes commonly altered within each group, such as activation of WNT pathway signaling in the S1 subclass, MYC and AKT activation in the S2 subclass, and increased cell growth and proliferation pathways in the S3 subclass. The more aggressive subclasses (S1 and S2) were associated with larger tumor size and worse differentiation, whereas the less aggressive subclass (S3) was more differentiated and had more retained overall liver function, likely related to increased expression of *CTNNB1*. Interestingly, S1 tumors were found to have increased vascular invasion and satellite tumors, which is likely the basis for this subclass's increased association with early recurrence.[48] Other large-scale gene expression analyses have validated these subclasses or suggested otherwise similar cohorts of tumors associated with patient outcomes and offer potential for future personalized medicine for patients with HCC.[49]

Currently Approved Targeted Therapies for Hepatocellular Carcinoma

Systemic therapy had historically had little benefit for patients diagnosed with advanced HCC, including negative results in trials of PIAF (cisplatin, interferon α2β, doxorubicin, and fluorouracil) and FOLFOX4 (fluorouracil, leucovorin, and oxaliplatin).[50,51] In 2007, sorafenib was found to have a significant survival benefit in 2 clinical trials for patients with advanced HCC, and this remained the only effective systemic therapy for some time.[52,53] However, recent major advancements of new systemic therapies have changed the landscape for patients with HCC in both the first and second line.

Lenvatinib, which is an oral inhibitor of VEGFR, FGFR1-4, RET, KIT, and PDGFRα, was shown to be noninferior to sorafenib for OS in a phase III trial (median 13.6 vs 12.3 months).[54] This resulted in lenvatinib being an alternative first-line treatment for patients with advanced HCC, except patients with main portal vein or greater than 50% liver involvement. In the landmark IMbrave150 trial, patients with advanced HCC received either sorafenib or the combination of atezolizumab [programmed death ligand 1 (PD-L1) inhibitor] with bevacizumab (vascular endothelial growth factor [VEGF] inhibitor).[55] The combination of atezolizumab and bevacizumab resulted in a 12-month OS of 67% compared to 55% for sorafenib, which lead to this regimen becoming standard of care first-line treatment for patients with advanced, unresectable HCC.[55] Later, improved survival was found with single-dose tremelimumab and regular interval durvalumab compared to single-agent durvalumab versus sorafenib in the HIMALAYA trial.[56]

Patients who undergo resection are at high risk for recurrence; however, no adjuvant therapy has shown an improvement in survival and there is no approved therapy in this setting yet. Sorafenib failed to improve RFS compared to placebo in the adjuvant setting.[57] With the improved survival found in the metastatic setting, combination atezolizumab with bevacizumab has been under investigation in the adjuvant setting following surgical resection or ablation for patients at high risk for recurrence in the IMbrave050 trial.[58] After interim analysis, the combination of atezolizumab and bevacizumab increased RFS by 28% compared to active surveillance.[59] These results make IMbrave050 the first phase III trial to show positive results in the adjuvant setting for HCC.

On the Horizon

Multiple clinical trials are ongoing in the adjuvant setting for patients who have undergone resection or ablation of HCC. The CheckMate-9DX trial (NCT03383458) is a phase III randomized placebo-controlled trial comparing adjuvant nivolumab to placebo with a primary endpoint of RFS.[60] Similarly, KEYNOTE-937 (NCT03867084) is a randomized, double-blind, phase III trial of pembrolizumab versus placebo in for patients with complete radiographic response after resection or ablation with co-primary endpoints of RFS and OS.[61] Further, EMERALD-2 (NCT03847428), comparing durvalumab ± bevacizumab versus placebo following resection or ablation, is also ongoing with a primary endpoint of RFS.[62] These trials may validate the role of both immunotherapy and anti-VEGF targeted therapy in the adjuvant setting for patients who undergo hepatectomy.

As the number of potentially efficacious therapies continues to increase for patients with HCC, there has been increasing interest in the use of these treatments in the neoadjuvant setting. Indeed, a small study of neoadjuvant nivolumab with the tyrosine kinase inhibitor cabozantinib given to 15 patients with high-risk HCC resulted in resection for 12 patients with 5 patients achieving major pathologic response.[63] In a trial of 21 patients with upfront resectable HCC, perioperative cemiplimab (2 cycles preoperatively, up to 8 additional cycles postoperatively) was tolerable with 20 patients undergoing resection with 4 patients achieving significant tumor necrosis, 3 of whom had a pathologic complete response (CR).[64] In a further trial of perioperative immunotherapy, 27 patients with resectable HCC from a single institution were randomized to receive either preoperative nivolumab followed by postoperative treatment for 2 years versus nivolumab plus ipilimumab preoperatively followed by the this regimen postoperatively with a primary endpoint of safety and tolerability.[65] Grade 3 to 4 adverse events were higher with the combination therapy; however, the authors found that both regimens were safe with no patients having their operations delayed due to adverse effects. Median PFS was 9.4 months with nivolumab and 19.53 months with nivolumab plus ipilimumab, supporting the use of perioperative immunotherapy for patients with resectable HCC.[65] Lastly, a phase II study of the neoadjuvant combination of atezolizumab with bevacizumab is ongoing for patients with resectable HCC with primary endpoints of safety and feasibility, as well as rates of pathologic CR (NCT04721132). Studies such as these will further inform the use of immunotherapy in the preoperative or perioperative period for patients with resectable HCC.

BILIARY TRACT CANCERS
Background

Biliary tract cancers (BTCs), comprised of both intrahepatic cholangiocarcinoma (iCCA) and extrahepatic CCA (eCCA) and gallbladder cancer (GBC), are epithelial cancers defined by their anatomic position within the biliary system. eCCA can be further subdivided into perihilar CCA (pCCA) and distal CCA (dCCA). Survival for all comers is overall quite depressing, with median survival of 6 months for iCCA and 9 months for eCCA.[66] Because of often being diagnosed at early stages and even incidentally, GBC has an improved survival, however, not significantly different from CCA at later stages. These cancers are often grouped together, particularly in large clinical trials, yet they have distinct biology that underpins individualized treatment strategies. Options for treatment for patients with BTCs are evolving rapidly, particularly for patients with actionable mutations (**Table 2**).

Table 2
Actionable mutations with available personalized therapies for patients with biliary tract cancers

Actionable Mutation	Available Drugs	Trial	Results
FGFR2	Pemigatinib[88]	FIGHT-202 (NCT03656536)	ORR 35.5%, mPFS 6.9 mo
	Futibatinib[89]	FOENIX-CCA2 (NCT02052778)	ORR 41.7%, mPFS 9 mo
	Derazantinib[91]	FIDES-01 (NCT03230318)	*Ongoing*
IDH1	Ivosidenib[97]	ClarIDHy (NCT02989857)	mPFS 2.7 mo
HER2	Trastuzumab + Pertuzumab[99]	MyPathway (NCT02091141)	ORR 23.1%, mPFS 4.0 mo
	Trastuzumab deruxtecan[102]	DESTINY PanTumor02 (NCT02564900)	ORR 22% Overall 56.3% in HER2 IHC 3+
		HERB Trial (JMA-IIA00423)	ORR 36.4%
NTRK	Larotrectinib[106]	LOXO-TRK-14001 (NCT02122913) SCOUT (NCT02637687) NAVIGATE (NCT02576431)	ORR 69%, mPFS 29.4%
	Entrectinib[21]	ALKA-372–0001 STARTRK-1 (NCT02097810) STARTRK-2 (NCT02568267)	ORR 61.3%, mPFS 13.8 mo
BRAF/MEK	Dabrafenib + Trametinib	ROAR Trial[108]	ORR 51%, mPFS 9 mo

Abbreviations: mPFS, median progression-free survival; ORR, objective response rate.

Molecular Pathogenesis

The development of CCA is commonly associated with mutations that may be associated with anatomic location of the disease. Mutations that are commonly found in other solid organ cancers, particularly mutations in KRAS and TP53, result in continued progression to carcinoma within an inflammatory environment. Further, large duct iCCA has been shown to have mutations in KRAS and TP53, whereas small duct iCCA is commonly found to have mutations in isocitrate dehydrogenase (IDH) 1/2 and fusions in fibroblast growth factor 2 (FGFR2).[67–69] eCCA and GBC are much less likely to harbor targetable alterations, such as IDH1/2 mutations or FGFR2 fusions, and commonly harbor deleterious mutations in KRAS and TP53.[70,71] Mutations in BRAF are rare across BTCs, as are mismatch repair deficient (dMMR)/microsatellite instability high (MSI-H) tumors, but both represent important therapeutic targets.[71]

Molecular Subtypes

There have been tremendous advancements in recent years in genomic and molecular profiling for patients with CCA that have led to more precise prognostication and individualized, targeted treatment strategies. Interestingly, deep sequencing studies have revealed that different anatomic locations of CCA have variation in mutational profiles, and characterization of these profiles are beginning to reveal classifications of tumors that are associated with response to therapy and prognosis. For example, after transcriptomic profiling of 104 resected CCA specimens from western countries, Andersen and colleagues[72] were able to classify patients into 2 subclasses associated 5-year OS, time to recurrence and the presence of mutations in KRAS. From there, these clusters were able to be subdivided into 4 survival subgroups based upon survival within each prognostic cluster, and expression analysis was able to identify genes that distinguished individual subgroups from each other and associated with prognosis.[72] Further, a 238-gene classifier distinguished the 2 prognostic subclasses and further network analysis of the classifier genes that distinguished these 2 subclasses were enriched in VEGF/ERBB, CTNNB1/MYC, and TNF pathways.[72] In a subsequent investigation, Sia and colleagues[73] performed integrative analyses on iCCA tumors from 149 patients and identified an inflammation class (38% of tumors) and proliferation class (62% of tumors) associated with outcomes. The proliferation class had worse survival outcomes and was characterized by expression signatures commonly associated with poor outcomes in other cancers, such as activation of oncogenic MAPK and MET pathways, specific DNA amplifications, and mutations in KRAS or BRAF.[73] The inflammatory class was marked by activation of inflammatory signaling pathways and cytokines, as well as increased activation of STAT3.[73] Further, these authors also identified a gene expression signature that was associated with worse survival outcomes and this signature was associated with the proliferation class of iCCA.[73] In a further integrative analysis of 38 liver fluke-negative CCAs, Farshidfar and colleagues[74] were able to stratify tumors into 2 distinct groups, one of which is enriched with IDH1 mutations. This IDH1-mutation–enriched subtype had decreased chromatin modifier gene expression, which may be a result of epigenetic silencing of ARID1A expression.[74] Integrative analyses that reveal molecular classifications such as these may allow for individualized treatment strategies for patients with CCA.

Current Broad Systemic Therapy Options

A broad treatment algorithm for patients with BTC is illustrated in **Fig. 1**. For patients with resectable BTC, complete surgical resection is the only chance for cure. However, recurrence risk is high for patients with resected BTC, which may be as high as

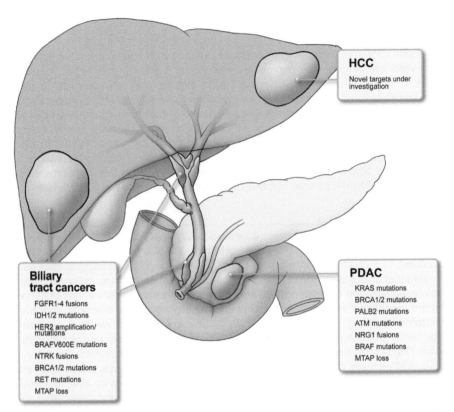

Fig. 1. Management of biliary tract cancers. GemCis, gemcitabine plus cisplatin. (Copyright used with the permission of The Board of Regents of the University of Texas System through The University of Texas MD Anderson Cancer Center.)

80% at 2 years postoperatively.[75–77] Therefore, adjuvant systemic therapy is reasonable for patients with BTC and is currently the standard of care. However, for patients with unresectable or metastatic BTC, gemcitabine with cisplatin (Gem + Cis) is the standard of care following the ABC-02 trial. In the ABC-02 trial, Gem + Cis resulted in a 3.6 month improvement in median OS compared to gemcitabine alone (11.7 months vs 8.1 months, $P<.001$).[78] Building on this backbone, the addition of nab-paclitaxel (Abraxane) to Gem + Cis resulted in a median PFS of 11.8 months and median OS of 19.2 months in a phase II trial; however, it failed to demonstrate a statistically significant improvement in median OS in a recently completed phase III study.[79] Recently, the TOPAZ-1 trial revealed that Gem + Cis with the addition of durvalumab resulted in a 1.3 month increase in median OS compared to Gem + Cis plus placebo (12.8 vs 11.5 months, $P = .02$).[80] These trials serve as the foundation for adjuvant therapy trials as well as emerging neoadjuvant regimens.

Multiple trials have failed to demonstrate survival advantage for systemic therapy following resection of BTC. For example, PRODIGE-12/ACCORD-18 failed to show a significant improvement in relapse-free or OS for gemcitabine plus oxaliplatin compared to surveillance following resection of BTC.[81] The Bile Duct Cancer Adjuvant Trial (BCAT) was a phase III trial that compared gemcitabine to surveillance following complete resection of eCCA and did not find a difference in relapse-free or OS.[82] However, the multicenter phase III BILCAP trial included patients with all

BTCs who underwent curative-intent resection and randomized to 8 cycles of post-operative capecitabine versus surveillance.[83] After initially failing to meet the trials primary endpoint of OS in an intention-to-treat analysis, there was a significant OS benefit when analyzed per-protocol (53 vs 36 months, adjusted HR 0.75, 95% CI 0.58–0.97, P = .028).[83] This has led to adjuvant capecitabine being standard-of-care treatment for patients undergoing curative-intent resection of BTC.

Following the encouraging results of the addition of nab-paclitaxel to GemCis with improved survival outcomes in phase II studies for patients with advanced BTC, there was support for the addition of this regimen in the preoperative setting for patients with resectable iCCA with high-risk features. In the multi-institutional phase II NEO-GAP study, patients with resectable iCCA with tumors greater than 5 cm, multiple tumors, major vascular invasion, or positive lymph nodes received 4 cycles of preoperative GemCis + nab-paclitaxel with a primary endpoint of completion of preoperative therapy and complete resection.[84] Among 30 total patients enrolled, 73% completed all chemotherapy and resection with a disease control rate of 90%, RFS of 7.1 months, and a median OS of 24 months.[84] This study supports the feasibility of a neoadjuvant approach for these patients along with the safety of GemCis + nab-paclitaxel in the preoperative setting.

Targeted and Tumor-Specific Treatment Options

Fibroblast growth factor receptor mutations
Approximately 15% to 20% of patients with iCCA harbor an alteration in fibroblast growth factor receptor (FGFR) pathway.[85,86] The FGFR is a transmembrane tyrosine kinase receptor family with signaling that leads to downstream activation of the oncogenic MAPK, JAK-STAT, and PI3K-AKT-mTOR pathways.[87] The family has 4 subtypes (1, 2, 3, and 4) and majority of alterations are fusions of *FGFR2* in BTCs, particularly iCCA.

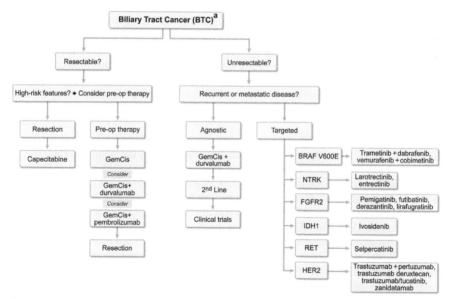

Fig. 2. Actionable mutations for hepatopancreatobiliary cancers by anatomic location. HCC, hepatocellular carcinoma; PDAC, pancreatic ductal adenocarcinoma. [a]Recommend tumor mutations profiling at time of diagnosis. (Copyright used with the permission of The Board of Regents of the University of Texas System through The University of Texas MD Anderson Cancer Center.)

Currently, patients with unresectable or metastatic BTC with *FGFR2* fusions or rearrangements are candidates for multiple targeted oral agents, such as pemigatinib, infigratinib, and futibatinib (**Fig. 2**). Pemigatinib is a selective inhibitor of FGFR1-3 that is FDA approved for patients with unresectable locally advanced or metastatic CCA with *FGFR2* fusions on rearrangements. In a phase II trial, 146 patients with advanced or metastatic CCA progressing on at least 1 previous treatment received pemigatinib, which resulted in an objective response rate of 35.5% (of which 3 were CRs) for patients harboring *FGFR2* fusions.[88] Next, the irreversible FGFR1-4 inhibitor futibatinib resulted in an ORR of 41.7% and a median PFS of 9 months in the phase II FOENIX-CCA2 trial, leading to FDA approval of futibatinib for patients with previously treated, unresectable locally advanced or metastatic iCCA with *FGFR2* fusions/rearrangements.[89] The oral FGFR 1, 2, and 3 inhibitor infigratinib, which resulted in a 23.1% ORR in a phase II trial of patients with previously treated metastatic CCA, had also been granted accelerated approved, but its development has now been stopped and distribution halted permanently in the United States.[90] Further, the anti-FGFR1-3 inhibitor derazantinib has shown promising results on interim analysis of the ongoing phase II FIDES-01 study.[91] Interestingly, acquired resistance to these FGFR inhibitors is common and via secondary mutations in the FGFR2 kinase domain, and futibatinib may have efficacy for patients who progress on the reversible FGFR inhibitors (pemigatinib, infigratinib).[92,93] Additional and novel agents, as well as agents that overcome common resistance mechanisms, are an active area of research for patients with FGFR2-altered CCA.[94]

Isocitrate dehydrogenase 1 mutations

Mutations in IDH1 are found in 13% to 20% of iCCA and less than 1% of pCCA or dCCA and result in the accumulation of 2-hydroxyglutarate, which results in uncontrolled cellular growth and differentiation.[71,95,96] In a phase III trial, the small molecule inhibitor of mutated *IDH1*, ivosidenib, improved PFS from a median of 1.4 months to 2.7 months, compared to placebo.[97] OS was not significantly improved by ivosidenib in the trial, yet this result is difficult to interpret because 70% of patients who progressed on placebo were able to cross over to receive ivosidenib. Ivosidenib was approved by the FDA in 2021 for the treatment of CCA that has failed prior chemotherapy following these results. Many other IDH1 inhibitors are currently being studied in trials, as well as PARP inhibitors due to IDH1's role in DNA damage repair.

HER2 (ErbB2) alterations

Alterations in HER2 have been identified and exploited in many cancers, including BTCs. Alterations in HER2 occur in 5% to 19% of BTC, most commonly in eCCA (17%) and GBC (19%), and less frequently in iCCA (5%). A phase II study of folinic acid, 5-fluorouracil, and oxaliplatin (FOLFOX) plus trastuzumab for previously treated HER2-positive BTCs resulted in a median PFS of 5.1 months and OS of 10.7 months.[98] Trastuzumab plus pertuzumab, both anti-HER2 antibodies, have been incorporated into National Cancer Center Network guidelines for previously treated BTC that are HER2 positive since the phase II MyPathway basket study.[99] In this study, this combination resulted in an ORR of 23% and a median PFS of 4 months. In the phase I trial expansion, HER2 bispecific antibody zanidatamab demonstrated a 38% ORR in HER2-positive BTC.[100] In the pivotal HERIZON-BTC-01 trial, zanidatamab demonstrated confirmed objective responses in 41·3% of patients with BTC with HER2 IHC 3+ or 2+ cancer.[101] In the phase II DESTINY PanTumor02 study, HER2 antibody drug conjugate trastuzumab deruxtecan demonstrated an ORR of 22% in patients with BTC enrolled with HER2 3+ or 2+ disease, and an ORR of 56.3% in patients with centrally confirmed HER2 3+ BTC.[102]

Similarly, an ORR of 36% with trastuzumab deruxtecan was seen in the phase II HERB trial that included 32 patients with HER2-expressing BTCs.[103] Therefore, multiple trials have not demonstrated that HER2 is an actionable alteration in HER2-expressing BTC.

Neurotrophic tropomyosin receptor kinase fusions

Neurotrophic tropomyosin receptor kinase (NTRK1, 2, and 3) are genes for receptor tyrosine kinases (TRKA, TRKB, TRKC) that are involved in neuronal differentiation and development and activation of these receptors results in signaling cascades that result in growth and survival pathways.[104] Although actionable, mutations in these oncogenes occur in 0.20% to 0.25% of BTCs.[104,105] The TRK inhibitors entrectenib and larotrectinib are approved in the first-line and following progression for tumors with *NTRK* gene fusions.[21,106]

B-type Raf oncogene V600 E mutations

The *BRAF* is a member of the mitogen-activated protein kinase (MAPK) pathway, which when constitutively activated results in uncontrolled cellular survival, growth, and differentiation via ERK signaling. Mutations in *BRAF* are found in up to 5% of BTCs, particularly iCCA, and mainly *V600 E* point mutations.[95,107] Dual inhibition of the MAPK pathway with the BRAF inhibitor dabrafenib in combination with the MEK inhibitor trametinib resulted in an ORR of 47% and median PFS of 9 months in the phase II ROAR trial, which included 43 patients with advanced or metastatic *BRAFV600E*-mutated BTC.[108] Dabrafenib in combination with trametinib has been FDA approved for patients with BRAF V600E-mutant tumors in a tumor agnostic fashion. The combination of BRAF inhibitor vemurafenib and MEK inhibitor cobimetinib has also shown tumor agnostic activity, with an objective response rate of 57% in the TAPUR study, with responses seen in multiple tumor types including CCA; this regimen is being explored in additional tumor agnostic studies.[109]

Genomic testing and circulating tumor deoxyribonucleic acid testing

Given the number of established targets for genomically informed therapy for BTCs, genomic testing is recommended for treatment planning for patients with advanced BTC. Notably although tissue-based genomic testing is preferred for initial profiling, available tissue may be insufficient and tumors may not be safely accessible for biopsy. Therefore, liquid biopsies with circulating tumor DNA (ctDNA) sequencing is emerging as an alternate option, with over 70% concordance with sequencing results of ctDNA and metastatic tumor biopsies.[110,111] There is also growing interest in liquid biopsies to assess early molecular response and minimal residual disease. Notably, longitudinal liquid biopsies have already been shown to be an important tool to discover mechanisms of acquired resistance to targeted therapy, such as *FGFR2* mutations and MAPK pathway mutations in patients with CCA with *FGFR* fusions being treated with FGFR inhibitors.[112]

Impact of Precision Oncology on Patient Outcomes in Biliary Tract Cancers

The impact of molecularly matched therapy in BTC was assessed by Okamura and colleagues[110] in the PREDICT study. Among the 121 patients with BTC, 80 patients had systemic therapies initiated after the molecular profiling in locally advanced or metastatic disease setting, and 34 (43%) of 80 were administered at least 1 drug matched to their profiling results. RECIST evaluation was available in 76 (95%) of the 80 treated patients, and the PR rate was significantly higher in patients that received a molecularly matched regimen versus those that received an unmatched regimen (24% vs 4.7%, *P*=.02). Further, Kaplan-Meier analysis demonstrated that the matched regimen had a significantly longer PFS than the unmatched regimen (median PFS, 4.3 vs 3.0 months, P=.04). Importantly, receiving a matched regimen remained significantly associated with better PFS even upon multivariate analysis.

Immunotherapy

The indications for immunotherapy for patients with BTC have been extensively explored in recent times. Indeed, immunotherapy may be offered to patients based on specific tumor deficiency in mismatch repair (dMMR), MSI-H, or high tumor mutational burden (TMB) or in a nonspecific indication for advanced disease. For example, patients with MSI-H tumors are candidates to receive pembrolizumab, an antibody against PD-1, as treatment with pembrolizumab resulted in a 53% ORR in a study of 86 patients with dMRR or MSI-H solid tumors.[113] Impressively, 21% of patients in the study had a CR.[113] Further, KEYNOTE-158 was a phase II trial with multiple cohorts of solid tumors that received pembrolizumab and this resulted in a 30.8% ORR across many different MSI-H/dMMR tumor types with durable responses to a median of 47.5 months.[114] Specifically, 22 patients with CCA were included in cohort K had an ORR of 40.8%, median PFS of 4.2 months, and median OS of 19.4 months.[114] Pembrolizumab is also an option for patients with high TMB.[115] Indeed, the immune checkpoint inhibitor (ICI) pembrolizumab is approved for MSI-H/dMMR or high TMB tumors; however, less than 5% of CCAs are found to be candidates.[94] In a separate cohort of KEYNOTE-158, pembrolizumab monotherapy had much more meager response with ORR of only 5.8% and median PFS of only 2 months.[116] Responses in the phase II KEYNOTE-158 and phase 1b KEYNOTE-028 revealed that PD-L1 expression did not necessarily improve responses.[116]

Since these studies, interest has increased for the addition of ICI with cytotoxic chemotherapy. For example, a phase II study from Korea randomized patients with treatment-naïve, advanced BTC to standard first-line GemCis plus durvalumab (PD-L1 inhibitor) with or without tremelimumab (CTLA-4 inhibitor) and found a 72% ORR for patients who received GemCis plus durvalumab.[117] Interestingly, the ORR was similar for patients who received tremelimumab (ORR 70%).[117] This served as the impetus for the phase III TOPAZ-1 trial, where patients with treatment naïve unresectable or metastatic BTC or recurrent BTC were randomized to receive durvalumab or placebo in combination with GemCis for up to 8 cycles, followed by durvalumab or placebo monotherapy.[118] In TOPAZ-1, the addition of durvalumab to GemCis improved OS compared to GemCis alone with a median OS of 12.8 months versus 11.5 months and 24.9% 2-year OS for patients receiving triplet therapy compared to 10.4% for GemCis alone.[118] In the recently published KEYNOTE-966 trial, 1069 patients with previously untreated, unresectable or metastatic BTC were randomized to receive either GemCis plus pembrolizumab or GemCis plus placebo.[119] In this study, the found statistically significant difference in median OS for patients who received GemCis plus pembrolizumab was 12.7 months compared to 10.9 months in the GemCis alone group, resulting in yet another option for patients with advanced BTC.[119] Among the 40 patients with matched ctDNA and tissue-DNA sequencing, concordance was high between the ctDNA and metastatic tumor profiling (78%). Among 80 patients who received molecularly matched therapies based on genomic profiling, significantly longer PFS was observed. (HR: 0.6, [0.37–0.99]).

On the horizon

Over the next few years, we expect a large amount of research in biomarker-driven therapy in BTC. There are several emerging targets including *KRAS* mutations,

MTAP loss, *MDM2* amplification, and DNA damage repair alterations. In addition, cell surface biomarkers present additional opportunities for antibodies, antibody drug conjugates, T cell engagers, CAR-T, and CAR-NK strategies.

For patients with surgically resectable BTC, the application of regimens with activity in the metastatic or advanced disease space may be applicable as a neoadjuvant treatment paradigm. Indeed, this approach is attractive as rates of disease recurrence are high following resection of BTC with curative-intent. Furthermore, there may be rationale for preoperative immunotherapy over adjuvant therapy due to neoantigen presence, the robustness of the immune response in the preoperative setting rather than postoperative immunosuppression due to surgical stress, and an intact local immune-tumor environment. Therefore, multiple trials of neoadjuvant and perioperative therapy including immunotherapy are ongoing or planned (NCT04308174; NCT05967182; NCT04989218). Currently, it remains unclear which patients benefit from neoadjuvant therapy and which patients benefit from immunotherapy/chemotherapy combinations; thus, neoadjuvant trials are likely to give unique insights. Further, perioperative targeted therapy trials are in planning.

SUMMARY

In summary, there are well-established targets for BTC, with exciting new targets emerging in PDAC and potential targets in HCC. Taken together, these data suggest an important role for molecular profiling for personalizing cancer therapy in advanced disease and the need for design of novel neoadjuvant studies to leverage these novel therapeutics perioperatively in the surgical patient.

CLINICS CARE POINTS

- Currently several genomic alterations are proven therapeutic targets in advanced disease including *FGFR2* fusions, *IDH* mutations, and BRAF V600 E mutations and *HER2* in BTC demonstrating the importance of genomic profiling including assessment of mutations, copy number changes, and fusions.

- Transcriptional profiling may identify therapeutic targets such as fusions as well as provide important insights such as assessing prognostic subtypes in PDAC; however, further work is needed for use of therapeutic subtypes in clinical decision-making.

- Immunotherapy has emerged as an important therapeutic modality for the treatment of HCC and BTC and is being further studied in the neoadjuvant setting.

- Further work is needed to determine how to transition these therapeutic targets into the management of operable disease.

ACKNOWLEDGMENTS

Special thanks to Jordan Pietz, MA, CMI from the MD Anderson Biomedical Visualization team for his assistance in creating the visual artwork.

DISCLOSURE

T.E. Newhook and S. Tsai report no disclosures. F. Meric-Bernstam reports Consulting fees from AbbVie, Aduro BioTech Inc., Alkermes, AstraZeneca, Daiichi Sankyo Co. Ltd., Calibr (a division of Scripps Research), DebioPharm, Ecor1 Capital, eFFECTOR Therapeutics, F. Hoffman-La Roche Ltd., GT Apeiron, Genentech Inc., Harbinger Health, IBM

Watson, Incyte, Infinity Pharmaceuticals, Jackson Laboratory, Kolon Life Science, LegoChem Bio, Lengo Therapeutics, Menarini Group, OrigiMed, PACT Pharma, Parexel International, Pfizer Inc., Protai Bio Ltd, Samsung Bioepis, Seattle Genetics Inc., Tallac Therapeutics, Tyra Biosciences, Xencor, Zymeworks; serves on Advisory Committees for Black Diamond, Biovica, Eisai, FogPharma, Immunomedics, Inflection Biosciences, Karyopharm Therapeutics, Loxo Oncology, Mersana Therapeutics, OnCusp Therapeutics, Puma Biotechnology Inc., Seattle Genetics, Sanofi, Silverback Therapeutics, Spectrum Pharmaceuticals, Theratechnologies, Zentalis; receives Sponsored Research (to her institution) from Aileron Therapeutics, United States. AstraZeneca, United Kingdom, Bayer Healthcare Pharmaceutical, Calithera Biosciences, United States, Curis Inc., CytomX Therapeutics Inc., Daiichi-Sankyo, Japan, Debiopharm International, eFFECTOR Therapeutics, United States, Genentech, United States, Guardant Health Inc., Klus Pharma, Takeda Pharmaceutical, Novartis, Switzerland, Puma Biotechnology, United States, Taiho Pharmaceutical Co., Japan; has received Honoraria from Dava Oncology, and nonfinancial support and reasonable reimbursement for travel from European Organisation for Research and Treatment of Cancer (EORTC), Belgium, European Society for Medical Oncology (ESMO), Switzerland, Cholangiocarcinoma Foundation, United States, Dava Oncology.

REFERENCES

1. Marcus L, Lemery SJ, Keegan P, et al. FDA Approval Summary: Pembrolizumab for the Treatment of Microsatellite Instability-High Solid Tumors. Clin Cancer Res 2019;25(13):3753–8.
2. Balachandran VP, DeMatteo RP. Gastrointestinal stromal tumors: who should get imatinib and for how long? Adv Surg 2014;48(1):165–83.
3. Network NCC. Pancreatic Adenocarcinoma. Available at: https://www.nccn.org/professionals/physician_gls/pdf/pancreatic.pdf. Published 2023. Accessed September 24, 23, 2023.
4. Jones S, Zhang X, Parsons DW, et al. Core signaling pathways in human pancreatic cancers revealed by global genomic analyses. Science 2008;321(5897):1801–6.
5. Collisson EA, Sadanandam A, Olson P, et al. Subtypes of pancreatic ductal adenocarcinoma and their differing responses to therapy. Nat Med 2011;17(4):500–3.
6. Moffitt RA, Marayati R, Flate EL, et al. Virtual microdissection identifies distinct tumor- and stroma-specific subtypes of pancreatic ductal adenocarcinoma. Nat Genet 2015;47(10):1168–78.
7. Bailey P, Chang DK, Nones K, et al. Genomic analyses identify molecular subtypes of pancreatic cancer. Nature 2016;531(7592):47–52.
8. Feldmann G, Beaty R, Hruban RH, et al. Molecular genetics of pancreatic intraepithelial neoplasia. J Hepatobiliary Pancreat Surg 2007;14(3):224–32.
9. Aung KL, Fischer SE, Denroche RE, et al. Genomics-Driven Precision Medicine for Advanced Pancreatic Cancer: Early Results from the COMPASS Trial. Clin Cancer Res 2018;24(6):1344–54.
10. Rashid NU, Peng XL, Jin C, et al. Purity independent subtyping of tumors (PurIST), a clinically robust, single-sample classifier for tumor subtyping in pancreatic cancer. Clinical Cancer Research 2020;26(1):82–92.
11. Tiriac H, Belleau P, Engle DD, et al. Organoid Profiling Identifies Common Responders to Chemotherapy in Pancreatic Cancer. Cancer Discov 2018;8(9):1112–29.

12. Chantrill LA, Nagrial AM, Watson C, et al. Precision Medicine for Advanced Pancreas Cancer: The Individualized Molecular Pancreatic Cancer Therapy (IMPaCT) Trial. Clin Cancer Res 2015;21(9):2029–37.

13. Pishvaian MJ, Bender RJ, Halverson D, et al. Molecular Profiling of Patients with Pancreatic Cancer: Initial Results from the Know Your Tumor Initiative. Clin Cancer Res 2018;24(20):5018–27.

14. Qian ZR, Rubinson DA, Nowak JA, et al. Association of Alterations in Main Driver Genes With Outcomes of Patients With Resected Pancreatic Ductal Adenocarcinoma. JAMA Oncol 2018;4(3):e173420.

15. Waters AM, Der CJ. KRAS: The Critical Driver and Therapeutic Target for Pancreatic Cancer. Cold Spring Harb Perspect Med 2018;8(9).

16. Wolpin BM, Hezel AF, Abrams T, et al. Oral mTOR inhibitor everolimus in patients with gemcitabine-refractory metastatic pancreatic cancer. J Clin Oncol 2009; 27(2):193–8.

17. Bedard PL, Tabernero J, Janku F, et al. A phase Ib dose-escalation study of the oral pan-PI3K inhibitor buparlisib (BKM120) in combination with the oral MEK1/2 inhibitor trametinib (GSK1120212) in patients with selected advanced solid tumors. Clin Cancer Res 2015;21(4):730–8.

18. Bekaii-Saab TS, Spira AI, Yaeger R, et al. KRYSTAL-1: Updated activity and safety of adagrasib (MRTX849) in patients (Pts) with unresectable or metastatic pancreatic cancer (PDAC) and other gastrointestinal (GI) tumors harboring a KRASG12C mutation. J Clin Oncol 2022;40(4_suppl):519.

19. Singhi AD, George B, Greenbowe JR, et al. Real-Time Targeted Genome Profile Analysis of Pancreatic Ductal Adenocarcinomas Identifies Genetic Alterations That Might Be Targeted With Existing Drugs or Used as Biomarkers. Gastroenterology 2019;156(8):2242–2253 e4.

20. Schram AM, Goto K, Kim D-W, et al. Efficacy and safety of zenocutuzumab, a HER2 x HER3 bispecific antibody, across advanced NRG1 fusion (NRG1+) cancers. J Clin Oncol 2022;40(16_suppl):105.

21. Doebele RC, Drilon A, Paz-Ares L, et al. Entrectinib in patients with advanced or metastatic NTRK fusion-positive solid tumours: integrated analysis of three phase 1-2 trials. Lancet Oncol 2020;21(2):271–82.

22. Hendifar A, Blais EM, Wolpin B, et al. Retrospective Case Series Analysis of RAF Family Alterations in Pancreatic Cancer: Real-World Outcomes From Targeted and Standard Therapies. JCO Precision Oncology 2021;(5):1325–38.

23. Conroy T, Desseigne F, Ychou M, et al. FOLFIRINOX versus gemcitabine for metastatic pancreatic cancer. N Engl J Med 2011;364(19):1817–25.

24. Von Hoff DD, Goldstein D, Renschler MF. Albumin-bound paclitaxel plus gemcitabine in pancreatic cancer. N Engl J Med 2014;370(5):479–80.

25. Kaufman B, Shapira-Frommer R, Schmutzler RK, et al. Olaparib monotherapy in patients with advanced cancer and a germline BRCA1/2 mutation. J Clin Oncol 2015;33(3):244–50.

26. O'Reilly EM, Lowery MA, Segal MF, et al. Phase IB trial of cisplatin (C), gemcitabine (G), and veliparib (V) in patients with known or potential BRCA or PALB2-mutated pancreas adenocarcinoma (PC). J Clin Oncol 2014;32(15).

27. Golan T, Hammel P, Reni M, et al. Maintenance Olaparib for Germline BRCA-Mutated Metastatic Pancreatic Cancer. N Engl J Med 2019;381(4):317–27.

28. O'Reilly EM, Lee JW, Zalupski M, et al. Randomized, Multicenter, Phase II Trial of Gemcitabine and Cisplatin With or Without Veliparib in Patients With Pancreas Adenocarcinoma and a Germline BRCA/PALB2 Mutation. J Clin Oncol 2020; 38(13):1378–88.

29. Golan T, O'Kane GM, Denroche RE, et al. Genomic Features and Classification of Homologous Recombination Deficient Pancreatic Ductal Adenocarcinoma. Gastroenterology 2021;160(6):2119–32.e9.

30. Aguirre AJ, Nowak JA, Camarda ND, et al. Real-time Genomic Characterization of Advanced Pancreatic Cancer to Enable Precision Medicine. Cancer Discov 2018;8(9):1096–111.

31. Casolino R, Paiella S, Azzolina D, et al. Homologous Recombination Deficiency in Pancreatic Cancer: A Systematic Review and Prevalence Meta-Analysis. J Clin Oncol 2021;39(23):2617–31.

32. Van Cutsem E, Tempero MA, Sigal D, et al. Randomized Phase III Trial of Pegvorhyaluronidase Alfa With Nab-Paclitaxel Plus Gemcitabine for Patients With Hyaluronan-High Metastatic Pancreatic Adenocarcinoma. J Clin Oncol 2020; 38(27):3185–94.

33. Jiang H, Hegde S, Knolhoff BL, et al. Targeting focal adhesion kinase renders pancreatic cancers responsive to checkpoint immunotherapy. Nat Med 2016; 22(8):851–60.

34. De Jesus-Acosta A, Sugar EA, O'Dwyer PJ, et al. Phase 2 study of vismodegib, a hedgehog inhibitor, combined with gemcitabine and nab-paclitaxel in patients with untreated metastatic pancreatic adenocarcinoma. Br J Cancer 2020; 122(4):498–505.

35. Llovet JM, Kelley RK, Villanueva A, et al. Hepatocellular carcinoma. Nat Rev Dis Primers 2021;7(1):6.

36. Fujiwara N, Friedman SL, Goossens N, et al. Risk factors and prevention of hepatocellular carcinoma in the era of precision medicine. J Hepatol 2018;68(3): 526–49.

37. Huang DQ, El-Serag HB, Loomba R. Global epidemiology of NAFLD-related HCC: trends, predictions, risk factors and prevention. Nat Rev Gastroenterol Hepatol 2021;18(4):223–38.

38. Kanwal F, Kramer J, Asch SM, et al. Risk of Hepatocellular Cancer in HCV Patients Treated With Direct-Acting Antiviral Agents. Gastroenterology 2017; 153(4):996–1005.e1.

39. Pinna AD, Yang T, Mazzaferro V, et al. Liver Transplantation and Hepatic Resection can Achieve Cure for Hepatocellular Carcinoma. Ann Surg 2018;268(5): 868–75.

40. Tsilimigras DI, Bagante F, Moris D, et al. Defining the chance of cure after resection for hepatocellular carcinoma within and beyond the Barcelona Clinic Liver Cancer guidelines: A multi-institutional analysis of 1,010 patients. Surgery 2019;166(6):967–74.

41. Zucman-Rossi J, Villanueva A, Nault JC, et al. Genetic Landscape and Biomarkers of Hepatocellular Carcinoma. Gastroenterology 2015;149(5): 1226–1239 e1224.

42. Llovet JM, Pinyol R, Kelley RK, et al. Molecular pathogenesis and systemic therapies for hepatocellular carcinoma. Nat Cancer 2022;3(4):386–401.

43. Schulze K, Imbeaud S, Letouze E, et al. Exome sequencing of hepatocellular carcinomas identifies new mutational signatures and potential therapeutic targets. Nat Genet 2015;47(5):505–11.

44. Llovet JM, Montal R, Sia D, et al. Molecular therapies and precision medicine for hepatocellular carcinoma. Nat Rev Clin Oncol 2018;15(10):599–616.

45. Torrecilla S, Sia D, Harrington AN, et al. Trunk mutational events present minimal intra- and inter-tumoral heterogeneity in hepatocellular carcinoma. J Hepatol 2017;67(6):1222–31.

46. Lee JS, Chu IS, Heo J, et al. Classification and prediction of survival in hepato-cellular carcinoma by gene expression profiling. Hepatology 2004;40(3): 667–76.

47. Kim SM, Leem SH, Chu IS, et al. Sixty-five gene-based risk score classifier predicts overall survival in hepatocellular carcinoma. Hepatology 2012;55(5): 1443–52.

48. Hoshida Y, Nijman SM, Kobayashi M, et al. Integrative transcriptome analysis reveals common molecular subclasses of human hepatocellular carcinoma. Cancer Res 2009;69(18):7385–92.

49. Cancer Genome Atlas Research Network. Electronic address wbe, Cancer Genome Atlas Research N. Comprehensive and Integrative Genomic Characterization of Hepatocellular Carcinoma. Cell 2017;169(7):1327–41.e3.

50. Qin S, Bai Y, Lim HY, et al. Randomized, multicenter, open-label study of oxaliplatin plus fluorouracil/leucovorin versus doxorubicin as palliative chemotherapy in patients with advanced hepatocellular carcinoma from Asia. J Clin Oncol 2013;31(28):3501–8.

51. Yeo W, Mok TS, Zee B, et al. A randomized phase III study of doxorubicin versus cisplatin/interferon alpha-2b/doxorubicin/fluorouracil (PIAF) combination chemotherapy for unresectable hepatocellular carcinoma. J Natl Cancer Inst 2005;97(20):1532–8.

52. Llovet JM, Ricci S, Mazzaferro V, et al. Sorafenib in advanced hepatocellular carcinoma. N Engl J Med 2008;359(4):378–90.

53. Cheng AL, Kang YK, Chen Z, et al. Efficacy and safety of sorafenib in patients in the Asia-Pacific region with advanced hepatocellular carcinoma: a phase III randomised, double-blind, placebo-controlled trial. Lancet Oncol 2009;10(1): 25–34.

54. Kudo M, Finn RS, Qin S, et al. Lenvatinib versus sorafenib in first-line treatment of patients with unresectable hepatocellular carcinoma: a randomised phase 3 non-inferiority trial. Lancet 2018;391(10126):1163–73.

55. Finn RS, Qin S, Ikeda M, et al. Atezolizumab plus Bevacizumab in Unresectable Hepatocellular Carcinoma. N Engl J Med 2020;382(20):1894–905.

56. Abou-Alfa GK, Lau G, Kudo M, et al. Tremelimumab plus Durvalumab in Unresectable Hepatocellular Carcinoma. NEJM Evidence 2022;1(8). EVIDoa2100070.

57. Bruix J, Takayama T, Mazzaferro V, et al. Adjuvant sorafenib for hepatocellular carcinoma after resection or ablation (STORM): a phase 3, randomised, double-blind, placebo-controlled trial. Lancet Oncol 2015;16(13):1344–54.

58. Hack SP, Spahn J, Chen M, et al. IMbrave 050: a Phase III trial of atezolizumab plus bevacizumab in high-risk hepatocellular carcinoma after curative resection or ablation. Future Oncol 2020;16(15):975–89.

59. Chow P CM, Cheng AL, Kaseb AO, et al. IMbrave050: Phase 3 study of adjuvant atezolizumab + bevacizumab versus active surveillance in patients with hepatocellular carcinoma (HCC) at high risk of disease recurrence following resection or ablation. Paper presented at: 114th Annual Meeting of the American Association for Cancer Research; April 14-19, 2023; Orlando, FL.

60. Jimenez Exposito MAM, Alvarez J, Assenate E, et al. Abstract No. 526 CheckMate-9DX: phase 3, randomized, double-blind study of adjuvant nivolumab vs placebo for patients with hepatocellular carcinoma (HCC) at high risk of recurrence after curative resection or ablation. J Vasc Intervent Radiol 2019;30(3):S227–8.

61. Vogel AZA, Cheng AL, Yau T, et al. 1017TiP KEYNOTE-937 trial in progress: adjuvant pembrolizumab in patients with hepatocellular carcinoma (HCC) and complete radiologic response after surgical resection or local ablation. Ann Oncol 2020;31:S703.

62. Knox JCA, Cleary S, Galle P, et al. A phase 3 study of durvalumab with or without bevacizumab as adjuvant therapy in patients with hepatocellular carcinoma at high risk of recurrence after curative hepatic resection or ablation: EMERALD-2. Ann Oncol 2019;30:IV59–60.

63. Ho WJ, Zhu Q, Durham J, et al. Neoadjuvant Cabozantinib and Nivolumab Converts Locally Advanced HCC into Resectable Disease with Enhanced Antitumor Immunity. Nat Cancer 2021;2(9):891–903.

64. Marron TU, Fiel MI, Hamon P, et al. Neoadjuvant cemiplimab for resectable hepatocellular carcinoma: a single-arm, open-label, phase 2 trial. Lancet Gastroenterol Hepatol 2022;7(3):219–29.

65. Kaseb AO, Hasanov E, Cao HST, et al. Perioperative nivolumab monotherapy versus nivolumab plus ipilimumab in resectable hepatocellular carcinoma: a randomised, open-label, phase 2 trial. Lancet Gastroenterol Hepatol 2022; 7(3):208–18.

66. Kang MJ, Lim J, Han SS, et al. Distinct prognosis of biliary tract cancer according to tumor location, stage, and treatment: a population-based study. Sci Rep 2022;12(1):10206.

67. Valle JW, Kelley RK, Nervi B, et al. Biliary tract cancer. Lancet 2021;397(10272): 428–44.

68. Nakamura H, Arai Y, Totoki Y, et al. Genomic spectra of biliary tract cancer. Nat Genet 2015;47(9):1003–10.

69. Borger DR, Tanabe KK, Fan KC, et al. Frequent mutation of isocitrate dehydrogenase (IDH)1 and IDH2 in cholangiocarcinoma identified through broad-based tumor genotyping. Oncol 2012;17(1):72–9.

70. Fontugne J, Augustin J, Pujals A, et al. PD-L1 expression in perihilar and intrahepatic cholangiocarcinoma. Oncotarget 2017;8(15):24644–51.

71. Scott AJ, Sharman R, Shroff RT. Precision Medicine in Biliary Tract Cancer. J Clin Oncol 2022;40(24):2716–34.

72. Andersen JB, Spee B, Blechacz BR, et al. Genomic and genetic characterization of cholangiocarcinoma identifies therapeutic targets for tyrosine kinase inhibitors. Gastroenterology 2012;142(4):1021–31.e5.

73. Sia D, Hoshida Y, Villanueva A, et al. Integrative molecular analysis of intrahepatic cholangiocarcinoma reveals 2 classes that have different outcomes. Gastroenterology 2013;144(4):829–40.

74. Farshidfar F, Zheng S, Gingras MC, et al. Integrative Genomic Analysis of Cholangiocarcinoma Identifies Distinct IDH-Mutant Molecular Profiles. Cell Rep 2017;19(13):2878–80.

75. Jarnagin WR, Ruo L, Little SA, et al. Patterns of initial disease recurrence after resection of gallbladder carcinoma and hilar cholangiocarcinoma: implications for adjuvant therapeutic strategies. Cancer 2003;98(8):1689–700.

76. Doussot A, Gonen M, Wiggers JK, et al. Recurrence Patterns and Disease-Free Survival after Resection of Intrahepatic Cholangiocarcinoma: Preoperative and Postoperative Prognostic Models. J Am Coll Surg 2016;223(3):493–505 e492.

77. Li J, Rocha FG, Mayo SC. Past, Present, and Future Management of Localized Biliary Tract Malignancies. Surg Oncol Clin N Am 2023;32(1):83–99.

78. Valle J, Wasan H, Palmer DH, et al. Cisplatin plus gemcitabine versus gemcitabine for biliary tract cancer. N Engl J Med 2010;362(14):1273–81.

79. Shroff RT, Guthrie KA, Scott AJ, et al. SWOG 1815: A phase III randomized trial of gemcitabine, cisplatin, and nab-paclitaxel versus gemcitabine and cisplatin in newly diagnosed, advanced biliary tract cancers. J Clin Oncol 2023; 41(4_suppl):LBA490.

80. Oh D-Y, He AR, Qin S, et al. A phase 3 randomized, double-blind, placebo-controlled study of durvalumab in combination with gemcitabine plus cisplatin (GemCis) in patients (pts) with advanced biliary tract cancer (BTC): TOPAZ-1. J Clin Oncol 2022;40(4_suppl):378.

81. Edeline J, Benabdelghani M, Bertaut A, et al. Gemcitabine and Oxaliplatin Chemotherapy or Surveillance in Resected Biliary Tract Cancer (PRODIGE 12-ACCORD 18-UNICANCER GI): A Randomized Phase III Study. J Clin Oncol 2019;37(8):658–67.

82. Ebata T, Hirano S, Konishi M, et al. Randomized clinical trial of adjuvant gemcitabine chemotherapy versus observation in resected bile duct cancer. Br J Surg 2018;105(3):192–202.

83. Primrose JN, Fox RP, Palmer DH, et al. Capecitabine compared with observation in resected biliary tract cancer (BILCAP): a randomised, controlled, multicentre, phase 3 study. Lancet Oncol 2019;20(5):663–73.

84. Maithel SK, Keilson JM, Cao HST, et al. NEO-GAP: A Single-Arm, Phase II Feasibility Trial of Neoadjuvant Gemcitabine, Cisplatin, and Nab-Paclitaxel for Resectable, High-Risk Intrahepatic Cholangiocarcinoma. Ann Surg Oncol 2023;30(11):6558–66.

85. Helsten T, Elkin S, Arthur E, et al. The FGFR Landscape in Cancer: Analysis of 4,853 Tumors by Next-Generation Sequencing. Clin Cancer Res 2016;22(1): 259–67.

86. Lamarca A, Barriuso J, McNamara MG, et al. Molecular targeted therapies: Ready for "prime time" in biliary tract cancer. J Hepatol 2020;73(1):170–85.

87. Dienstmann R, Rodon J, Prat A, et al. Genomic aberrations in the FGFR pathway: opportunities for targeted therapies in solid tumors. Ann Oncol 2014;25(3):552–63.

88. Abou-Alfa GK, Sahai V, Hollebecque A, et al. Pemigatinib for previously treated, locally advanced or metastatic cholangiocarcinoma: a multicentre, open-label, phase 2 study. Lancet Oncol 2020;21(5):671–84.

89. Goyal L, Meric-Bernstam F, Hollebecque A, et al. Futibatinib for FGFR2-Rearranged Intrahepatic Cholangiocarcinoma. N Engl J Med 2023;388(3): 228–39.

90. Javle M, Roychowdhury S, Kelley RK, et al. Infigratinib (BGJ398) in previously treated patients with advanced or metastatic cholangiocarcinoma with FGFR2 fusions or rearrangements: mature results from a multicentre, open-label, single-arm, phase 2 study. Lancet Gastroenterol Hepatol 2021;6(10):803–15.

91. Javle MM, Abou-Alfa GK, Macarulla T, et al. Efficacy of derazantinib in intrahepatic cholangiocarcinoma patients with FGFR2 mutations or amplifications: Interim results from the phase 2 study FIDES-01. J Clin Oncol 2022; 40(4_suppl):427.

92. Goyal L, Shi L, Liu LY, et al. TAS-120 Overcomes Resistance to ATP-Competitive FGFR Inhibitors in Patients with FGFR2 Fusion-Positive Intrahepatic Cholangiocarcinoma. Cancer Discov 2019;9(8):1064–79.

93. Meric-Bernstam F, Bahleda R, Hierro C, et al. Futibatinib, an Irreversible FGFR1-4 Inhibitor, in Patients with Advanced Solid Tumors Harboring FGF/FGFR Aberrations: A Phase I Dose-Expansion Study. Cancer Discov 2022;12(2):402–15.

94. Ilyas SI, Affo S, Goyal L, et al. Cholangiocarcinoma - novel biological insights and therapeutic strategies. Nat Rev Clin Oncol 2023;20(7):470–86.

95. Valle JW, Lamarca A, Goyal L, et al. New Horizons for Precision Medicine in Biliary Tract Cancers. Cancer Discov 2017;7(9):943–62.

96. Boscoe AN, Rolland C, Kelley RK. Frequency and prognostic significance of isocitrate dehydrogenase 1 mutations in cholangiocarcinoma: a systematic literature review. J Gastrointest Oncol 2019;10(4):751–65.

97. Abou-Alfa GK, Macarulla T, Javle MM, et al. Ivosidenib in IDH1-mutant, chemotherapy-refractory cholangiocarcinoma (ClarIDHy): a multicentre, randomised, double-blind, placebo-controlled, phase 3 study. Lancet Oncol 2020;21(6): 796–807.

98. Lee CK, Chon HJ, Cheon J, et al. Trastuzumab plus FOLFOX for HER2-positive biliary tract cancer refractory to gemcitabine and cisplatin: a multi-institutional phase 2 trial of the Korean Cancer Study Group (KCSG-HB19–14). Lancet Gastroenterol Hepatol 2023;8(1):56–65.

99. Javle M, Borad MJ, Azad NS, et al. Pertuzumab and trastuzumab for HER2-positive, metastatic biliary tract cancer (MyPathway): a multicentre, open-label, phase 2a, multiple basket study. Lancet Oncol 2021;22(9):1290–300.

100. Meric-Bernstam F, Beeram M, Hamilton E, et al. Zanidatamab, a novel bispecific antibody, for the treatment of locally advanced or metastatic HER2-expressing or HER2-amplified cancers: a phase 1, dose-escalation and expansion study. Lancet Oncol 2022;23(12):1558–70.

101. Harding JJ, Fan J, Oh DY, et al. Zanidatamab for HER2-amplified, unresectable, locally advanced or metastatic biliary tract cancer (HERIZON-BTC-01): a multicentre, single-arm, phase 2b study. Lancet Oncol 2023;24(7):772–82.

102. Meric-Bernstam F, Makker V, Oaknin A, et al. Efficacy and Safety of Trastuzumab Deruxtecan in Patients With HER2-Expressing Solid Tumors: Primary Results From the DESTINY-PanTumor02 Phase II Trial. J Clin Oncol 2023;JCO2302005.

103. Ohba A, Morizane C, Kawamoto Y, et al. Trastuzumab deruxtecan (T-DXd; DS-8201) in patients (pts) with HER2-expressing unresectable or recurrent biliary tract cancer (BTC): An investigator-initiated multicenter phase 2 study (HERB trial). J Clin Oncol 2022;40(16_suppl):4006.

104. Farha N, Dima D, Ullah F, et al. Precision Oncology Targets in Biliary Tract Cancer. Cancers 2023;15(7).

105. Westphalen CB, Krebs MG, Le Tourneau C, et al. Genomic context of NTRK1/2/3 fusion-positive tumours from a large real-world population. npj Precis Oncol 2021;5(1):69.

106. Drilon A, Laetsch TW, Kummar S, et al. Efficacy of Larotrectinib in TRK Fusion-Positive Cancers in Adults and Children. N Engl J Med 2018;378(8):731–9.

107. Hyman DM, Puzanov I, Subbiah V, et al. Vemurafenib in Multiple Nonmelanoma Cancers with BRAF V600 Mutations. N Engl J Med 2015;373(8):726–36.

108. Subbiah V, Lassen U, Elez E, et al. Dabrafenib plus trametinib in patients with BRAF(V600E)-mutated biliary tract cancer (ROAR): a phase 2, open-label, single-arm, multicentre basket trial. Lancet Oncol 2020;21(9):1234–43.

109. Meric-Bernstam F, Rothe M, Garrett-Mayer E, et al. Cobimetinib plus vemurafenib (C+V) in patients (Pts) with solid tumors with BRAF V600E/d/k/R mutation: Results from the targeted agent and profiling utilization registry (TAPUR) study. J Clin Oncol 2022;40(16_suppl):3008.

110. Okamura R, Kurzrock R, Mallory RJ, et al. Comprehensive genomic landscape and precision therapeutic approach in biliary tract cancers. Int J Cancer 2021; 148(3):702–12.

111. DiPeri TP, Zhao M, Evans KW, et al. Convergent MAPK pathway alterations mediate acquired resistance to FGFR inhibitors in FGFR2 fusion-positive cholangiocarcinoma. J Hepatol 2023;S0168-8278(23)05274-1.

112. Goyal L, Saha SK, Liu LY, et al. Polyclonal Secondary FGFR2 Mutations Drive Acquired Resistance to FGFR Inhibition in Patients with FGFR2 Fusion-Positive Cholangiocarcinoma. Cancer Discov 2017;7(3):252–63.

113. Le DT, Durham JN, Smith KN, et al. Mismatch repair deficiency predicts response of solid tumors to PD-1 blockade. Science 2017;357(6349):409–13.

114. Maio M, Ascierto PA, Manzyuk L, et al. Pembrolizumab in microsatellite instability high or mismatch repair deficient cancers: updated analysis from the phase II KEYNOTE-158 study. Ann Oncol 2022;33(9):929–38.

115. Marabelle A, Fakih M, Lopez J, et al. Association of tumour mutational burden with outcomes in patients with advanced solid tumours treated with pembrolizumab: prospective biomarker analysis of the multicohort, open-label, phase 2 KEYNOTE-158 study. Lancet Oncol 2020;21(10):1353–65.

116. Piha-Paul SA, Oh DY, Ueno M, et al. Efficacy and safety of pembrolizumab for the treatment of advanced biliary cancer: Results from the KEYNOTE-158 and KEYNOTE-028 studies. Int J Cancer 2020;147(8):2190–8.

117. Oh DY, Lee KH, Lee DW, et al. Gemcitabine and cisplatin plus durvalumab with or without tremelimumab in chemotherapy-naive patients with advanced biliary tract cancer: an open-label, single-centre, phase 2 study. Lancet Gastroenterol Hepatol 2022;7(6):522–32.

118. Oh DYHA, Qin S, Chen LT, et al, for the TOPAZ-1 Investigators. Durvalumab plus Gemcitabine and Cisplatin in Advanced Biliary Tract Cancer. NEJM Evidence 2022;1(8).

119. Kelley RK, Ueno M, Yoo C, et al. Pembrolizumab in combination with gemcitabine and cisplatin compared with gemcitabine and cisplatin alone for patients with advanced biliary tract cancer (KEYNOTE-966): a randomised, double-blind, placebo-controlled, phase 3 trial. Lancet 2023;401(10391):1853–65.

Precision Oncology in Melanoma and Skin Cancer Surgery

Shoshana Levi, MD[a], Hannah Bank, MD, PhD[a], John Mullinax, MD[b], Genevieve Boland, MD, PhD[a,c],*

KEYWORDS

- Cutaneous oncology • Melanoma • Merkel cell carcinoma • Immunotherapy
- Targeted therapy

KEY POINTS

- The treatment of patients with cutaneous melanoma requires personalization based on tumor factors which predict response to a wide array of both targeted therapy and immunotherapy approaches.
- There have been significant advances in the treatment of metastatic melanoma in the last decade due to intrinsic tumor features such as specific gene mutation or immune response.
- Despite significant efficacy for some patients, immunotherapy approaches have significant and specific toxicity profiles. Physicians need to be alert and aware of the novel clinical presentations for these unique toxicities.
- The role of the surgeon in the treatment of advanced melanoma is rapidly changing due to personalized systemic treatment options. Optimal surgical timing and degree of resection is evolving rapidly.

TARGETED THERAPY

Historically, the treatment of metastatic melanoma was limited to single-agent chemotherapy regimens with DNA damaging agents such as dacarbazine (DTIC) or temozolomide, and cytokine immunotherapy with high-dose interleukin IL-2. These therapies yielded limited responses of around 12% to 16%,[1,2] leaving a large proportion of patients in need of more effective treatments. The use of precision medicine and next-generation sequencing (NGS) has led to the development of newer therapies by identification of tumor-specific driver mutations in *BRAF*, *NRAS*, and *KIT*.

[a] Department of Surgery, MGH, Boston, MA, USA; [b] Sarcoma Department, Moffitt Cancer Center, Tampa, FL, USA; [c] Department of Surgery, Massachusetts General Hospital (MGH) Cancer Center, Harvard Medical School (HMS), Boston, MA, USA
* Corresponding author. 55 Fruit Street, Yawkey 7B, Boston, MA 02114.
E-mail address: GMBOLAND@MGH.HARVARD.EDU

Surg Oncol Clin N Am 33 (2024) 369–385
https://doi.org/10.1016/j.soc.2023.12.017
1055-3207/24/© 2023 Elsevier Inc. All rights reserved.

Identification and characterization of these mutations has made it possible to personalize patient's treatment regimens based on the molecular drivers of their cancer.

BRAF

The most common mutation found in cutaneous melanoma is in the BRAF gene, with approximately 50% of melanomas harboring an activating BRAF mutation. The vast majority of these BRAF mutations (>90%) occur at codon 600, and the majority of those (>90%) result in a substitution of glutamic acid for valine, so termed BRAF V600 E.[3] The pathogenesis from this common mutation comes predominantly from the constitutive activation of the MAPK/ERK pathway, allowing tumor cells to become self-sufficient and unregulated in growth signals.[4] The prevalence of the BRAF V600 E mutation and its importance in tumor progression made it an attractive option for targeted therapeutic development.

Ultimately, the development of vemurafenib, a BRAF kinase inhibitor specific for mutant BRAF, led to a turning point in the treatment of metastatic melanoma. The promising results of phase 1 and 2 studies[5,6] led to the landmark trial that validated the use of vemurafenib in the treatment of metastatic melanoma.[7] This phase 3 randomized clinical study (BRIM-3) compared vemurafenib to standard-of-care DTIC in patients with previously untreated metastatic melanoma with the BRAFV600 E mutation. Response rates to vemurafenib were 48% compared with only 5% in patients treated with DTIC. Furthermore, the overall survival at 6 months was noted to be superior in the vemurafenib group (84% vs 64%).[7] These results led to the development of additional BRAF kinase inhibitors such as dabrafenib, with similarly dramatic responses found.[8–10] In the phase 3 randomized clinical study (BREAK-3) comparing dabrafenib to DTIC in patients with unresectable stage III or IV BRAF V600 E melanoma, the response rates were 50% in the dabrafenib group compared with 6% in the DTIC group. Moreover, the overall survival hazard ratio (HR) was 0.61 (95% CI 0.25–1.48) in favor of dabrafenib.[10]

Although initial results of BRAF inhibition were very promising, the challenge of drug resistance was quickly encountered. Through the use of NGS techniques, mechanisms of either acquired or intrinsic resistance to BRAF inhibition were proposed and validated including activation of alternative survival pathways,[11,12] reactivation of the MAPK pathway via NRAS or MEK mutations,[11,13] and dimerization of BRAF V600 E.[14] The scope of the problem was later illustrated in the long-term outcomes reported from the BRIM-3 trial which showed that only 36 of 336 (10.7%) patients treated with vemurafenib had not experienced disease progression at 5 years.[15] Similarly, long-term outcomes from the BREAK-3 trial showed a 5-year progression-free survival (PFS) of only 12% in the dabrafenib arm.[16] Given the limitations of monotherapy and the mechanisms of drug resistance described, alternative targets of the MAPK/ERK pathway such as MEK inhibition offered an attractive treatment strategy. Multiple studies confirmed the effectiveness of MEK inhibition in the treatment of BRAF-mutated melanoma, either as monotherapy or more notably as combination therapy with BRAF inhibition.[17–20] Results from the CoBRIM trial which compared combination BRAF/MEK inhibition with cobimetinib and vemurafenib to monotherapy vemurafenib showed increased PFS (12.3 months vs 7.2 months [HR 0.58; 95% CI 0.42–0.72; P < .0001]) and overall survival (OS) (22.3 months vs 17.4 months [HR 0.70; 95% CI 0.55–0.90; P=.005]) in the combination therapy group.[20,21] Extended follow-up at 5 years reported consistent outcomes, demonstrating long-term benefit.[22] Similarly, combination therapy with dabrafenib, another BRAF V600 E inhibitor, and trametinib was found to have improved overall survival compared with dabrafenib alone (COMBI-D trial)[23] or vemurafenib alone (COMBI-V trial).[24]

The history of BRAF/MEK inhibition highlights the importance of precision medicine in identifying therapeutic targets, studying their limitations, and finding alternative therapies to address these limitations. In these ways, precision medicine has and will continue to advance cancer care forward.

KIT

Oncogenic *KIT* mutations are identified in ~3% of cutaneous melanomas, although they are enriched in non-cutaneous melanomas (36% of acral melanomas, 39% mucosal melanomas, and 28% on chronically sun-damaged skin). Efforts focused on targeting *KIT* mutations have been approached via imatinib,[25] nilotinib,[26] dasatinib,[27] and sunitinib[28] with modest efficacy.

NRAS

To date, no approved NRAS-targeted therapies are approved in melanoma. However, strategies using MEK inhibitors alone or in combination have been studied in this patient population.[29]

TARGETED THERAPIES FOR OTHER SKIN CANCERS

Although surgical excision remains the primary treatment modality for most nonmelanoma skin cancers, a subset of these basal and squamous cell carcinomas (SCCs) can metastasize or be locally invasive requiring systemic therapy for treatment.

Basal Cell Carcinoma

The hedgehog (HH) pathway is normally suppressed in normal adult tissues, but activating mutations in the smoothened (*SMO*) proto-oncogene of the HH pathway, can lead to basal cell carcinomas (BCCs) formation. Because SMO is a downstream activator of the HH pathway, it can be inhibited with drugs such as vismodegib, sonidegib, oatidegib, and taladegib in the rare cases of metastatic BCC not amenable to surgical resection.[30]

Squamous Cell Carcinoma

In rare subset of nonsurgical patients with advanced SCC, immune checkpoint inhibitors (ICIs) have also showed efficacy. Approved agents include cemiplimab [31] and pembrolizumab.[32] There are ongoing trials using the combination nivolumab and ipilimumab.

Dermatofibrosarcoma Protuberans

This rare sarcoma which arises from the skin may be effectively treated with imatinib, a tyrosine kinase inhibitor which targets platelet derived growth factor subunit B (PDGFRB). This is because dermatofibrosarcoma protuberans (DFSP) contains a specific translocation, *COL1A1-PDGFB* which results in constitutive activation of PDGFRB. In patients with either locally advanced or metastatic disease, imatinib is an effective treatment in the neoadjuvant setting or as monotherapy, respectively.[33,34] In the neoadjuvant setting, treatment with imatinib was associated with a 57% overall response rate (ORR, 7% complete response [CR] + 50% partial response [PR]) which makes this an effective strategy for locally advanced disease. This effect is typically restricted to DFSP without fibrosarcomatous (FS) change because with DFSP-FS, the genomic events driving malignancy are not restricted to the unique *COL1A1-PDGFB* translocation. Therefore, the efficacy of imatinib is limited because PDGFR-B activity contributes less to the aggressive nature. In one report describing efficacy in the metastatic setting, imatinib had more limited effect with a median PFS of less than 1 year.[34] Despite this limitation, 50% of patients treated were able to undergo metastectomy given the limited burden of disease. Thus, based on these data, imatinib should be considered the treatment of patients with oligometastatic disease that harbor a COLO1A1-PDGFB translocation.

IMMUNOTHERAPY
Immune Checkpoint Blockade

The development of ICIs revolutionized treatment paradigms for several malignancies, with melanoma being one of the first solid tumors to demonstrate marked responses to such agents (**Table 1**). The US Food and Drug Administration (FDA) approvals were quickly followed by integration into national guidelines that recommended first-line use of ICI as standard of care. The widespread utilization of ICI in melanoma, and other cancer subtypes, has led to durable responses and long-term survival in many patients who previously had limited options.

Immune checkpoints refer to molecules or receptors that are responsible for regulation of the immune system. Immune cells such as T cells contain various immune checkpoints that regulate immune cell activation status and function. One of the hallmarks of cancer biology is evasion of the immune system. For instance, interaction of the PD-1 protein on T cells and the PD-L1 protein on tumor cells results in downregulation of the immune system by decreasing T-cell proliferation and activation, activating apoptosis of antigen-specific T cells, and inhibiting apoptosis of regulatory T cells.[35] Thus, immune checkpoint such as PD-1/PD-L1, CTLA-4, LAG-3, TIM3, and TIGIT offered to be promising targets in cancer immunotherapy. Investigation into these targets has led to the development and approval of multiple ICI, for various cancer histologies, in both the adjuvant and neoadjuvant settings.

The first ICI to be approved by the food and drug administration (FDA) was ipilimumab, a humanized antibody against CTLA-4. Interactions between CTLA-4 on T cells and its ligand, CD80, which is present on antigen-presenting cells, result in both the dampening of effector T-cell function and the enhancement of regulatory T-cell inhibitory function, resulting in immunosuppression.[36] Anti-CTLA-4 monotherapy has been extensively studied and shown to provide clinical benefit in the treatment of advanced melanoma. In a pooled analysis of 1861 patients treated with ipilimumab, the median OS was 11.4 months with a 3-year survival rate of 22%, which compared favorably to a historical median OS of 8 to 10 months and 5-year survival rates of 10% with previously approved therapies.[37]

Table 1		
Selected practice changing immunotherapy trials		
Adjuvant		
Stage IIB and IIC		
Trial	KEYNOTE-716	CheckMate-76K
Agent	Pembrolizumab	Nivolumab
Microscopic Stage III		
Trial	Checkmate 238	KEYNOTE-054	COMBI-AD
Agent	Nivolumab	Pembrolizumab	Dabrafenib + trametinib
Neoadjuvant		
Macroscopic Stage III		
Trial	SWOG 1808	OpACIN-neo, PRADO
Agent	Pembrolizumab	Nivolumab + ipilimumab

The use of anti-PD-1/PD-L1 monotherapy yielded more dramatic results, not just in the treatment of melanoma, but across multiple tumor subtypes.[38] Two notable studies looking at the efficacy of nivolumab, a monoclonal PD-1 antibody, are the CheckMate 066 and CheckMate 037 studies which demonstrated improved response rates compared with chemotherapy in treatment naïve and previously treated patients, respectively.[39,40] In the CheckMate 066 study, a randomized controlled trial comparing nivolumab to DTIC in previously untreated patients with metastatic melanoma, the 1-year OS, and ORR of the nivolumab group was 72.9% and 40%, respectively, compared with 42.1% (HR 0.42; 95% CI 0.25–0.73, $P < .001$) and 13.9% (odds ratio 4.06, $P < .001$) in the DTIC group, respectively.[39] The randomized controlled CheckMate 037 trial evaluated the efficacy of nivolumab versus investigator choice chemotherapy in patients with progressive disease after ipilimumab or ipilimumab with a BRAF inhibitor. Response rates to nivolumab were 31.7% compared with only 10.6% in the chemotherapy group.[40] Future analyses of OS did not show a difference between the two groups; however, there was a significant crossover rate as 41% of patients in the chemotherapy group subsequently received an anti-PD-1/PD-L1 agent.[41] Similar results were shown with pembrolizumab, another monoclonal PD-1 antibody, in the KEYNOTE-002 and KEYNOTE-006 studies which compared pembrolizumab to investigator choice chemotherapy and ipilimumab, respectively.[42–45] The KEYNOTE-002 study comparing pembrolizumab (2 and 10 mg/kg) to chemotherapy showed superior response rates (21% and 25% vs 4%, $P < .0001$) and PFS (HR 0.57 and 0.50, $P < .0001$) in the pembrolizumab groups.[42] As was the case in the CheckMate 037 trial, there was no statistical difference in overall survival between the groups, likely due to a 55% crossover rate in the chemotherapy group.[43] The KEYNOTE-006 trial comparing pembrolizumab (every 2 weeks and every 3 weeks) to ipilimumab showed prolonged 6-month PFS (47.3% and 46.6% vs 26.5%, $P < .001$) and 24-month overall survival (55% vs 43%, HR 0.68, $P=.0009$).[44,45]

CTLA-4 is involved in the early stages of antigen presentation and priming, whereas PD-1 operates during the effector phase of the immune response. Given the distinct mechanisms of these two classes of ICI, combination therapy was the next logical approach, with results showing unprecedented durable responses. Long-term follow-up from the CheckMate 067 trial at 6.5 years has shown improved median OS in patients with unresectable stage III or IV treated with combination nivolumab and ipilimumab compared with either nivolumab or ipilimumab monotherapy (72.1 vs 36.9 vs 19.9 months with 6.5-year OS rates of 49% vs 42% vs 23%, respectively).[46]

More recent studies have evaluated the efficacy of dual checkpoint inhibitor therapy with nivolumab and relatlimab, a first-in-class LAG-3 antibody.[47] LAG-3 is a protein expressed on the cell surface of immune cells that negatively regulates T-cell proliferation and effector function. In the RELATIVITY-047 trial, patients with untreated unresectable or metastatic melanoma were found to benefit more from combination nivolumab and relatlimab compared with nivolumab alone with improved median PFS of 10.1 months versus 4.6 months (HR 0.75, 95% CI 0.62–0.92, $P=.006$).[47] Of note, grade 3 or 4 treatment-related adverse events occurred in only 18.9% of patients in the nivolumab plus relatlimab group. Although this is a much lower event rate compared with the 59% reported for the nivolumab plus ipilimumab group in the CheckMate 067 trial, there is a significant discrepancy in the rate of grade 3 or 4 events for the nivolumab group between the two trials—9.7% in the RELATIVITY-047 trial versus 21% in the CheckMate 067 trial.[47,48] Nevertheless, combination nivolumab and relatlimab may offer a high-efficacy regimen with a more tolerable toxicity profile than ipilimumab and nivolumab.

Adjuvant and Neoadjuvant Therapy

Adjuvant

Given the high rates of recurrence seen after resection of stage III melanoma and the efficacy of immunotherapy, it is unsurprising that the application of immunotherapies extended into the adjuvant setting for high-risk resectable melanoma. The EORTC-18071 and KEYNOTE-054 trials evaluated the use of ipilimumab and pembrolizumab, respectively, as adjuvant treatment for resected stage III melanoma and demonstrated significant improvements in recurrence-free survival (RFS) and distant metastasis-free survival (DMFS) when compared with placebo.[49–52] A comparison of nivolumab to ipilimumab as adjuvant therapy in the CheckMate 238 trial revealed that treatment with nivolumab resulted in longer RFS at 12 months (70.5% vs 60.8%; HR 0.65, 95% CI 0.51–0.83, $P < .001$) and was associated with less grade 3 or 4 adverse events (14.4% vs 45.9%) when compared with ipilimumab.[53]

Neoadjuvant

The next logical step in the evolution of ICI use was in the neoadjuvant setting as it offers several advantages over adjuvant administration including increased antigen presentation and thus an increased immune response, ability to assess pathologic response to therapy which is known to correlate with RFS, and downstaging of disease leading to less extensive resections.[54] Several early phase clinical trials have evaluated the feasibility of neoadjuvant immunotherapy for resectable melanoma. The phase 2 OpACIN trial compared neoadjuvant to adjuvant administration of ipilimumab plus pembrolizumab and noted high pathologic response rates of 78% and increased expansion of tumor-resident T-cell clones in the neoadjuvant arm.[55] Although the rates of pathologic response were promising, the rates of grade 3 or 4 toxicities were higher than expected at 90% in both arms. The OpACIN-neo trial identified a tolerable neoadjuvant dosing schedule without compromising pathologic response.[56] The recently published SWOG 1801 trial compared combination neoadjuvant and adjuvant pembrolizumab to adjuvant pembrolizumab alone in patients with stage IIIB to IVC melanoma and found that the neoadjuvant–adjuvant group had a longer event-free survival (EFS) of 72% compared with 49% in the adjuvant group ($P=.004$).[57]

Perioperative toxicity

There are two hallmark surgical considerations for patients that have received ICI in either the neoadjuvant or adjuvant setting, both of which are related to the unique autoimmune side effect profile of this therapy. For those that have received neoadjuvant ICI in the immediate preoperative period, adrenal insufficiency should be at the forefront of concern for any patient with hypotension, altered mental status, or severe fatigue in the postoperative period. Patients may have underlying adrenal insufficiency associated with iatrogenic steroid use or even primary adrenal insufficiency from the ICI treatment itself which becomes uncompensated under the physiologic stress of the perioperative period. In either scenario, rapid recognition of the clinical signs and confirmation with laboratory testing is crucial to use corticosteroid supplementation. A random serum cortisol level of less than 20 mcg/dL should prompt initiation of corticosteroids in patients exhibiting any sign of adrenal insufficiency.

Another critical concern for the surgeon is the development of colitis in some patients while under treatment with ICI. This is seen most commonly during treatment with ipilimumab and most commonly in patients receiving ipilimumab in the adjuvant setting. This specific toxicity can present as peritonitis with perforated viscus or simply as vague abdominal pain. Prompt surgical intervention for the patient with peritonitis should be undertaken with liberal resection based on gross appearance of bowel. Any patient presenting with abdominal pain and radiographic evidence of colonic inflammation should have surgical consultation early to ensure serial abdominal examinations can be followed with rapid intervention if deterioration is noted. Validated clinical guidelines for the management of perioperative ICI toxicity have been published by the National Comprehensive Cancer Network and the Society for the Immunotherapy of Cancer.[58,59]

The toxicity profile of ICI is the primary concern with the timing of administration around the time of surgical intervention. In the OpACIN trial, patients received their last dose of ICI 3 weeks before lymphadenectomy, a timing chosen to allow for any acute toxicity to appear before impacting the operation. With this strategy, of the 89 patients enrolled, only 3 (3.3%) required a delay in the operation due to immune-related adverse events (irAEs) associated with ICI before the operation. This time interval has been thus advocated as the optimal approach to operate following neoadjuvant ICI. Similarly, a time interval of 3 weeks postoperatively is a minimum interval before initiating adjuvant ICI therapy. This time interval allows for appropriate pathologic review of the resected specimen regarding degree of lymph node involvement and for any acute postoperative complications (ie, surgical site infection, seroma, lymphocele) to be diagnosed.

Pathologic response
Pathologic response to neoadjuvant therapy may help inform subsequent surgical and adjuvant decision-making. The PRADO trial, an extension of the OpACIN-neo study, omitted therapeutic lymph node dissection and additional adjuvant therapy in patients with major pathologic responses to neoadjuvant treatment (<10% viable tumor) and found a 2-year RFS rate of 93.3% and DMFS rate of 100%.[60] However, longer follow-up is need to determine the durability of this treatment approach.

Biomarkers for Predicting Response and Toxicity to Immunotherapy

As various immunotherapy agents have become widely applied in clinical practice, there has been a robust research effort to identify biomarkers of response and resistance. Early trials using melanoma exomes and transcriptomes from patients treated with CTLA-4 antibodies found that mutational load, neoantigen load, and expression of cytolytic markers were associated with the degree of clinical benefit.[61,62] A large meta-analysis including 12,450 patients from 117 clinical trials has illustrated the positive association between tumor mutational burden (TMB) and clinical response to anti-CTLA-4, anti-PD-1/PD-L1, and combination ICI.[63] TMB is reported as the number of coding somatic mutations per megabase pair and is a continuous variable that represents the tremendous spectrum of heterogeneity in solid tumors. Solid tumor diagnoses with TMB greater than 10 mutations/MB (ie, cutaneous melanoma and non-small cell lung cancer) are generally considered to be "high," whereas those with less than 5 mutations/MB (ie, ocular melanoma and sarcoma) are considered to have a "low" TMB.

Although numerous studies have shown the association between TMB and response to immunotherapy, TMB alone is not an accurate enough biomarker to guide patient selection in clinical practice. Furthermore, incorporation of TMB into clinical practice, which relies on whole exome sequencing (WES), would be cost prohibitive. Surrogates such as cancer gene panels have been shown to have similar predictive value to WES,[64] but clinically available predictive tools are still needed to better guide patient selection for immunotherapy. More recent studies have developed and shown an IFN-γ signature to be a predictive biomarker for pathologic response in patients receiving neoadjuvant immunotherapy.[65,66] Subsequently, the DOMINI trial, a study evaluating the efficacy of domatinostat, a class I histone deacetylase inhibitor, found that the IFN-γ signature adequately predicted which patients would benefit from nivolumab alone.[67] These results may lead to more individualized treatment regimens and allow clinicians to either escalate or de-escalate treatment regimens to optimize the risk–benefit balance of immunotherapy administration.

Given that the mechanisms of immunotherapies rely on upregulation of the immune system to induce tumor targeting, it is unsurprising that the attributable toxicities are irAEs. These toxicities can be severe and may require discontinuation of treatment or necessitate the use of glucocorticoids or other immune suppressants, which in turn can limit the effectiveness of the immunotherapy.[68] Aside from patients with preexisting autoimmune diseases, identifying patients at high risk of developing irAE has remained a challenge. There has been extensive research of biologic markers that may predict risk of severe autoimmune toxicity associated with immunotherapy. A recent study evaluating cytokine expression identified 11 cytokines that were significantly upregulated at baseline and early during treatment in patients with melanoma treated with combination anti-CTLA-4 and anti-PD-1 antibodies who developed severe immune toxicity. The 11 cytokines were integrated into a toxicity score (CYTOX) which demonstrated relatively low AUC scores of 0.68 and 0.7 for pretreatment and early-treatment using ROC analysis.[69] Additional studies have used multi-omic approaches to identify other factors associated with development of irAEs such as T-cell characteristics before treatment,[70] immune signatures after initiation of treatment,[71] or the presence of certain antibodies.[72] Although the results from such studies are promising, they are not easily integrated into clinical practice and, thus far, no biomarkers have been validated for clinical use in predicting immune toxicities.[73]

Combination Immunotherapy and Targeted Therapy

Given the groundbreaking results of treatment with dual checkpoint inhibitors and BRAF/MEK targeted therapies, subsequent research has looked at combination immunotherapy and targeted therapy. The randomized controlled trial IMspire150 compared triple therapy atezolizumab (a PD-L1 inhibitor), vemurafenib, and cobimetinib (MEK inhibitor) with placebo plus vemurafenib and cobimetinib in patients with treatment naïve unresectable stage III and IV melanoma. Triple therapy was found to provide prolonged median PFS of 15.1 versus 10.6 months in the control group (HR 0.78, 95 CI 0.63–0.97, P=.025).[74] In an interim analysis, median OS in the triple therapy group was 39 months compared with 25.8 months in the control group. However, this did not reach statistical significance with P=.14, and longer term analysis is needed.[75] Another study that evaluated the efficacy of combined immunotherapy and targeted therapy for advanced melanoma was the KEYNOTE-022 study. In this study, combination pembrolizumab plus dabrafenib and trametinib provided improved median PFS, duration of response (DOR), and OS compared with placebo plus dabrafenib and trametinib (median PFS: 16.9 vs 10.7 months, HR 0.5; 95% CI 0.34–0.83, DOR: 25.1 vs 12.1 months, median OS: not-reached vs 26.3 months, HR 0.64; 95% CI 0.38–1.06).[76]

ADOPTIVE CELL TRANSFER

Adoptive cell transfer (ACT) is a form of personalized cancer immunotherapy which uses tumor-infiltrating lymphocytes (TIL) harvested from a patient's tumor that are ex vivo expanded and activated to be administered as a "living drug" after lymphodepletion. There are several methods in which ACT can be carried out, namely with TIL, chimeric antigen receptor T cells (CAR-T), or T-cell receptor transduced T cells. Each of these methods is a highly personalized therapy that uses a patient's own immune cells to target their cancer, but only TIL ACT requires involvement of a surgeon in the treatment regimen.

The consultant surgeon plays an integral role on the treatment team for patients receiving TIL ACT because the T cells in the infusion product are derived from a surgical specimen. Working closely with the primary treating oncologist, the surgeon should be involved early when TIL ACT is considered as a treatment option because the eligibility for TIL ACT may not align with the fitness of the patient for the operating room. The morbidity of the proposed metastasectomy is of paramount importance in the surgical decision-making process because the intent of the operation is nontherapeutic and therefore all efforts should be made to eliminate risk by not undertaking a complex operation. Tumor-bearing lymph nodes, subcutaneous metastases, small peripheral lung metastases, and superficial liver metastases are the most appropriate lesions to target with a surgical resection for TIL expansion.[77,78] In the latter two scenarios, all efforts should be made to conduct the operation in a minimally invasive fashion (ie, VATS, laparoscopic, or robotic-assisted). The patient needs to recover completely from the operation during the relatively short manufacturing time—from 21 to 42 days, depending on the specific process—to receive lymphodepleting chemotherapy regimen and post-infusion IL-2.

TIL ACT for the treatment of patients with metastatic melanoma was piloted and initially described in the 1980s by Rosenberg and colleagues at the Surgery Branch of the National Cancer Institute (NCI). They illustrated the specific tumor-lysis capabilities of autologous TIL and their promise as a personalized therapy after in vitro expansion and reinfusion to the patient.[79,80] Preliminary results from a Phase I study published in 1988 showed a 55% ORR in patients with metastatic melanoma who received TIL in combination with IL-2, after a cyclophosphamide lymphodepletion regimen, compared with 15% in patients treated with cyclophosphamide and IL-2 alone.[80] Of note, the implementation of lymphodepletion before TIL infusion is necessary for durable responses as it eliminates regulatory T cells and competition for homeostatic cytokines.[81] Subsequent studies evaluating the efficacy of TIL in the treatment of metastatic melanoma were carried out at multiple institutions which demonstrated durable objective responses ranging from 38% to 72%.[82–91] A recent retrospective analysis of 226 patients with metastatic melanoma who were treated with TIL at the NCI demonstrated an ORR of 51% with a complete response rate of 22%.[92]

Although response rates were demonstrated to be higher in patients with treatment naïve melanoma, particularly in the case of prior anti-PD-1 therapy, patients with anti-PD-1 refractory disease were still observed to have ORR of 24% to 26% to TIL therapy.[92,93] These findings are of particular importance as primary and acquired resistance to immune checkpoint blockade leaves up to two-thirds of patients in need of additional therapy.[94] The utility of TIL therapy as a salvage therapy has been further demonstrated in a phase II open-label, multicenter study designed and sponsored by Iovance Biotherapeutics, Inc.[95] In this trial, 66 patients with unresectable or metastatic melanoma (stage IIIC or IV) with progressive disease on ICB were treated with lifileucel, an autologous, centrally manufactured TIL product, in combination with a lymphodepletion regimen and IL-2. The ORR was noted to be 36% with a disease control rate of 80% and a 1-year DOR rate of 69%. Similar results were reported from the full analysis set which included four cohorts composed of 153 patients treated with lifileucel; the ORR was 31.4% with 41.7% of responses maintained for ≥18 months.[96] These results led Iovance Biotherapeutics, Inc to submit a

Biologics License Application to the FDA in March 2023. The FDA has since granted lifileucel priority review with a target action date set for February 2024.

SUMMARY

Precision therapy based on the patient-specific genomic alterations of solid tumors has produced meaningful improvements in the treatment of advanced cancer over the past decade. This is especially true for patients with stage III and stage IV melanoma. Many of these successful treatments leverage the innate immunogenicity or the shared driver mutations of cutaneous melanoma. Effective precision therapy can be used in the perioperative period for patients with locally advanced disease and result in the conversion to resectable disease, thereby rendering a patient tumor-free. The toxicity of these treatments is not insignificant and can present in unique fashion relative to conventional cytotoxic chemotherapy regimens, requiring hyperacuity in the perioperative period. The role of the surgeon in the management of advanced melanoma has changed dramatically in the context of these new treatments where the timing, extent, and even candidacy for surgical resection are now more fluid than ever. Close collaboration among a multidisciplinary team as genomic-based treatment choices are made is absolutely essential to the safe and effective treatment of these patients.

DISCLOSURE

GMB has sponsored research agreements through her institution with: Olink Proteomics, Teiko Bio, InterVenn Biosciences, Palleon Pharmaceuticals. She served on advisory boards for: Iovance, Merck, Nektar Therapeutics, Novartis, and Ankyra Therapeutics. She consults for: Merck, InterVenn Biosciences, Iovance, and Ankyra Therapeutics. She holds equity in Ankyra Therapeutics.

REFERENCES

1. Yang AS, Chapman PB. The History and Future of Chemotherapy for Melanoma. 2009.
2. Atkins MB, Lotze MT, Dutcher JP, et al. High-dose recombinant interleukin 2 therapy for patients with metastatic melanoma: Analysis of 270 patients treated between 1985 and 1993. J Clin Oncol 1999;17(7). https://doi.org/10.1200/jco.1999.17.7.2105.
3. Ascierto PA, Kirkwood JM, Grob JJ, et al. The role of BRAF V600 mutation in melanoma. 2012.
4. Cantwell-Dorris ER, O'Leary JJ, Sheils OM. BRAFV600E: Implications for carcinogenesis and molecular therapy. Published online 2011.
5. Flaherty KT, Puzanov I, Kim KB, et al. Inhibition of Mutated, Activated BRAF in Metastatic Melanoma. N Engl J Med 2010;363(9). https://doi.org/10.1056/nejmoa1002011.
6. Ribas A, Kim KB, Schuchter LM, et al. BRIM-2: An open-label, multicenter phase II study of vemurafenib in previously treated patients with BRAF V600E mutation-positive metastatic melanoma. J Clin Oncol 2011;29(15_suppl). https://doi.org/10.1200/jco.2011.29.15_suppl.8509.
7. Chapman PB, Hauschild A, Robert C, et al. Improved Survival with Vemurafenib in Melanoma with BRAF V600E Mutation. N Engl J Med 2011;364(26). https://doi.org/10.1056/nejmoa1103782.
8. Kefford R, Arkenau H, Brown MP, et al. Phase I/II study of GSK2118436, a selective inhibitor of oncogenic mutant BRAF kinase, in patients with metastatic

melanoma and other solid tumors. J Clin Oncol 2010;28(15_suppl). https://doi.org/10.1200/jco.2010.28.15_suppl.8503.

9. Trefzer U, Minor D, Ribas A, et al. BREAK-2: a phase IIA trial of the selective BRAF kinase inhibitor GSK2118436 in patients with BRAF mutation-positive (V600E/K) metastatic melanoma. Pigment Cell Res 2011;24(abstr. LBA1-1):1020.

10. Hauschild A, Grob JJ, Demidov LV, et al. Dabrafenib in BRAF-mutated metastatic melanoma: A multicentre, open-label, phase 3 randomised controlled trial. Lancet 2012;(9839):380. https://doi.org/10.1016/S0140-6736(12)60868-X.

11. Nazarian R, Shi H, Wang Q, et al. Melanomas acquire resistance to B-RAF(V600E) inhibition by RTK or N-RAS upregulation. Nature 2010;468(7326). https://doi.org/10.1038/nature09626.

12. Shi H, Hugo W, Kong X, et al. Acquired resistance and clonal evolution in melanoma during BRAF inhibitor therapy. Cancer Discov 2014;4(1). https://doi.org/10.1158/2159-8290.CD-13-0642.

13. Wagle N, Emery C, Berger MF, et al. Dissecting therapeutic resistance to RAF inhibition in melanoma by tumor genomic profiling. J Clin Oncol 2011;29(22). https://doi.org/10.1200/JCO.2010.33.2312.

14. Poulikakos PI, Persaud Y, Janakiraman M, et al. RAF inhibitor resistance is mediated by dimerization of aberrantly spliced BRAF(V600E). Nature 2011;(7377):480. https://doi.org/10.1038/nature10662.

15. Chapman PB, Robert C, Larkin J, et al. Vemurafenib in patients with BRAFV600 mutation-positive metastatic melanoma: Final overall survival results of the randomized BRIM-3 study. Ann Oncol 2017;28(10). https://doi.org/10.1093/annonc/mdx339.

16. Hauschild A, Ascierto PA, Schadendorf D, et al. Long-term outcomes in patients with BRAF V600-mutant metastatic melanoma receiving dabrafenib monotherapy: Analysis from phase 2 and 3 clinical trials. European Journal of Cancer 2020;125. https://doi.org/10.1016/j.ejca.2019.10.033.

17. Kim KB, Kefford R, Pavlick AC, et al. Phase II study of the MEK1/MEK2 inhibitor trametinib in patients with metastatic BRAF-mutant cutaneous melanoma previously treated with or without a BRAF inhibitor. J Clin Oncol 2013;31(4). https://doi.org/10.1200/JCO.2012.43.5966.

18. Flaherty KT, Robert C, Hersey P, et al. Improved Survival with MEK Inhibition in BRAF-Mutated Melanoma. N Engl J Med 2012;367(2). https://doi.org/10.1056/nejmoa1203421.

19. Flaherty KT, Infante JR, Daud A, et al. Combined BRAF and MEK Inhibition in Melanoma with BRAF V600 Mutations. N Engl J Med 2012;367(18). https://doi.org/10.1056/nejmoa1210093.

20. Larkin J, Ascierto PA, Dréno B, et al. Combined Vemurafenib and Cobimetinib in BRAF -Mutated Melanoma. N Engl J Med 2014;(20):371. https://doi.org/10.1056/nejmoa1408868.

21. Ascierto PA, McArthur GA, Dréno B, et al. Cobimetinib combined with vemurafenib in advanced BRAFV600-mutant melanoma (coBRIM): updated efficacy results from a randomised, double-blind, phase 3 trial. Lancet Oncol 2016;17(9). https://doi.org/10.1016/S1470-2045(16)30122-X.

22. Ascierto PA, Dreno B, Larkin J, et al. 5-year outcomes with cobimetinib plus vemurafenib in BRAFV600 mutation⫫positive advanced melanoma: Extended follow-up of the coBRIM study. Clin Cancer Res 2021;27(19). https://doi.org/10.1158/1078-0432.CCR-21-0809.

23. Long GV, Stroyakovskiy D, Gogas H, et al. Dabrafenib and trametinib versus dabrafenib and placebo for Val600 BRAF-mutant melanoma: A multicentre, double-

blind, phase 3 randomised controlled trial. Lancet 2015;(9992):386. https://doi.org/10.1016/S0140-6736(15)60898-4.

24. Robert C, Karaszewska B, Schachter J, et al. Improved Overall Survival in Melanoma with Combined Dabrafenib and Trametinib. N Engl J Med 2015;372(1). https://doi.org/10.1056/nejmoa1412690.

25. Curtin JA, Busam K, Pinkel D, et al. Somatic activation of KIT in distinct subtypes of melanoma. J Clin Oncol 2006;24(26):4340–6.

26. Delyon J, Chevret S, Jouary T, et al. STAT3 Mediates Nilotinib Response in KIT-Altered Melanoma: A Phase II Multicenter Trial of the French Skin Cancer Network. J Invest Dermatol 2018;138(1):58–67.

27. Kalinsky K, Lee S, Rubin KM, et al. A phase 2 trial of dasatinib in patients with locally advanced or stage IV mucosal, acral, or vulvovaginal melanoma: A trial of the ECOG-ACRIN Cancer Research Group (E2607). Cancer 2017;123(14):2688–97.

28. Decoster L, Vande Broek I, Neyns B, et al. Biomarker Analysis in a Phase II Study of Sunitinib in Patients with Advanced Melanoma. Anticancer Res 2015;35(12):6893–9. https://www.ncbi.nlm.nih.gov/pubmed/26637913.

29. Johnson DB, Puzanov I. Treatment of NRAS-mutant melanoma. Curr Treat Options Oncol 2015;16(4):15.

30. Bendell J, Andre V, Ho A, et al. Phase I Study of LY2940680, a Smo Antagonist, in Patients with Advanced Cancer Including Treatment-Naïve and Previously Treated Basal Cell Carcinoma. Clin Cancer Res 2018;24(9):2082–91.

31. Migden MR, Rischin D, Schmults CD, et al. PD-1 Blockade with Cemiplimab in Advanced Cutaneous Squamous-Cell Carcinoma. N Engl J Med 2018;379(4):341–51.

32. Hughes BGM, Munoz-Couselo E, Mortier L, et al. Pembrolizumab for locally advanced and recurrent/metastatic cutaneous squamous cell carcinoma (KEYNOTE-629 study): an open-label, nonrandomized, multicenter, phase II trial. Ann Oncol 2021;32(10):1276–85.

33. Ugurel S, Mentzel T, Utikal J, et al. Neoadjuvant Imatinib in Advanced Primary or Locally Recurrent Dermatofibrosarcoma Protuberans: A Multicenter Phase II De-COG Trial with Long- term Follow-up. Clin Cancer Res 2014;20(2):499–510. https://doi.org/10.1158/1078-0432.CCR-13-1411.

34. Stacchiotti A, Pantaleo MA, Negri T, et al. Efficacy and Biological Activity of Imatinib in Metastatic Dermatofibrosarcoma Protuberans(DFSP). Clin Cancer Res 2016 Feb 15;22(4):837–46. Epub 2015 Aug 10.

35. Han Y, Liu D, Li L. PD-1/PD-L1 pathway: current researches in cancer. Am J Cancer Res 2020;10(3).

36. Pardoll DM. The blockade of immune checkpoints in cancer immunotherapy. Nat Rev Cancer 2012;12(4):252–64.

37. Schadendorf D, Hodi FS, Robert C, et al. Pooled analysis of long-term survival data from phase II and phase III trials of ipilimumab in unresectable or metastatic melanoma. J Clin Oncol 2015;33(17). https://doi.org/10.1200/JCO.2014.56.2736.

38. Zhao B, Zhao H, Zhao J. Efficacy of PD-1/PD-L1 blockade monotherapy in clinical trials. Therapeutic Advances in Medical Oncology 2020;12. https://doi.org/10.1177/1758835920937612.

39. Robert C, Long GV, Brady B, et al. Nivolumab in Previously Untreated Melanoma without BRAF Mutation. N Engl J Med 2015;372(4). https://doi.org/10.1056/nejmoa1412082.

40. Weber JS, D'Angelo SP, Minor D, et al. Nivolumab versus chemotherapy in patients with advanced melanoma who progressed after anti-CTLA-4 treatment

(CheckMate 037): A randomised, controlled, open-label, phase 3 trial. Lancet Oncol 2015;16(4). https://doi.org/10.1016/S1470-2045(15)70076-8.

41. Larkin J, Minor D, D'Angelo S, et al. Overall survival in patients with advanced melanoma who received nivolumab versus investigator's choice chemotherapy in CheckMate 037: A Randomized, Controlled, Open-Label Phase III Trial. J Clin Oncol 2018;36:383–90. https://doi.org/10.1200/JCO.2016.71.8023. American Society of Clinical Oncology.

42. Ribas A, Puzanov I, Dummer R, et al. Pembrolizumab versus investigator-choice chemotherapy for ipilimumab-refractory melanoma (KEYNOTE-002): A randomised, controlled, phase 2 trial. Lancet Oncol 2015;16(8). https://doi.org/10.1016/S1470-2045(15)00083-2.

43. Hamid O, Puzanov I, Dummer R, et al. Final overall survival for KEYNOTE-002: pembrolizumab (pembro) versus investigator-choice chemotherapy (chemo) for ipilimumab (ipi)-refractory melanoma. Ann Oncol 2016;27. https://doi.org/10.1093/annonc/mdw379.02.

44. Robert C, Schachter J, Long GV, et al. Pembrolizumab versus Ipilimumab in Advanced Melanoma. N Engl J Med 2015;372(26). https://doi.org/10.1056/nejmoa1503093.

45. Schachter J, Ribas A, Long GV, et al. Pembrolizumab versus ipilimumab for advanced melanoma: final overall survival results of a multicentre, randomised, open-label phase 3 study (KEYNOTE-006). Lancet 2017;390(10105). https://doi.org/10.1016/S0140-6736(17)31601-X.

46. Wolchok JD, Chiarion-Sileni V, Gonzalez R, et al. Long-Term Outcomes With Nivolumab Plus Ipilimumab or Nivolumab Alone Versus Ipilimumab in Patients With Advanced Melanoma. J Clin Oncol 2022;40(2). https://doi.org/10.1200/JCO.21.02229.

47. Tawbi HA, Schadendorf D, Lipson EJ, et al. Relatlimab and Nivolumab versus Nivolumab in Untreated Advanced Melanoma. N Engl J Med 2022;386(1). https://doi.org/10.1056/nejmoa2109970.

48. Wolchok JD, Chiarion-Sileni V, Gonzalez R, et al. Overall Survival with Combined Nivolumab and Ipilimumab in Advanced Melanoma. N Engl J Med 2017;377(14). https://doi.org/10.1056/nejmoa1709684.

49. Eggermont AMM, Chiarion-Sileni V, Grob JJ, et al. Adjuvant ipilimumab versus placebo after complete resection of high-risk stage III melanoma (EORTC 18071): A randomised, double-blind, phase 3 trial. Lancet Oncol 2015;16(5). https://doi.org/10.1016/S1470-2045(15)70122-1.

50. Eggermont AMM, Chiarion-Sileni V, Grob JJ, et al. Adjuvant ipilimumab versus placebo after complete resection of stage III melanoma: long-term follow-up results of the European Organisation for Research and Treatment of Cancer 18071 double-blind phase 3 randomised trial. European Journal of Cancer 2019;119. https://doi.org/10.1016/j.ejca.2019.07.001.

51. Eggermont AMM, Blank CU, Mandala M, et al. Adjuvant Pembrolizumab versus Placebo in Resected Stage III Melanoma. N Engl J Med 2018;378(19). https://doi.org/10.1056/nejmoa1802357.

52. Eggermont AMM, Blank CU, Mandalà M, et al. Adjuvant pembrolizumab versus placebo in resected stage III melanoma (EORTC 1325-MG/KEYNOTE-054): distant metastasis-free survival results from a double-blind, randomised, controlled, phase 3 trial. Lancet Oncol 2021;22(5). https://doi.org/10.1016/S1470-2045(21)00065-6.

53. Weber J, Mandala M, Del Vecchio M, et al. Adjuvant Nivolumab versus Ipilimumab in Resected Stage III or IV Melanoma. N Engl J Med 2017;377(19). https://doi.org/10.1056/nejmoa1709030.

54. Witt RG, Erstad DJ, Wargo JA. Neoadjuvant therapy for melanoma: rationale for neoadjuvant therapy and pivotal clinical trials. Ther Adv Med Oncol 2022. https://doi.org/10.1177/17588359221083052.

55. Blank CU, Rozeman EA, Fanchi LF, et al. Neoadjuvant versus adjuvant ipilimumab plus nivolumab in macroscopic stage III melanoma. Nat Med 2018;24(11): 1655–61.

56. Rozeman EA, Menzies AM, van Akkooi ACJ, et al. Identification of the optimal combination dosing schedule of neoadjuvant ipilimumab plus nivolumab in macroscopic stage III melanoma (OpACIN-neo): a multicentre, phase 2, randomised, controlled trial. Lancet Oncol 2019;20(7). https://doi.org/10.1016/S1470-2045(19)30151-2.

57. Patel SP, Othus M, Chen Y, et al. Neoadjuvant–Adjuvant or Adjuvant-Only Pembrolizumab in Advanced Melanoma. N Engl J Med 2023;388(9). https://doi.org/10.1056/nejmoa2211437.

58. Brahmer JR, Abu-Sbeih H, Ascierto PA, et al. Society for immunotherapy of cancer (sitc) clinical practice guideline on immune checkpoint inhibitor-related adverse events. Journal for ImmunoTherapy of Cancer 2021;9(6). https://doi.org/10.1136/jitc-2021-002435.

59. Thompson JA, Schneider BJ, Brahmer J, et al. Management of Immunotherapy-Related Toxicities, Version 1.2022, NCCN Clinical Practice Guidelines in Oncology. J Natl Compr Cancer Netw 2022;20(4). https://doi.org/10.6004/jnccn.2022.0020.

60. Blank CU, Reijers ILM, Saw RPM, et al. Survival data of PRADO: A phase 2 study of personalized response-driven surgery and adjuvant therapy after neoadjuvant ipilimumab (IPI) and nivolumab (NIVO) in resectable stage III melanoma. J Clin Oncol 2022;40(16_suppl). https://doi.org/10.1200/jco.2022.40.16_suppl.9501.

61. Snyder A, Makarov V, Merghoub T, et al. Genetic Basis for Clinical Response to CTLA-4 Blockade in Melanoma. N Engl J Med 2014;371(23). https://doi.org/10.1056/nejmoa1406498.

62. Van Allen EM, Miao D, Schilling B, et al. Genomic correlates of response to CTLA-4 blockade in metastatic melanoma. Science 2015;350(6257). https://doi.org/10.1126/science.aad0095.

63. Osipov A, Lim SJ, Popovic A, et al. Tumor Mutational Burden, Toxicity, and Response of Immune Checkpoint Inhibitors Targeting PD(L)1, CTLA-4, and Combination: A Meta-regression Analysis. Clin Cancer Res 2020;26(18). https://doi.org/10.1158/1078-0432.CCR-20-0458.

64. Campesato LF, Barroso-Sousa R, Jimenez L, et al. Comprehensive cancer-gene panels can be used to estimate mutational load and predict clinical benefit to PD-1 blockade in clinical practice. Oncotarget 2015;6(33). https://doi.org/10.18632/oncotarget.5950.

65. Ayers M, Lunceford J, Nebozhyn M, et al. IFN-γ-related mRNA profile predicts clinical response to PD-1 blockade. J Clin Invest 2017;127(8). https://doi.org/10.1172/JCI91190.

66. Rozeman EA, Hoefsmit EP, Reijers ILM, et al. Survival and biomarker analyses from the OpACIN-neo and OpACIN neoadjuvant immunotherapy trials in stage III melanoma. Nat Med 2021;27(2). https://doi.org/10.1038/s41591-020-01211-7.

67. Reijers ILM, Rao D, Versluis JM, et al. IFN-γ signature enables selection of neo-adjuvant treatment in patients with stage III melanoma. J Exp Med 2023;(5):220. https://doi.org/10.1084/jem.20221952.

68. Bai X, Hu J, Betof Warner A, et al. Early Use of High-Dose Glucocorticoid for the Management of irAE Is Associated with Poorer Survival in Patients with Advanced Melanoma Treated with Anti-PD-1 Monotherapy. Clin Cancer Res 2021;27(21): 5993–6000.

69. Lim SY, Lee JH, Gide TN, et al. Circulating cytokines predict immune-related toxicity in melanoma patients receiving anti-PD-1–based immunotherapy. Clin Cancer Res 2019;25(5). https://doi.org/10.1158/1078-0432.CCR-18-2795.

70. Lozano AX, Chaudhuri AA, Nene A, et al. T cell characteristics associated with toxicity to immune checkpoint blockade in patients with melanoma. Nat Med 2022;28(2). https://doi.org/10.1038/s41591-021-01623-z.

71. Nuñez NG, Berner F, Friebel E, et al. Immune signatures predict development of autoimmune toxicity in patients with cancer treated with immune checkpoint inhibitors. Med 2023;4(2). https://doi.org/10.1016/j.medj.2022.12.007.

72. Shen L, Brown JR, Johnston SA, et al. Predicting response and toxicity to immune checkpoint inhibitors in lung cancer using antibodies to frameshift neoantigens. J Transl Med 2023;21(1). https://doi.org/10.1186/s12967-023-04172-w.

73. Les I, Martínez M, Pérez-Francisco I, et al. Predictive Biomarkers for Checkpoint Inhibitor Immune-Related Adverse Events. Cancer (Basal) 2023. https://doi.org/10.3390/cancers15051629.

74. Gutzmer R, Stroyakovskiy D, Gogas H, et al. Atezolizumab, vemurafenib, and cobimetinib as first-line treatment for unresectable advanced BRAFV600 mutation-positive melanoma (IMspire150): primary analysis of the randomised, double-blind, placebo-controlled, phase 3 trial. Lancet 2020;395(10240). https://doi.org/10.1016/S0140-6736(20)30934-X.

75. Ascierto PA, Stroyakovskiy D, Gogas H, et al. Overall survival with first-line atezolizumab in combination with vemurafenib and cobimetinib in BRAFV600 mutation-positive advanced melanoma (IMspire150): second interim analysis of a multicentre, randomised, phase 3 study. Lancet Oncol 2023;24(1). https://doi.org/10.1016/S1470-2045(22)00687-8.

76. Ferrucci PF, Di Giacomo AM, Del Vecchio M, et al. KEYNOTE-022 part 3: A randomized, double-blind, phase 2 study of pembrolizumab, dabrafenib, and trametinib in BRAF-mutant melanoma. Journal for ImmunoTherapy of Cancer 2020; 8(2). https://doi.org/10.1136/jitc-2020-001806.

77. Crompton JG, Klemen N, Kammula US. Metastasectomy for Tumor-Infiltrating Lymphocytes: An Emerging Operative Indication in Surgical Oncology. Ann Surg Oncol 2018;25(2). https://doi.org/10.1245/s10434-017-6266-8.

78. Mullinax JE, Egger ME, McCarter M, et al. Surgical Considerations for Tumor Tissue Procurement to Obtain Tumor-Infiltrating Lymphocytes for Adoptive Cell Therapy. Cancer J 2022.

79. Muul LM, Spiess PJ, Director EP, et al. Identification of specific cytolytic immune responses against autologous tumor in humans bearing malignant melanoma. J Immunol 1987;138(3). https://doi.org/10.4049/jimmunol.138.3.989.

80. Rosenberg SA, Packard BS, Aebersold PM, et al. Use of tumor-infiltrating lymphocytes and interleukin-2 in the immunotherapy of patients with metastatic melanoma. A preliminary report [see comments]. N Engl J Med 1988;319(25).

81. Gattinoni L, Finkelstein SE, Klebanoff CA, et al. Removal of homeostatic cytokine sinks by lymphodepletion enhances the efficacy of adoptively transferred tumor-

specific CD8+ T cells. J Exp Med 2005;202(7). https://doi.org/10.1084/jem.20050732.

82. Kradin RL, Lazarus DS, Dubinett SM, et al. Tumour-infiltrating lymphocytes and interleukin-2 in treatment of advanced cancer. Lancet 1989. https://doi.org/10.1016/S0140-6736(89)91609-7.

83. Rosenberg SA, Yannelli JR, Yang JC, et al. Treatment of patients with metastatic melanoma with autologous tumor-infiltrating lymphocytes and interleukin 2. J Natl Cancer Inst 1994. https://doi.org/10.1093/jnci/86.15.1159.

84. Dudley ME, Wunderlich JR, Yang JC, et al. A Phase I Study of Nonmyeloablative Chemotherapy and Adoptive Transfer of Autologous Tumor Antigen-Specific T Lymphocytes in Patients With Metastatic Melanoma. J Immunother 2002. https://doi.org/10.1097/00002371-200205000-00007.

85. Dudley ME, Wunderlich JR, Yang JC, et al. Adoptive cell transfer therapy following non-myeloablative but lymphodepleting chemotherapy for the treatment of patients with refractory metastatic melanoma. J Clin Oncol 2005. https://doi.org/10.1200/JCO.2005.00.240.

86. Dudley ME, Yang JC, Sherry R, et al. Adoptive cell therapy for patients with metastatic melanoma: Evaluation of intensive myeloablative chemoradiation preparative regimens. J Clin Oncol 2008;26(32). https://doi.org/10.1200/JCO.2008.16.5449.

87. Rosenberg SA, Yang JC, Sherry RM, et al. Durable complete responses in heavily pretreated patients with metastatic melanoma using T-cell transfer immunotherapy. Clin Cancer Res 2011. https://doi.org/10.1158/1078-0432.CCR-11-0116.

88. Pilon-Thomas S, Kuhn L, Ellwanger S, et al. Efficacy of adoptive cell transfer of tumor-infiltrating lymphocytes after lymphopenia induction for metastatic melanoma. J Immunother 2012. https://doi.org/10.1097/CJI.0b013e31826e8f5f.

89. Besser MJ, Shapira-Frommer R, Itzhaki O, et al. Adoptive transfer of tumor-infiltrating lymphocytes in patients with metastatic melanoma: Intent-to-treat analysis and efficacy after failure to prior immunotherapies. Clin Cancer Res 2013. https://doi.org/10.1158/1078-0432.CCR-13-0380.

90. Goff SL, Dudley ME, Citrin DE, et al. Randomized, prospective evaluation comparing intensity of lymphodepletion before adoptive transfer of tumor-infiltrating lymphocytes for patients with metastatic melanoma. J Clin Oncol 2016. https://doi.org/10.1200/JCO.2016.66.7220.

91. Sarnaik A, Khushalani NI, Chesney JA, et al. Safety and efficacy of cryopreserved autologous tumor infiltrating lymphocyte therapy (LN-144, lifileucel) in advanced metastatic melanoma patients who progressed on multiple prior therapies including anti-PD-1. J Clin Oncol 2019;37(15_suppl). https://doi.org/10.1200/jco.2019.37.15_suppl.2518.

92. Seitter SJ, Sherry RM, Yang JC, et al. Impact of prior treatment on the efficacy of adoptive transfer of tumor-infiltrating lymphocytes in patients with metastatic melanoma. Clin Cancer Res 2021;27(19). https://doi.org/10.1158/1078-0432.ccr-21-1171.

93. Levi ST, Copeland AR, Nah S, et al. Neoantigen Identification and Response to Adoptive Cell Transfer in Anti–PD-1 Naïve and Experienced Patients with Metastatic Melanoma. Clin Cancer Res 2022;28(14). https://doi.org/10.1158/1078-0432.CCR-21-4499.

94. Gide TN, Wilmott JS, Scolyer RA, et al. Primary and acquired resistance to immune checkpoint inhibitors in metastatic melanoma. Clin Cancer Res 2018.

95. Sarnaik AA, Hamid O, Khushalani NI, et al. Lifileucel, a Tumor-Infiltrating Lympho-cyte Therapy, in Metastatic Melanoma. J Clin Oncol 2021;39(24). https://doi.org/10.1200/JCO.21.00612.

96. Chesney J, Lewis KD, Kluger H, et al. Efficacy and safety of lifileucel, a one-time autologous tumor-infiltrating lymphocyte (TIL) cell therapy, in patients with advanced melanoma after progression on immune checkpoint inhibitors and tar-geted therapies: pooled analysis of consecutive cohorts of the C-144-01 study. Journal for immunotherapy of cancer 2022;10(12). https://doi.org/10.1136/jitc-2022-005755.

Precision Oncology in Soft Tissue Sarcomas and Gastrointestinal Stromal Tumors

Adam M. Fontebasso, MD, PhD[a,b,c,1], Jeffrey D. Rytlewski, MD[d,1], Jean-Yves Blay, MD, PhD[e], Rebecca A. Gladdy, MD, PhD[a,b,c], Breelyn A. Wilky, MD[d,*]

KEYWORDS

- Gastrointestinal stromal tumor • Precision medicine • Precision oncology • Sarcoma
- Tumor biology

KEY POINTS

- Precision oncology can help tailor therapy for individual sarcoma patients.
- Molecular profiling of soft tissue sarcoma (STS) and gastrointestinal stromal tumor (GIST) may lead to better treatment outcomes.
- The interplay between precision oncology and surgery in a multidisciplinary setting is critical to improving outcomes of patients with STS and GIST.

INTRODUCTION

Sarcomas represent a diverse group of mesenchymal tumors with highly variable biologic behavior. Although they are rare entities and represent only 1% of adult cancers, the World Health Organization has described more than 100 histologic types of sarcoma,[1] making pathologic classification, diagnosis, and prognostication challenging. Soft tissue sarcomas (STSs) can occur throughout the body. This adds to the clinical complexity of treating these patients with unique surgical considerations based on anatomy as well as accentuates the importance for multidisciplinary care. In fact, distinct genetic fusions and molecular alterations have greatly aided in the diagnosis

[a] Division of Surgical Oncology, Department of Surgery, University of Toronto, 700 University Avenue, 7th Floor, Ontario Power Generation Building, Toronto, Ontario, Canada; [b] Department of Surgery, Mount Sinai Hospital, Sinai Health Systems, 600 University Avenue Room 6-445.10 Surgery, Toronto, Ontario M5G 1X5, Canada; [c] Princess Margaret Cancer Centre, University Health Network, Toronto, Ontario, Canada; [d] University of Colorado School of Medicine, 12801 East 17th Avenue, Mailstop 8117, Aurora, CO 80045, USA; [e] Centre Léon Bérard, 28, rue Laennec, 69373 cedex 08. Lyon, France
[1] These authors contributed equally to this work.
* Corresponding author. 12801 East 17th Avenue, Mailstop 8117, Aurora, CO 80045.
E-mail address: Breelyn.Wilky@cuanschutz.edu

Surg Oncol Clin N Am 33 (2024) 387–408
https://doi.org/10.1016/j.soc.2023.12.018
1055-3207/24/© 2024 Elsevier Inc. All rights reserved.
surgonc.theclinics.com

and treatment of certain types of STS.[2] In many cases, identification of these molecular alterations is linked to a precision oncology approach using molecularly matched targeted therapies.[2]

Overall, understanding the biologic behavior of sarcomas is paramount to harmonize the optimal management of these rare tumors across specialties. In this review, the authors focus on key examples of molecular drivers in STS and gastrointestinal stromal tumor (GIST) that have helped guide clinical management in the field to date and have facilitated a precision medicine with targeted therapies in this complex family of tumors.

Soft Tissue Sarcomas

Expert pathologic diagnosis is central to sarcoma care

Given the rarity and heterogeneity of STS, initial determination of the histologic type is critical and requires experienced pathologists. In fact, one study showed that the initial diagnosis can overturned in up to 40% of cases following expert review.[3] One example of how accurate pathologic classification directly impacts clinical decision-making is for retroperitoneal sarcoma (RPS), where distinct patterns of recurrence occur across diverse STS types.[4] Subgroup analysis from the multi-institutional STRASS trial showed that preoperative radiotherapy was associated with improved abdominal recurrence-free survival (ARFS), but only in well-differentiated liposarcoma (WDLPS).[5] These results were supported by the STREXIT trial for patients treated at STRASS centers, but not enrolled in STRASS. In this study, better ARFS was seen following preoperative radiotherapy for patients with primary WDLPS and grade 1 to 2 dedifferentiated liposarcoma (DDLPS).[6] The ongoing STRASS2 trial aims to expand these findings, by enrolling patients with high-grade DDLPS and leiomyosarcoma (LMS), histologies that demonstrate elevated risk for metastatic disease. In this study, patients will be randomized to surgery alone or preoperative chemotherapy followed by surgery.[7] Taken together, with more than 100 histologic types of sarcoma that can present with three different tumor grades, the heterogeneity of these cancers is vast. Therefore, optimal care requires proper diagnosis to determine the best treatment approach.

Principles of soft tissue sarcoma management

Surgical resection is the cornerstone of curative intent treatment for patients with localized STS.[8,9] Radiation therapy is considered when assessing the individual patient risk of local recurrence.[10] Common factors that drive local recurrence risk and the use of radiation therapy include anatomic site, histologic type, tumor grade, and margin-positive resection.[11] Importantly, certain sarcoma types are more chemosensitive with standard of care treatment including traditional cytotoxic chemotherapy before local surgical control. Examples include Ewing sarcoma family tumors, rhabdomyosarcomas, osteosarcomas, and synovial sarcomas.[12–15]

For localized primary extremity STS, only doxorubicin-containing regimens have data established in the adjuvant space, with modestly improved progression-free survival (PFS) and overall survival (OS) seen with doxorubicin/ifosfamide/mesna (AIM) to a greater degree than single-agent doxorubicin.[16–18] Subsequent studies have optimized the number of cycles and patient populations benefiting most from adjuvant regimens.[19,20] Preoperatively, chemotherapy may also be used in the neoadjuvant setting to improve the likelihood of an R0 resection following tumor shrinkage and necrosis.[21] Additional benefits of neoadjuvant therapy include early targeting of micro-metastatic disease and in vivo assessment of chemotherapy efficacy. This was seen in a study by Delaney and colleagues who reported a distant metastasis-free survival improvement in those who received neoadjuvant chemotherapy.[22] Overall, there remains a proven role for systemic treatment in patients with STS.

However, we are beginning to see a shift from this paradigm. In contrast to the one-size-fits-all approach of prior studies of adjuvant chemotherapy, more contemporary studies have now created a better precision medicine approach to further selection of patients most likely to benefit from treatment. The "Sarculator" nomogram incorporates age, tumor size, grade, and histologic type to predict 5- and 10-year rates of distant metastasis and OS with resection alone.[23] Application of the nomogram to the EORTC-STBSG 62931 study of more than 350 patients randomized to AIM versus observation revealed that the low-predicted OS group (10 year predicted OS $\leq$ 51%) achieved a 21.3% absolute risk reduction in OS at 8 years with AIM treatment.[24] Even though this should formally require prospective or real-world evidence confirmation to increase the level of evidence, extremity STS with intermediate or high risk of recurrence based on the predicted 10 year OS rates can now be more rationally stratified for likely benefit from chemotherapy. Additional attempts to customize chemotherapy for specific sarcoma types showed alternative regimens (gemcitabine/docetaxel for undifferentiated pleomorphic sarcoma [UPS], high-dose ifosfamide for synovial sarcoma, etoposide/ifosfamide for malignant peripheral nerve sheath tumor [MPNST], and gemcitabine/dacarbazine for LMS) were inferior to anthracycline–ifosfamide regimens, with the exception of myxoid liposarcoma which showed equivalent outcomes with trabectedin.[25] Unfortunately, these data have largely been confined to extremity sarcomas, with ongoing quandary about approaches for RPS. The aforementioned STRASS 2 trial (NCT04031677) will hopefully establish rationale for neoadjuvant chemotherapy in at least a subset of RPS patients. Ultimately, it has been through subsetting patients that we have begun to further improve care and will continue to identify novel treatments for patients. The authors describe the examples of soft tissue tumors and their evolving precision oncology treatment strategies in defined disease types in the following.

Key examples of treatment-changing paradigms from precision oncology

Desmoid fibromatosis. Desmoid fibromatosis (DF) is caused by either somatic *CTNNB1* mutations or germline *APC* gene mutations that drive Wnt/beta-catenin signaling. In recent years, the management guidelines have dramatically shifted for this benign, but locally invasive soft tissue tumor. International working group recommendations have now transitioned management largely to active surveillance and avoiding upfront surgical resection. For highly symptomatic patients as well as those patients with an immediate threat to life or limb who are not candidates for observation, medical therapy is now the primary approach.[26–28] This is due to the ability of DF to remain dormant or even regress. This was confirmed in a randomized phase 2 trial of sorafenib versus placebo where an objective response rate (ORR) of 20% was observed in the placebo arm. On the failure of active surveillance, surgical resection is preferred for sporadic DF of the abdominal wall, and medical therapy is preferred for sporadic DF in all other locations.[26] Imatinib, sorafenib, and pazopanib are tyrosine kinase inhibitors (TKIs) with activity in DF, with imatinib demonstrating a comparatively lower response rate compared with sorafenib and pazopanib.[29–31]

The Notch pathway intersects with the Wnt/beta-catenin pathway. Thus, Notch pathway gamma secretase inhibitors, specifically nirogacestat, are a newer treatment modality available to treat DF. A phase III international double-blinded study by Gounder and colleagues enrolled 142 progressing DF patients to either nirogacestat or placebo with the primary endpoint of PFS.[32] Results were favorable in the nirogacestat arm, with event-free survival (EFS) at 1 year (85% vs 53%) and 2 years

(76% vs 44%) demonstrating superiority of nirogacestat to placebo. Total events were not reached in the nirogacestat arm, and as such, the EFS endpoint was unable to be statistically assessed.[32] Nirogacestat is now approved by the US Food and Drug Administration. Overall, DF is a key example of the evolving relationship of surgery and medical therapy, both taking a second line to an active surveillance approach. Further, medical therapies have been shown to significantly impact PFS and as such the role of surgical resection is able to be reserved for only the most emergent circumstances.

Dedifferentiated liposarcomas. Liposarcomas exist on a spectrum from well-differentiated to dedifferentiated (Grades 1–3), characterized by a supernumerary ring and giant marker chromosomes that harbor mouse double minute 2 homolog (*MDM2*) and *CDK4* gene amplifications.[33] As with most sarcomas, the front-line approach to treatment involves surgical resection if possible. However, recurrence remains problematic with cumulative surgical risk and morbidity being important factors to consider. Because responses to anthracycline-based chemotherapy are poor, there is high unmet need for better outcomes with targeted therapies.

One emerging treatment approach for DDLPS is to inhibit the *CDK4* oncogene amplification, most commonly with the CDK4/6 inhibitors, palbociclib and abemaciclib. The single-arm phase II study performed by Dickson and colleagues reported a 12-week PFS of 66% and median PFS of 17.9 weeks for palbociclib; in the phase II single-arm study for abemaciclib, Dickson and colleagues reported a 12-week PFS of 76% and median PFS of 30.9 weeks.[34,35] Both of these trials lend credence to a role for CDK4/6 inhibitors in DDLPS, with abemaciclib being the more potent CDK4 inhibitor and possible more efficacious.[35] In fact, there has been a case report of a near pathologic complete response in a DDLPS patient treated with abemaciclib. Because further studies are warranted for this targeted approach, SARC41 is an ongoing phase 3 trial of abemaciclib versus placebo for progressing DDLPS (NCT04967521).

MDM2-targeted therapies seem to have similar promise. An initial trial of a first-generation MDM2 inhibitor demonstrated clinical benefit in the neoadjuvant setting.[36] Gounder and colleagues published an early study of milademetan, where median disease-free survival was 7.2 months.[37] Unfortunately, a phase III trial comparing milademetan to trabectedin did not meet the primary endpoint with median PFS of 3.6 months with milademetan compared with 2.2 months with trabectedin.[38] However, recent results from a phase 1 study of the MDM2 inhibitor brigimadlin showed an ORR of 19%, and disease control rate of 84.8% in 79 heavily treated DDLPS patients.[39,40] Thus, brigimadlin is being studied in several ongoing trials including BRIGHTLINE-1, which compares brigimadlin to doxorubicin in patients with inoperable DDLPS (NCT05118499).[41] Finally, another intriguing study combined the MDM2 inhibitor siremadlin and ribociclib, a CDK4/6 inhibitor, producing disease control in 41 of 74 (55.4%) patients (NCT NCT04116541).[42] Given the long-standing role of surgical resection in DDLPS, including repeated resections, these active agents will hopefully emerge as a strategy to downsize tumors or at least offer meaningful disease control between surgeries in the future.

Additional sarcomas and therapies. The examples above provide some perspective for the use of targeted therapies and precision medicine as a tool to develop personalized therapies for patients. **Table 1** depicts other key examples of driver genetic abnormalities, downstream protein targets, and corresponding therapies that are either approved or in late-stage clinical trials for non-GIST STS. **Table 2** summarizes the exciting early-phase studies investigating novel targets of interest.

Table 1
Selected examples of precision-matched targeted therapies for soft tissue sarcomas, bone sarcomas, and other soft tissue tumors

Sarcoma Histologic Subtype	Genetic Driver	Therapies
Dermatofibrosarcoma protuberans (including fibrosarcoma variants)	t(17;22) (fusion *COL1A1/PDGFB*) ➤ PDGF-B	Imatinib[43]
Alveolar soft part sarcoma	t(17;X) (fusion *ASPS1/TFE3*) ➤ VEGF and related mediators	**Atezolizumab,**[44] *anlotinib,*[45] cediranib,[46] sunitinib,[47] pazopanib,[48] axitinib/ pembrolizumab[49]
Perivascular epithelial cell tumor (PEComa)	TSC1/TSC2 mutations ➤ mTORCH1 activation	**Nab-sirolimus,**[50] temsirolimus[51]
Desmoid fibromatosis	NOTCH signaling	**Nirogacestat,**[32] *AL102*[52] Sorafenib[29]
Giant cell tumor of bone	RANK/RANK ligand overexpression	**Denosumab**[53]
Tenosynovial giant cell tumor (pigmented villonodular synovitis)	t(1;2) translocation (collagen/)*CSF1* ➤ CSF1	**Pexidartinib,***[54] vimseltinib,*[55] imatinib,[56] other CSF1 inhibitors
Inflammatory myofibroblastic tumor	ALK rearrangements, specific resistance mutations from lung cancer	Crizotinib,[57] alectinib,[58] brigatinib,[59] ceritinib,[60] lorlatinib[61]
Well-differentiated/dedifferentiated liposarcomas	*CDK4/MDM2* amplification	CDK4/6 inhibitor—Palbociclib,[34] *abemaciclib*[35] MDM2 inhibitor—*brigimadlin*[39]
Solitary fibrous tumor	*NAB2-STAT6* translocation ➤ VEGF	Temozolomide/bevacizumab,[62] pazopanib[63]
Epithelioid sarcoma	*SMARCB1/INI1* loss	**Tazemetostat**[64]
Chondrosarcomas	*IDH1/IDH2* mutations DR5 expression	Ivosidenib,[65] enasidenib[66] *INBRX-109 (DR5 agonist)*[67] pazopanib[68]
Ewing sarcoma	*EWS-FLI1* translocation DR5 expression	TK-216 (disrupts binding of fusion protein to RNA helicase A)
Synovial sarcoma	NY-ESO 1, MAGE-A4 expression ➤ Engineered T-cell receptor therapies	*Letetresgene-autoleucel,*[69] *afamitresgene-autoleucel*[70]

(continued on next page)

Table 1
(continued)

Sarcoma Histologic Subtype	Genetic Driver	Therapies
Metastasizing leiomyomata, uterine smooth muscle tumors of undetermined potential (STUMP), low-grade endometrial stromal sarcomas	Estrogen receptor (ER) expression	ER blockade, that is, tamoxifen, aromatase inhibitors, and so forth
Epithelioid hemangioendothelioma	WWTR1-CAMTA ▶ MEK upregulation, Hippo pathway	Trametinib[71]
Cutaneous angiosarcomas	UV signature, not always high TMB	Pembrolizumab,[72] ipilimumab/nivolumab[73]
Various subtypes including GIST, spindle cell neoplasms	*NTRK* fusions	**Entrectinib**,[74] **larotrectinib**[75]
Plexiform neurofibromas	*NF1* mutations	**Selumetinib**[76]
Various STS and bone sarcomas	High tumor mutational burden	**Pembrolizumab**[77]

Bolded agents are FDA-approved. Italicized agents are undergoing late-stage clinical trials.

Table 2
Selected examples of ongoing clinical trials using precision oncology in sarcoma

Target	Pharmaceutical Agent	Trial Number	Subtypes Included	Combined Therapy?
NGS informed FDA therapy	Multiple	NCT03784014	Any STS	No
		NCT05238831		No
KIT/PDGFRA	IDRX-42	NCT05489237	GIST	No
KIT/PDGFRA	NB003	NCT04936178	GIST	No
CDK4	Palbociclib	NCT03242382	CDK4-overexpressed sarcoma	No
DR5	IGM-8444	NCT04553692	Any sarcoma	No
DR5	INBRX-109	NCT03715933	Any sarcoma	Carboplatin/cisplatin
				Pemetrexed
				5-FU
				Irinotecan
				Temozolomide
SDHA/B/C/D	Temozolomide	NCT03556384	SDH-deficient GIST	No
Folate receptor A	ELU001	NCT05001282	Endometrial sarcomas	No
GSK-3B	9-ING-41	NCT03678883	Any sarcoma	No
HER2	Lapatinib	NCT01454479	Endometrial carcinosarcoma	Ixabepilone
	Trastuzumab/pertuzumab	NCT05256225	HER2+ endometrial carcinosarcoma	No
bFGF	Sulfatinib	NCT05590572	Osteosarcoma	No
FGFR	Rogaratinib	NCT04595747	Any sarcoma	No
			SDH-deficient GIST	
TRKA	Larotrectinib	NCT02576431	NTRK + tumors	No
DKK1	DKN-01	NCT03395080	Gynecologic sarcoma	Paclitaxel

(continued on next page)

Table 2
(continued)

Target	Pharmaceutical Agent	Trial Number	Subtypes Included	Combined Therapy?
HDAC	Vorinostat	NCT01879085	Any STS	Docetaxel Gemcitabine Vinorelbine Nivolumab Ipilimumab
	Mocetinostat	NCT04299113	Rhabdomyosarcoma	Doxorubicin
	Tazemetostat	NCT05407441	SAMRC-4-deficient tumor	No
	Abexinostat	NCT01027910	Any sarcoma	
	Romidepsin	NCT00112463	Any STS	
VEGFR2	Apatinib	NCT04447274	UPS ASPS	Carilizumab
		NCT05277480	Osteosarcoma	Ifosfamide Gemcitabine
		NCT03742193		Docetaxel Ifosfamide
		NCT04824352		Etoposide
		NCT04351308		MAPI Camrelizumab
VEGF	Bevacizumab	NCT02020707	Uterine sarcomas	Nab-paclitaxel Carboplatin
		NCT00989651	Uterine sarcomas	Paclitaxel Veliparib
Oncofetal fibronectin	Onfekafusp alpha	NCT04032964	Any STS	Doxorubicin
		NCT04650984		
		NCT02076620		
		NCT03420014	Leiomyosarcoma	
mTOR	Everolimus	NCT00767819	Any sarcoma	No
		NCT03245151	Ewing sarcoma Rhabdomyosarcoma	Lenvatinib

Target	Agent	NCT	Histology	Comparator/Combination
Pan-TKI	Pazopanib	NCT02357810	Any sarcoma	Topotecan
		NCT01532687	Any STS	Gemcitabine
	Sunitinib	NCT00753727	Any STS	Radiation
	Cabozantinib	NCT04551430	Any STS (excluding [Excl] ASPS)	Nivolumab Ipilimumab
		NCT04200443	Multiple STS	Temozolomide
		NCT05836571	UPS, Liposarcoma, Leiomyosarcoma, Myxoid Chondrosarcoma	Nivolumab Ipilimumab
	Lenvatinib	NCT05617859	Any sarcoma	No
		NCT04154189	Osteosarcoma	Ifosfamide Etoposide
		NCT03245151	Ewing sarcoma, Rhabdomyosarcoma, Osteosarcoma	Everolimus
		NCT02432274	Osteosarcoma	Ifosfamide Etoposide
PARP	Olaparib	NCT03880019	Uterine Leiomyosarcoma	Temozolomide
NTSR1	[225Ac]-FPI-2059 [111In]-FPI-2058	NCT05605522	NTSR1-expressing tumors	No
XPO-1	Selinexor	NCT06114004	MPNST, Leiomyosarcoma, UPS	Gemcitabine
		NCT04595994	Leiomyosarcoma, ASPS, Osteosarcoma	Gemcitabine
		NCT04138381	GIST	Imatinib

CLINICS CARE POINTS

- The multidisciplinary management of STS at expert centers is key to optimizing patient outcomes.
- Several examples of molecular-directed/biomarker-driven treatment exist in STS; however, there continues to be a vast unmet need for further precision oncology approaches in these diverse diseases.
- Clinical trials and international collaboration are essential for the future progress of STS.

Gastrointestinal Stromal Tumors

Gastrointestinal stromal tumors: risk stratification

GIST is the most common type of sarcoma and is postulated to arise from the interstitial cells of Cajal.[78] They can arise throughout the GI tract but most commonly occur in the stomach and small intestine.[78] GISTs have a wide spectrum of clinical behavior, ranging from indolent small lesions in the stomach to larger, rapidly growing high-risk lesions. Risk classifications have been shown to be useful in the management of GISTs, with several scoring systems developed that incorporate specific risk factors associated with higher risk of recurrence, including high tumor mitotic count, non-gastric locations, large size, and tumor rupture.[79] Small low-risk GISTs less than 2 cm arising in the stomach can be considered for active surveillance protocols. Resectable gastric GISTs larger than 2 cm or GISTs in non-gastric locations of the GI tract are typically managed with surgical resection as local therapy in the nonmetastatic setting is the cornerstone of treatment.

KIT- and PDGFRA-mutant gastrointestinal stromal tumor

GIST is pathologically diagnosed based on positive immunostaining for DOG1 and CD117 (KIT).[78] Although KIT immunostain does not imply a KIT mutation, genomic alterations in multiple exons of the KIT proto-oncogene have been shown to occur in up to 80% of GIST,[80] whereas a platelet derived growth factor receptor alpha (PDGFRA) mutations occur in about 10% to 15% of GIST.[81] These mutations result in constitutive activation of downstream growth factor pathways.[78] Somatic mutations in KIT most commonly occur within exon 11 (juxtamembrane domain) and exon 9 (extracellular domain), with primary mutations in exon 13/14 (ATP-binding domain) and 17/18 (activation loop domain) being less common.[82] Specific KIT mutations can be preferentially seen in different anatomic regions of the stomach and elsewhere in the GI tract (**Fig. 1**).[81,83] Interestingly, germline KIT mutations at similar hotspot mutations also have been identified in more than 30 familial kindreds with GIST (A Fontebasso and R Gladdy personal communication, 2024).[84,85] A variety of other mutations have been identified in very small proportions of GIST (see **Table 2**), including germline mutations in succinate dehydrogenase (SDH) subunit genes which will be discussed as follows.[84]

Targeted therapy with KIT inhibitors such as imatinib has been indispensable to the management of GIST patients. Imatinib is a small molecule inhibitor of the kinase domains of KIT- and PDGFRA, and it has been shown to be clinically effective in the neoadjuvant, adjuvant, and metastatic settings for GIST (**Fig. 2**).[81,86–88] The specific KIT mutation can determine sensitivity to TKIs, including imatinib, and may be factored into dosing for therapy.[82] KIT exon 9-mutated GIST typically occurs in the small bowel and requires higher dosing of imatinib in the metastatic setting for superior efficacy.[82] PDGFRA-mutant GIST remains sensitive to imatinib for most mutations occurring in exons 12, 14, and 18 (including D842 insertion/deletions); however, D842 V mutations

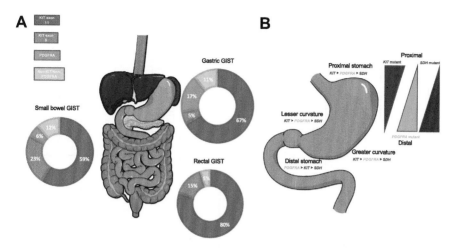

Fig. 1. Dominant driver mutations seen in GIST demonstrate anatomic specificity. (*A*) Relative frequency of mutations identified in GIST along the GI tract. (*B*) The relative frequency of driver mutations in GIST varies according to specific anatomic location in the stomach. (Source: Infographics for figure created using Mind the Graph platform (www. mindthegraph.com).)

in exon 18 are entirely resistant to imatinib.[81,89] For any patient who will receive TKI therapy, whether in the neoadjuvant, adjuvant, or metastatic setting, performing mutation testing is paramount to ensure that drug therapy is likely to be efficacious.

Targeting secondary resistance mutations

Unfortunately, the vast majority of patients develop imatinib resistance mutations after therapy in the ATP-binding pocket (KIT exons 13/14 mutations) or the activation loop (KIT exons 17/18 mutations), necessitating the development of next-generation TKIs (**Table 3**). Sunitinib has been approved as second-line therapy and regorafenib as

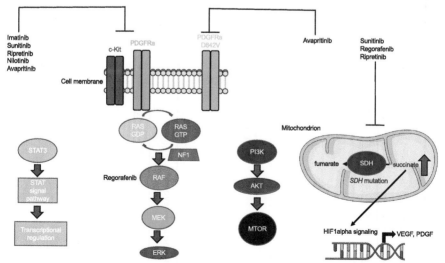

Fig. 2. The molecular basis of GIST driver mutations and their inhibition. (Source: Infographics for figure created using Mind the Graph platform (www.mindthegraph.com).)

Table 3
Current and future treatment landscape for unresectable/metastatic gastrointestinal stromal tumor

Line of Treatment	Mutation	Drug	Outcomes	Ongoing Trials
KIT or PDGFRA mutant (includes D842 indels; excludes D842 V mutations)				
First	Exon 11	Imatinib 400 mg	mPFS 18 mo[90]	
	Exon 9	Imatinib 800 mg	33% will achieve PR or SD with higher dose[90]	
Second	No resistance mutations	Sunitinib	mPFS 7.0 mo[91,96]	PEAK study
	Exon 13/14	Sunitinib	mPFS 15.1 mo[98]	
	Exon 17/18	Ripretinib	mPFS 14.2. mo[98]	INSIGHT trial
Third	No resistance mutations	Regorafenib	mPFS 4.8 mo[92]	
			mPFS 5.6 mo[97]	
	Exon 13/14	Regorafenib	mPFS 7.4 mo[99]	
	Exon 17/18	Regorafenib	mPFS 6.7 mo[99]	
		Avapritinib?	mPFS 4.7 mo[99]	
Fourth	No resistance mutations	Ripretinib 150 mg (activity with 150 mg twice daily on progression)	mPFS 6.0 mo[93,94]	
Fifth line and beyond				NB003 (NCT04936178)
				IDRX-42 (NCT05489237)
PDGFRA D842 V mutation (resistant to imatinib)				
		Avapritinib 300 mg	ORR 89%, PFS rate at 12 mo	
		Ripretinib (also has activity but not approved)	81%[95]	
SDH-mutant GIST (previously known as "wild-type")				
		Sunitinib		INBRX-109 DR5
		Regorefenib		agonist + temozolomide
		Ripretinib		Temozolomide
				Rogaratinib

Other potential driver alterations with histology agnostic FDA-approved therapies

BRAF V600 E	Dabrafenib + trametinib
NTRK fusion	Larotrectinib, entrectinib

Other potential mutations: Direct to clinical trials/targeted therapies above unless approved agents

NF1
RAS
PI3KCA
IGF-1R
FGFR fusion
Unclassified/"wild-type"

Abbreviations: mPFS, median progression free survival; PR, partial response.

third-line therapy in GIST, with activity in *KIT/PDGFRA*-mutant GIST, as well as some SDH-deficient GIST.[89] Avapritinib, which targets the active conformation of KIT/PDGFRA (unlike imatinib, sunitinib and regorafenib), has activity in *KIT*- and *PDGFRA*-mutant GIST and is the only agent approved for the imatinib-resistant *PDGFRA* D842 V mutation.[89] In addition, ripretinib, a broad spectrum TKI with dual mechanism of action through binding of the kinase switch pocket and the activation loop has demonstrated efficacy in inhibiting *PDGFRA*-mutant GIST.[89,100]

There is a great deal of interest in understanding whether specific resistance mutations are more likely to respond to different TKIs, further customizing treatment options for individual patients. Importantly, mutation data were captured for patients treated in two recent large phase 3 clinical trials where novel drugs did not show superiority over the approved agents. The INTRIGUE study compared ripretinib versus sunitinib in the second line, with median PFS for ripretinib of 8.3 months compared with 7.0 months for sunitinib, which was not significantly different.[96] In the VOYAGER trial, regorafenib versus avapritinib was compared in the third line and again showed no statistically significant difference with median PFS of 5.6 months for regorafenib compared with 4.2 months for avapritinib.[97] Correlative data from these negative trials investigated specific tumor mutations by circulating tumor DNA (ctDNA) using the Guardant platform. Remarkably, in the INTRIGUE trial, patients with *KIT* exon 11 and mutations in the ATP-binding pocket (exons 13/14) showed remarkably disparate outcomes, with a median PFS of 15.0 months with sunitinib compared with 4.0 months with ripretinib. There was similar improvement in OS, with median OS not reached for sunitinib compared with 24.5 months with ripretinib.[96,98] In contrast, patients with concurrent *KIT* exon 11 and activation loop resistance mutations (exons 17/18) showed the opposite trend, with median PFS of 14.2 months with ripretinib compared with 1.5 months with sunitinib, as well as median OS not reached for ripretinib compared with 17.5 months for sunitinib.[98] These findings are being validated in the prospective INSIGHT clinical trial, where patients with exon 17/18 mutations are randomized to sunitinib versus ripretinib (NCT05734105). Disparate findings were also reported in the VOYAGER study, where patients with ATP-binding pocket mutations by ctDNA exhibited median PFS with regorafenib of 7.4 months, compared with only 1.9 months with avapritinib. In contrast, patients with *KIT* exon 17/18 mutations had reasonable outcomes with avapritinib, with median PFS of 4.7 months compared with 6.7 months with regorafenib. Although regorafenib was still superior, outcomes with avapritinib may be clinically meaningful in this group of patients.[99] Although not yet ready for implementation, given limitations of ctDNA technology, these observations may eventually further stratify drug selection for patients with GIST in the later lines of therapy as provided in **Table 2**.[99]

SDHx-mutant gastrointestinal stromal tumor

Mutations in the SDH complex genes (*SDHA, SDHB, SDHC,* and *SDHD*) have also been associated with the development of SDH-deficient GIST.[83,101] Succinate dehydrogenase mutations (*SDHx*) germline mutations can lead to hereditary GIST in the Carney-Stratakis syndrome.[101] Interestingly, recent data have also pointed to the anatomic specificity of *SDHx*-mutant GIST within the distal stomach (see **Fig. 1**).[83] Surgery is the cornerstone of treatment of *SDHx*-mutant GIST, although decision-making for hereditary GIST syndromes can be quite challenging in the balance of risk of future development of GIST against the surgical morbidity of more extended resections.[84] Thus, total gastrectomy is not recommend for risk reduction in the patient population. Epigenetic modification patterns with DNA hypermethylation have been shown to be unique in *SDH*-mutant GIST, demonstrating that epigenetic changes can drive oncogenic programs in kinase wild-type GIST.

Until recently, treatment options for SDHx-mutant GIST have been very limited, with modest responses to standard TKIs used for *KIT*- and *PDGFRA*-mutant GIST. However, recently presented early results for clinical trials have renewed hope for better outcomes. Sicklick and colleagues successfully generated novel preclinical models for SDH-deficient GIST, and identified temozolomide as a promising agent to elicit DNA damage and apoptosis.[102] Excitingly, data presented from a phase 2 trial confirmed clinical benefit in patients, with a best response rate of 17.4%, and median PFS of 11 months.[103] In addition, an ongoing cohort is testing temozolomide in combination with a novel DR5 agonist (INBRX-109) for SDH-deficient GIST patients (NCT03715933). Finally, a phase 2 trial (NCT04595747) also recently reported initial results for SDH-deficient GIST treated with the pan-fibroblast growth factor (FGF) receptor inhibitor rogaratinib, based on evidence of the important of fibroblast growth factor receptor (FGFR) signaling in this subtype of GIST patients.[104] With 23 evaluable patients, the best overall response rate was 30%, with the median PFS not yet reached at the data cutoff point.[105]

Rarer gastrointestinal stromal tumor subtypes

Importantly, a very small proportion of GIST may have mutations in other clinically actionable genes, as summarized in **Table 3**. Recognition of the very rare neurotrophic tyrosine receptor kinase (NTRK) fusions and BRAF V600E mutations are critical to identify given the availability of histology agnostic approvals for agents targeting these drivers (ie, larotrectinib or entrectinib or dabrafenib/trametinib, respectively.) For other driver mutations, enrollment in molecularly driven basket trials, if available, may be the best option for these patients.

SUMMARY

We have taken a molecular lens in this review to visualize STS and GIST management. With multiple large-scale genomic studies helping to elucidate the biologic heterogeneity of specific types of STS and their differing clinical behavior, there remains a dire need for molecularly informed clinical trials. The advent of KIT inhibitors such as imatinib has revolutionized the oncologic treatment and multidisciplinary management of GIST. We firmly believe that without molecular information, we cannot move forward in this complex field of highly heterogenous rare tumor entities. Steps must be taken toward a molecular diagnosis for sarcomas with identified driver alterations and this information needs to be disseminated to the broader sarcoma community. The onus of care in sarcoma should not remain on the individual physician in the management of this disease, but rather the multidisciplinary cancer conference where cases should be presented and molecular information integrated as available in making treatment decisions. With this, we can properly manage patients according to their tumor biology and enact the goal of precision medicine for sarcoma.

CLINICS CARE POINTS

- GIST is best managed in the multidisciplinary setting by experienced centers.
- The interplay between medical oncology and surgical oncology in this disease is critical in determining optimal management of locally advanced, high-risk, unresectable or metastatic cases.
- Mutational profiling is key to determining the utility of adjuvant treatment given the differing mutation sensitivity to TKI.

DISCLOSURES

The following authors have conflicts of interest to disclose: J-Y. Blay receives research support from NETSARC+, INTERSARC+ and LYRICAN + grants from the French NCI (INCa). B.A. Wilky, is in a consulting or advisory role to Springworks, Deciphera, Epizyme, Adcendo, Polaris, Boehringer Ingelheim, AADi and receives research funding from Exelixis and receives travel, accommodation, and expenses from Agenus.

REFERENCES

1. Sbaraglia M, Bellan E, Dei Tos AP. The 2020 WHO Classification of Soft Tissue Tumours: news and perspectives. Pathologica 2021;113(2):70–84.
2. Wallander K, Öfverholm I, Boye K, et al. Sarcoma care in the era of precision medicine. J Intern Med 2023;294(6):690–707.
3. Rupani A, Hallin M, Jones RL, et al. Diagnostic Differences in Expert Second-Opinion Consultation Cases at a Tertiary Sarcoma Center. Sarcoma 2020; 2020:9810170.
4. Gronchi A, Strauss DC, Miceli R, et al. Variability in Patterns of Recurrence After Resection of Primary Retroperitoneal Sarcoma (RPS): A Report on 1007 Patients From the Multi-institutional Collaborative RPS Working Group. Ann Surg 2016; 263(5):1002–9.
5. Bonvalot S, Gronchi A, Péchoux CL, et al. Preoperative radiotherapy plus surgery versus surgery alone for patients with primary retroperitoneal sarcoma (EORTC-62092: STRASS): a multicentre, open-label, randomised, phase 3 trial. Lancet Oncol 2020;21(10):1366–77.
6. Callegaro D, Raut CP, Ajayi T, et al. Preoperative Radiotherapy in Patients With Primary Retroperitoneal Sarcoma: EORTC-62092 Trial (STRASS) Versus Off-trial (STREXIT) Results. Ann Surg 2023;278(1):127–34.
7. Lambdin J, Ryan C, Gregory S, et al. A Randomized Phase III Study of Neoadjuvant Chemotherapy Followed by Surgery Versus Surgery Alone for Patients with High-Risk Retroperitoneal Sarcoma (STRASS2). Ann Surg Oncol 2023; 30(8):4573–5.
8. Ng D, Swallow CJ. Decision-making for palliative versus curative intent treatment of retroperitoneal sarcoma (RPS). Chin Clin Oncol 2018;7(4):40.
9. Miwa S, Yamamoto N, Hayashi K, Takeuchi A, Igarashi K, Tsuchiya H. Therapeutic Targets for Bone and Soft-Tissue Sarcomas. International Journal of Molecular Sciences (Internet) 2019 (cited 2023 Nov 17);20(1). Available at: https://www.ncbi.nlm.nih.gov/pmc/articles/PMC6337155/.
10. Salerno KE. Radiation Therapy for Soft Tissue Sarcoma: Indications, Timing, Benefits, and Consequences. Surg Clin North Am 2022;102(4):567–82.
11. Cahlon O, Brennan MF, Jia X, et al. A Postoperative Nomogram for Local Recurrence Risk in Extremity Soft Tissue Sarcomas after Limb-Sparing Surgery Without Adjuvant Radiation. Ann Surg 2012;255(2):343–7.
12. Rathore R, Van Tine BA. Pathogenesis and Current Treatment of Osteosarcoma: Perspectives for Future Therapies. J Clin Med 2021;10(6):1182.
13. Biswas B, Bakhshi S. Management of Ewing sarcoma family of tumors: Current scenario and unmet need. World J Orthop 2016;7(9):527–38.
14. Makimoto A. Optimizing Rhabdomyosarcoma Treatment in Adolescents and Young Adults. Cancers 2022;14(9):2270.
15. Vining CC, Sinnamon AJ, Ecker BL, et al. Adjuvant chemotherapy in resectable synovial sarcoma. J Surg Oncol 2017;116(4):550–8.

16. Judson I, Verweij J, Gelderblom H, et al. Doxorubicin alone versus intensified doxorubicin plus ifosfamide for first-line treatment of advanced or metastatic soft-tissue sarcoma: a randomised controlled phase 3 trial. Lancet Oncol 2014;15(4):415–23.

17. Adjuvant chemotherapy for localised resectable soft-tissue sarcoma of adults: meta-analysis of individual data. Sarcoma Meta-analysis Collaboration. Lancet 1997;350(9092):1647–54.

18. Frustaci S, Gherlinzoni F, De Paoli A, et al. Adjuvant chemotherapy for adult soft tissue sarcomas of the extremities and girdles: results of the Italian randomized cooperative trial. J Clin Oncol 2001;19(5):1238–47.

19. Gronchi A, Frustaci S, Mercuri M, et al. Short, full-dose adjuvant chemotherapy in high-risk adult soft tissue sarcomas: a randomized clinical trial from the Italian Sarcoma Group and the Spanish Sarcoma Group. J Clin Oncol 2012;30(8): 850–6.

20. Pasquali S, Pizzamiglio S, Touati N, et al. The impact of chemotherapy on survival of patients with extremity and trunk wall soft tissue sarcoma: revisiting the results of the EORTC-STBSG 62931 randomised trial. Eur J Cancer 2019; 109:51–60.

21. Pasquali S, Gronchi A. Neoadjuvant chemotherapy in soft tissue sarcomas: latest evidence and clinical implications. Ther Adv Med Oncol 2017;9(6):415–29.

22. DeLaney TF, Spiro IJ, Suit HD, et al. Neoadjuvant chemotherapy and radiotherapy for large extremity soft-tissue sarcomas. Int J Radiat Oncol Biol Phys 2003;56(4):1117–27.

23. Voss RK, Callegaro D, Chiang YJ, et al. Sarculator is a Good Model to Predict Survival in Resected Extremity and Trunk Sarcomas in US Patients. Ann Surg Oncol 2022. https://doi.org/10.1245/s10434-022-11442-2.

24. Pasquali S, Palmerini E, Quagliuolo V, et al. Neoadjuvant chemotherapy in high-risk soft tissue sarcomas: A Sarculator-based risk stratification analysis of the ISG-STS 1001 randomized trial. Cancer 2022;128(1):85–93.

25. Gronchi A, Ferrari S, Quagliuolo V, et al. Histotype-tailored neoadjuvant chemotherapy versus standard chemotherapy in patients with high-risk soft-tissue sarcomas (ISG-STS 1001): an international, open-label, randomised, controlled, phase 3, multicentre trial. Lancet Oncol 2017;18(6):812–22.

26. Desmoid Tumor Working Group. The management of desmoid tumours: A joint global consensus-based guideline approach for adult and paediatric patients. Eur J Cancer 2020;127:96–107.

27. Penel N, Le Cesne A, Bonvalot S, et al. Surgical versus non-surgical approach in primary desmoid-type fibromatosis patients: A nationwide prospective cohort from the French Sarcoma Group. Eur J Cancer 2017;83:125–31.

28. Fiore M, Rimareix F, Mariani L, et al. Desmoid-type fibromatosis: a front-line conservative approach to select patients for surgical treatment. Ann Surg Oncol 2009;16(9):2587–93.

29. Gounder MM, Mahoney MR, Van Tine BA, et al. Sorafenib for Advanced and Refractory Desmoid Tumors. N Engl J Med 2018;379(25):2417–28.

30. Szucs Z, Messiou C, Wong HH, et al. Pazopanib, a promising option for the treatment of aggressive fibromatosis. Anti Cancer Drugs 2017;28(4):421–6.

31. Chugh R, Wathen JK, Patel SR, et al. Efficacy of imatinib in aggressive fibromatosis: Results of a phase II multicenter Sarcoma Alliance for Research through Collaboration (SARC) trial. Clin Cancer Res 2010;16(19):4884–91.

32. Gounder M, Ratan R, Alcindor T, et al. Nirogacestat, a γ-Secretase Inhibitor for Desmoid Tumors. N Engl J Med 2023;388(10):898–912.

33. Nishio J, Nakayama S, Nabeshima K, et al. Biology and Management of Dedifferentiated Liposarcoma: State of the Art and Perspectives. J Clin Med 2021; 10(15):3230.

34. Dickson MA, Tap WD, Keohan ML, et al. Phase II trial of the CDK4 inhibitor PD0332991 in patients with advanced CDK4-amplified well-differentiated or dedifferentiated liposarcoma. J Clin Oncol 2013;31(16):2024–8.

35. Dickson MA, Koff A, D'Angelo SP, et al. Phase 2 study of the CDK4 inhibitor abemaciclib in dedifferentiated liposarcoma. J Clin Orthod 2019;37(15_suppl): 11004.

36. Ray-Coquard I, Blay J-Y, Italiano A, et al. Effect of the MDM2 antagonist RG7112 on the P53 pathway in patients with MDM2-amplified, well-differentiated or dedifferentiated liposarcoma: an exploratory proof-of-mechanism study. Lancet Oncol 2012;13(11):1133–40.

37. Gounder MM, Bauer TM, Schwartz GK, et al. A First-in-Human Phase I Study of Milademetan, an MDM2 Inhibitor, in Patients With Advanced Liposarcoma, Solid Tumors, or Lymphomas. J Clin Oncol 2023;41(9):1714–24.

38. Milademetan Does Not Improve Survival Vs Trabectedin in Liposarcoma (Internet). Cancer Network. 2023 (cited 2023 Nov 11);Available at: https:// www.cancernetwork.com/view/milademetan-does-not-improve-survival-vs-trabectedin-in-liposarcoma.

39. LoRusso P, Yamamoto N, Patel MR, et al. The MDM2-p53 Antagonist Brigimadlin (BI 907828) in Patients with Advanced or Metastatic Solid Tumors: Results of a Phase Ia, First-in-Human, Dose-Escalation Study. Cancer Discov 2023;13(8): 1802–13.

40. Schöffski P, LoRusso P, Yamamoto N. A PHASE IA/IB, DOSE-ESCALATION/ EXPANSION STUDY OF THE MDM2-P53 ANTAGONIST BRIGIMADLIN (BI 907828) IN PATIENTS WITH SOLID TUMORS: SAFETY AND EFFICACY IN PATIENTS WITH LIPOSARCOMA. Presented at the Connective Tissue Oncology Society Annual Meeting. Dublin, Ireland. Paper 23. November 1, 2023.

41. Schöffski P, Lahmar M, Lucarelli A, et al. Brightline-1: phase II/III trial of the MDM2-p53 antagonist BI 907828 versus doxorubicin in patients with advanced DDLPS. Future Oncol 2023;19(9):621–9.

42. Abdul Razak AR, Bauer S, Suarez C, et al. Co-Targeting of MDM2 and CDK4/6 with Siremadlin and Ribociclib for the Treatment of Patients with Well-Differentiated or Dedifferentiated Liposarcoma: Results from a Proof-of-Concept, Phase Ib Study. Clin Cancer Res 2022;28(6):1087–97.

43. Rutkowski P, Klimczak A, Ługowska I, et al. Long-term results of treatment of advanced dermatofibrosarcoma protuberans (DFSP) with imatinib mesylate – The impact of fibrosarcomatous transformation. Eur J Surg Oncol 2017;43(6): 1134–41.

44. Chen AP, Sharon E, O'Sullivan-Coyne G, et al. Atezolizumab for Advanced Alveolar Soft Part Sarcoma. N Engl J Med 2023;389(10):911–21.

45. Chi Y, Fang Z, Hong X, et al. Safety and Efficacy of Anlotinib, a Multikinase Angiogenesis Inhibitor, in Patients with Refractory Metastatic Soft-Tissue Sarcoma. Clin Cancer Res 2018;24(21):5233–8.

46. Judson I, Morden JP, Kilburn L, et al. Cediranib in patients with alveolar soft-part sarcoma (CASPS): a double-blind, placebo-controlled, randomised, phase 2 trial. Lancet Oncol 2019;20(7):1023–34.

47. Stacchiotti S, Negri T, Zaffaroni N, et al. Sunitinib in advanced alveolar soft part sarcoma: evidence of a direct antitumor effect. Ann Oncol 2011;22(7):1682–90.

48. Stacchiotti S, Mir O, Le Cesne A, et al. Activity of Pazopanib and Trabectedin in Advanced Alveolar Soft Part Sarcoma. Oncol 2018;23(1):62–70.

49. Wilky BA, Trucco MM, Subhawong TK, et al. Axitinib plus pembrolizumab in patients with advanced sarcomas including alveolar soft-part sarcoma: a single-centre, single-arm, phase 2 trial. Lancet Oncol 2019;20(6):837–48.

50. Wagner AJ, Ravi V, Riedel RF, et al. Long-term follow-up for duration of response (DoR) after weekly nab-sirolimus in patients with advanced malignant perivascular epithelioid cell tumors (PEComa): Results from a registrational open-label phase II trial. AMPECT. JCO 2020;38(15_suppl):11516.

51. Benson C, Vitfell-Rasmussen J, Maruzzo M, et al. A retrospective study of patients with malignant PEComa receiving treatment with sirolimus or temsirolimus: the Royal Marsden Hospital experience. Anticancer Res 2014;34(7):3663–8.

52. Gounder MM, Jones RL, Chugh R, et al. RINGSIDE phase 2/3 trial of AL102 for treatment of desmoid tumors (DT): Phase 2 results. J Clin Orthod 2023; 41(16_suppl):11515.

53. Chawla S, Blay J-Y, Rutkowski P, et al. Denosumab in patients with giant-cell tumour of bone: a multicentre, open-label, phase 2 study. Lancet Oncol 2019; 20(12):1719–29.

54. Tap WD, Gelderblom H, Palmerini E, et al. Pexidartinib for advanced tenosynovial giant cell tumor: results of the randomized phase 3 ENLIVEN study. Lancet 2019;394(10197):478–87.

55. Tap WD, Sharma MG, Vallee M, et al. The MOTION study: a randomized, Phase III study of vimseltinib for the treatment of tenosynovial giant cell tumor. Future Oncol 2023. https://doi.org/10.2217/fon-2023-0238.

56. Verspoor FGM, Mastboom MJL, Hannink G, et al. Long-term efficacy of imatinib mesylate in patients with advanced Tenosynovial Giant Cell Tumor. Sci Rep 2019;9:14551.

57. Schöffski P, Kubickova M, Wozniak A, et al. Long-term efficacy update of crizotinib in patients with advanced, inoperable inflammatory myofibroblastic tumour from EORTC trial 90101 CREATE. Eur J Cancer 2021;156:12–23.

58. Peters S, Camidge DR, Shaw AT, et al. Alectinib versus Crizotinib in Untreated ALK-Positive Non–Small-Cell Lung Cancer. N Engl J Med 2017;377(9):829–38.

59. Sn G, La B, Cj L, et al. Activity and safety of brigatinib in ALK-rearranged non-small-cell lung cancer and other malignancies: a single-arm, open-label, phase 1/2 trial. The Lancet Oncology (Internet) 2016 (cited 2023 Nov 13);17(12). Available at: https://pubmed.ncbi.nlm.nih.gov/27836716/.

60. Mansfield AS, Murphy SJ, Harris FR, et al. Chromoplectic TPM3-ALK rearrangement in a patient with inflammatory myofibroblastic tumor who responded to ceritinib after progression on crizotinib. Ann Oncol 2016;27(11):2111–7.

61. Wong HH, Bentley H, Bulusu VR, et al. Lorlatinib for the treatment of inflammatory myofibroblastic tumour with TPM4-ALK fusion following failure of entrectinib. Anti Cancer Drugs 2020;31(10):1106.

62. Park MS, Patel SR, Ludwig JA, et al. Activity of temozolomide and bevacizumab in the treatment of locally advanced, recurrent, and metastatic hemangiopericytoma and malignant solitary fibrous tumor. Cancer 2011;117(21):4939–47.

63. Ebata T, Shimoi T, Bun S, et al. Efficacy and Safety of Pazopanib for Recurrent or Metastatic Solitary Fibrous Tumor. Oncology 2018;94(6):340–4.

64. Stacchiotti S, Schoffski P, Jones R, et al. Safety and efficacy of tazemetostat, a first-in-class EZH2 inhibitor, in patients (pts) with epithelioid sarcoma (ES) (NCT02601950). J Clin Orthod 2019;37(15_suppl):11003.

65. Tap WD, Villalobos VM, Cote GM, et al. Phase I Study of the Mutant IDH1 Inhibitor Ivosidenib: Safety and Clinical Activity in Patients With Advanced Chondrosarcoma. J Clin Oncol 2020;38(15):1693–701.

66. Stein EM, DiNardo CD, Pollyea DA, et al. Enasidenib in mutant IDH2 relapsed or refractory acute myeloid leukemia. Blood 2017;130(6):722–31.

67. Chawla SP, Wasp GT, Shepard DR, et al. A randomized, placebo-controlled, phase 2 trial of INBRX-109 in unresectable or metastatic conventional chondrosarcoma. J Clin Orthod 2022;40(16_suppl):TPS11582.

68. Chow W, Frankel P, Ruel C, et al. Results of a prospective phase 2 study of pazopanib in patients with surgically unresectable or metastatic chondrosarcoma. Cancer 2020;126(1):105–11.

69. D'Angelo SP, Druta M, Van Tine BA, et al. Safety and efficacy of letetresgene autoleucel (lete-cel; GSK3377794) in advanced myxoid/round cell liposarcoma (MRCLS) following high lymphodepletion (Cohort 2): Interim analysis. J Clin Orthod 2021;39(15_suppl):11521.

70. Van Tine BA, Ganjoo KN, Blay J-Y, et al. The SPEARHEAD-1 trial of afamitresgene autoleucel (afami-cel [formerly ADP-A2M4]): Analysis of overall survival in advanced synovial sarcoma. J Clin Orthod 2023;41(16_suppl):11563.

71. Schuetze S, Ballman KV, Ganjoo KN, et al. P10015/SARC033: A phase 2 trial of trametinib in patients with advanced epithelioid hemangioendothelioma (EHE). J Clin Orthod 2021;39(15_suppl):11503.

72. Florou V, Rosenberg AE, Wieder E, et al. Angiosarcoma patients treated with immune checkpoint inhibitors: a case series of seven patients from a single institution. J Immunother Cancer 2019;7(1):213.

73. Wagner MJ, Othus M, Patel SP, et al. Multicenter phase II trial (SWOG S1609, cohort 51) of ipilimumab and nivolumab in metastatic or unresectable angiosarcoma: a substudy of dual anti-CTLA-4 and anti-PD-1 blockade in rare tumors (DART). J Immunother Cancer 2021;9(8):e002990.

74. Doebele RC, Drilon A, Paz-Ares L, et al. Entrectinib in patients with advanced or metastatic NTRK fusion-positive solid tumours: integrated analysis of three phase 1–2 trials. Lancet Oncol 2020;21(2):271–82.

75. Drilon A, Laetsch TW, Kummar S, et al. Efficacy of Larotrectinib in TRK Fusion–Positive Cancers in Adults and Children. N Engl J Med 2018;378(8):731–9.

76. Gross AM, Wolters PL, Dombi E, et al. Selumetinib in Children with Inoperable Plexiform Neurofibromas. N Engl J Med 2020;382(15):1430–42.

77. Maio M, Ascierto PA, Manzyuk L, et al. Pembrolizumab in microsatellite instability high or mismatch repair deficient cancers: updated analysis from the phase II KEYNOTE-158 study. Ann Oncol 2022;33(9):929–38.

78. Serrano C, George S. Gastrointestinal Stromal Tumor: Challenges and Opportunities for a New Decade. Clin Cancer Res 2020;26(19):5078–85.

79. Joensuu H, Eriksson M, Hall KS, et al. Risk factors for gastrointestinal stromal tumor recurrence in patients treated with adjuvant imatinib. Cancer 2014; 120(15):2325–33.

80. Callegaro D, Roland CL, Raut CP. Relevant Trials Update in Sarcomas and Gastrointestinal Stromal Tumors: What Surgeons Should Know. Surg Oncol Clin N Am 2022;31(3):341–60.

81. Balachandran VP, DeMatteo RP. GIST tumors: Who should get imatinib and for how long? Adv Surg 2014;48(1):165–83.

82. Mechahougui H, Michael M, Friedlaender A. Precision Oncology in Gastrointestinal Stromal Tumors. Curr Oncol 2023;30(5):4648–62.

83. Sharma AK, de la Torre J, IJzerman NS, et al. Location of Gastrointestinal Stromal Tumor (GIST) in the Stomach Predicts Tumor Mutation Profile and Drug Sensitivity. Clin Cancer Res 2021;27(19):5334–42.

84. Kwak HV, Tardy KJ, Allbee A, et al. Surgical Management of Germline Gastrointestinal Stromal Tumor. Ann Surg Oncol 2023;30(8):4966–74.

85. Ricci R. Syndromic gastrointestinal stromal tumors. Hered Cancer Clin Pract 2016;14:15.

86. Reichardt P, Blay J-Y, Boukovinas I, et al. Adjuvant therapy in primary GIST: state-of-the-art. Ann Oncol 2012;23(11):2776–81.

87. Joensuu H, Eriksson M, Sundby Hall K, et al. Survival Outcomes Associated With 3 Years vs 1 Year of Adjuvant Imatinib for Patients With High-Risk Gastrointestinal Stromal Tumors. JAMA Oncol 2020;6(8):1–6.

88. Joensuu H, Eriksson M, Sundby Hall K, et al. One vs three years of adjuvant imatinib for operable gastrointestinal stromal tumor: a randomized trial. JAMA 2012;307(12):1265–72.

89. Bauer S, George S, von Mehren M, et al. Early and Next-Generation KIT/PDGFRA Kinase Inhibitors and the Future of Treatment for Advanced Gastrointestinal Stromal Tumor. Front Oncol 2021;11:672500.

90. Heinrich MC, Owzar K, Corless CL, et al. Correlation of Kinase Genotype and Clinical Outcome in the North American Intergroup Phase III Trial of Imatinib Mesylate for Treatment of Advanced Gastrointestinal Stromal Tumor: CALGB 150105 Study by Cancer and Leukemia Group B and Southwest Oncology Group. J Clin Oncol 2008;26(33):5360–7.

91. Demetri GD, van Oosterom AT, Garrett CR, et al. Efficacy and safety of sunitinib in patients with advanced gastrointestinal stromal tumour after failure of imatinib: a randomised controlled trial. Lancet 2006;368(9544):1329–38.

92. Demetri GD, Reichardt P, Kang Y-K, et al. Efficacy and safety of regorafenib for advanced gastrointestinal stromal tumours after failure of imatinib and sunitinib (GRID): an international, multicentre, randomised, placebo-controlled, phase 3 trial. Lancet 2013;381(9863):295–302.

93. Blay J-Y, Serrano C, Heinrich MC, et al. Ripretinib in patients with advanced gastrointestinal stromal tumours (INVICTUS): a double-blind, randomised, placebo-controlled, phase 3 trial. Lancet Oncol 2020;21(7):923–34.

94. George S, Chi P, Heinrich MC, et al. Ripretinib intrapatient dose escalation after disease progression provides clinically meaningful outcomes in advanced gastrointestinal stromal tumour. Eur J Cancer 2021;155:236–44.

95. Heinrich MC, Jones RL, von Mehren M, et al. Avapritinib in advanced PDGFRA D842V-mutant gastrointestinal stromal tumour (NAVIGATOR): a multicentre, open-label, phase 1 trial. Lancet Oncol 2020;21(7):935–46.

96. Serrano C, Bauer S, Gómez-Peregrina D, et al. Circulating tumor DNA analysis of the phase III VOYAGER trial: KIT mutational landscape and outcomes in patients with advanced gastrointestinal stromal tumor treated with avapritinib or regorafenib. Ann Oncol 2023;34(7):615–25.

97. Sun Y, Yue L, Xu P, et al. An overview of agents and treatments for PDGFRA-mutated gastrointestinal stromal tumors. Front Oncol 2022;12:927587.

98. Bauer S, Jones RL, Blay J-Y, et al. Ripretinib Versus Sunitinib in Patients With Advanced Gastrointestinal Stromal Tumor After Treatment With Imatinib (INTRIGUE): A Randomized, Open-Label, Phase III Trial. J Clin Oncol 2022; 40(34):3918–28.

99. Kang Y-K, George S, Jones RL, et al. Avapritinib Versus Regorafenib in Locally Advanced Unresectable or Metastatic GI Stromal Tumor: A Randomized, Open-Label Phase III Study. J Clin Oncol 2021;39(28):3128–39.

100. Bauer S, Jones RL, George S, et al. Mutational heterogeneity of imatinib resistance and efficacy of ripretinib vs sunitinib in patients with gastrointestinal stromal tumor: ctDNA analysis from INTRIGUE. J Clin Orthod 2023;41(36_suppl):397784.

101. Burgoyne AM, Somaiah N, Sicklick JK. Gastrointestinal stromal tumors in the setting of multiple tumor syndromes. Curr Opin Oncol 2014;26(4):408–14.

102. Yebra M, Bhargava S, Kumar A, et al. Establishment of Patient-Derived Succinate Dehydrogenase-Deficient Gastrointestinal Stromal Tumor Models for Predicting Therapeutic Response. Clin Cancer Res 2022;28(1):187–200.

103. Burgoyne A, Heinrich MC, von Mehren M, et al. Paper 83. Connective Tissue Oncology Society Annual Meeting. November 4, 2023. Dublin, Ireland: 2023.

104. Flavahan WA, Drier Y, Johnstone SE, et al. Altered chromosomal topology drives oncogenic programs in SDH-deficient GISTs. Nature 2019;575(7781):229–33.

105. Merriam P, Mazzola E, Chi P, et al. Paper 84. Connective Tissue Oncology Society Annual Meeting. November 4, 2023. Dublin, Ireland: 2023.

Precision Oncology in Pediatric Cancer Surgery

William G. Lee, MD[a], Eugene S. Kim, MD[b],*

KEYWORDS

- Precision oncology • Precision medicine • Pediatric cancer • Molecular profiling
- Gene sequencing • Targeted therapy • Basket trial

KEY POINTS

- Large-scale ongoing "basket trials" recruit pediatric patients and allocate targeted therapies based on molecular alterations, as opposed to tumor type, increasing access to clinical trials and providing a framework for clinical implementation.
- Pediatric precision oncology offers a promising treatment option for recurrent and treatment-refractory pediatric solid tumors, where prognosis remains dismal despite exhaustive multimodal therapy (chemotherapy, radiotherapy, and surgery).
- Although uncommon, immunotherapy and small molecule inhibitors are associated with impaired wound healing, coagulopathy, and spontaneous gastrointestinal perforation in children.
- Future research focuses on optimizing targeted treatment efficacy (eg, combination therapy) and improving biopsy strategies (eg, "liquid biopsy").

INTRODUCTION
Overview of Precision Medicine in Pediatric Population

Precision medicine incorporates the unique genetic alterations of a patient's disease to guide their therapy. One of the earliest well-known examples of precision medicine in the pediatric population is the targeted treatment of children with G551D-CFTR mutation positive cystic fibrosis with the CFTR potentiator ivacaftor, which led to improved lung function.[1] Within pediatric oncology, the strong link between genetic aberrations, tumorigenesis, and cancer biology creates an ideal model for the application of precision medicine—aptly termed precision oncology. Precision oncology is a developing multidisciplinary approach to personalized cancer treatment where therapies target

[a] Department of Surgery, Cedars-Sinai Medical Center, 116 North Robertson Boulevard, Suite PACT 700, Los Angeles, CA 90048, USA; [b] Division of Pediatric Surgery, Department of Surgery, Cedars-Sinai Medical Center, 116 North Robertson Boulevard, Suite PACT 700, Los Angeles, CA 90048, USA
* Corresponding author.
E-mail address: eugene.kimx@cshs.org
Twitter: @william_ghh_lee (W.G.L.); @dreskim (E.S.K.)

Surg Oncol Clin N Am 33 (2024) 409–446
https://doi.org/10.1016/j.soc.2023.12.008
1055-3207/24/© 2023 Elsevier Inc. All rights reserved.

surgonc.theclinics.com

specific molecular or genetic alterations (**Fig. 1**). In this article, the authors review the current role of precision oncology in the treatment of pediatric cancer—with a focus on pediatric solid tumors—and the surgical implications of these novel targeted therapies.

Overview of Pediatric Oncology

Cancer is one of the leading causes of non-accidental death in children after infancy ultimately leading to death in 20% of all children diagnosed with cancer.[2,3] Although improvements in local treatment and cytotoxic chemotherapy have drastically improved 5-year survival from 58% in the 1970s to 85% in 2022, progress has plateaued and prognosis remains dismal for patients with recurrent/refractory disease or particular high-risk biological features (eg, high-risk neuroblastoma [HR-NB]).[4,5] In addition, posttreatment morbidity among cancer survivors is especially common in the pediatric population due to longer life expectancy relative to their adult counterparts. Survivors of pediatric cancer are susceptible to an increased risk for end-organ damage from cytotoxic therapies (eg, ototoxicity, cardiomyopathy, nephropathy, and impaired fertility), impaired growth and development, decreased quality of life, and increased rates of secondary malignancies.[4] Thus, the goals of pediatric precision oncology are to use targeted therapies to not only increase survival but also decrease the long-term toxicity and morbidity associated with current cytotoxic therapies.

Although there is significant overlap between pediatric and adult oncology, there are many unique characteristics of pediatric cancers that limit the crossover from adult precision oncology to the pediatric world. In contrast to adult cancers, pediatric cancers and their subtypes are rare and often characterized by single driver mutations

Conventional Therapy

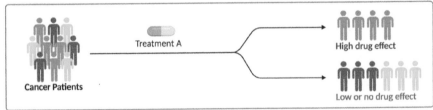

Precision Cancer Therapy

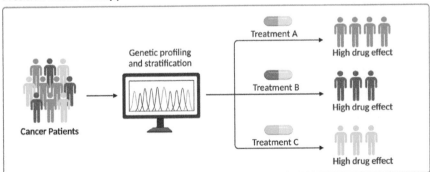

Fig. 1. Precision oncology process. (Created with BioRender.com.)

with relatively few somatic mutations.[6–10] In addition to a lower mutational burden, only 30% to 45% of known pediatric cancer mutations overlap with adult cancer mutations, which have limited the adoption of established targeted therapies currently being used for adult cancers.[11,12] Thus, fewer targetable somatic mutations have led to fewer available therapies and active clinical trials for pediatric patients, which highlights the need for ongoing pediatric-specific precision oncology studies to identify targetable genomic alterations.

IMPACT OF DISCOVERY SEQUENCING STUDIES IN PEDIATRIC ONCOLOGY
Overview of Genomic Alterations

Genomic alterations can occur due to single-nucleotide variations (eg, base pair insertions, deletions, or substitutions), copy number variation (eg, deletions or duplications of genomic segments), structural alteration (eg, chromoplexy, chromothripsis), loss of heterozygosity, or gene fusion products. Epigenetic modifications can also occur, such as chromatin remodeling, DNA methylation, or histone modification, which can affect downstream gene expression.[13] Next-generation sequencing (NGS), such as whole genome sequencing (WGS) or whole exome sequencing (WES), has allowed us to begin to understand the complexity of tumorigenesis and disease progression. The addition of transcriptomics (ie, RNA sequencing [RNAseq]) and proteomics has also allowed us to elucidate the downstream effects and identify potential targets or pathways for intervention. Although commercially available gene panels can be used to detect known deleterious mutations (eg, Oncomine Dx, FoundationOne CDx, and TruSight), discovery sequencing studies are increasingly combining tumor-specific gene sequencing panels with RNAseq or epigenetic studies to identify clinically actionable mutations.

Discovery Sequencing Studies

Discovery sequencing studies aim to identify recurrent mutations within a specific cancer type. Association of these recurrent mutations with clinical outcomes data can provide prognostic relevance and lead to further molecular risk stratification (eg, *MYCN* amplification and HR-NB). They may also provide a therapeutic target for an available FDA-approved or investigational drug currently being used for a different indication. This is particularly useful in refractory or difficult-to-treat rare tumors where no effective therapy exists. Thus, over the past 2 decades, a multitude of discovery sequencing studies in pediatric oncology have been performed to achieve these aims (**Table 1**).

Prior discovery sequencing studies have provided insight into the heterogeneity of genomic alterations that exist across pediatric cancers. Sequencing of tumors sampled at different time points has shown that mutational events can change with increasing age[14] and with variable retention of targetable mutations at later time points.[6,15] For example, in HR-NB, genomic alterations in the anaplastic lymphoma kinase (ALK) gene occurred in 10.5% of cases at diagnosis, but increased by 70% at the time of relapse.[16] In the setting of low somatic mutational burden, even in high-risk cancer subtypes, germline mutations, mutations of upstream regulators (ie, hijacking),[17] gene fusions,[18] and epigenetic modifications have also been identified as significant events in tumorigenesis.[19–22]

More importantly, these studies have demonstrated the feasibility of performing precision oncology in the clinical setting by translating biopsy samples into clinically actionable data that have been used to alter or refine diagnoses, identify and apply targeted therapies, and detect increased familial risk. Most of these studies are being

Table 1
Summary of discovery sequencing studies in pediatric oncology (2015–2023)

Study Name	Country	Year Published	Successful Samples Analyzed (No)	Tumor Types	Method of Genomic Analysis	Study Definition of Actionable Mutation	Actionable Mutations (%)	Actionable Mutation with Available Targeted Drug (%)	Genomic Analysis Altered Diagnosis (%)
Peds-MiOncoSeq	USA	2015	91	Relapsed/ refractory, primary high-risk, rare	WES, RNAseq	Targetable with current drug, altered diagnosis or risk stratification, altered plan for patient/ family counseling	46	23	2
ClinOmics	USA	2016	59	Relapsed/ refractory	WES, RNAseq, SNP array	Known pathogenic mutation, altered diagnosis, targetable with an approved/ investigational drug	51	41	7

BASIC3	USA	2016	121	Relapsed/ refractory, primary high risk	WES	Established clinical utility (known diagnostic or prognostic value, or therapeutic target), potential utility (within known targetable cancer pathway)	39	NR	NR
iCAT	USA	2016	89	Relapsed/ refractory	NGS panel, aCGH	Targetable with an approved/ investigational drug	31	31	3
PMTB	USA	2016	39	Primary high risk	Hybrid capture-based DNA sequencing assay, RNAseq, WES, NGS panel	Targetable with an approved/ investigational drug	73	73	NR
Molecular Biology Tumor Board (MBB)	France	2016	58	Relapsed/ refractory, primary high risk (poor prognosis at time of diagnosis)	NGS panel, aCGH	Targetable with an approved/ investigational drug	40	40	NR

(continued on next page)

Table 1
(continued)

Study Name	Country	Year Published	Successful Samples Analyzed (No)	Tumor Types	Method of Genomic Analysis	Study Definition of Actionable Mutation	Actionable Mutations (%)	Actionable Mutation with Available Targeted Drug (%)	Genomic Analysis Altered Diagnosis (%)
MOSCATO-01	France	2017	69	Relapsed/refractory	aCGH, NGS panel, WES, RNAseq	Targetable with an approved/investigational drug	61	61	4
PIPseq	USA	2017	50	Relapsed/refractory	WES, RNAseq	Led to change in assessment or management of patient (diagnosis, prognosis, therapeutic plan, genetic counseling plan)	90	80	34
TARGET	Australia	2017	27	Primary high risk (expected survival <30%)	NGS panel, RNAseq	Known pathogenic mutations	59	41	NR
UCSF	USA	2017	31	Central nervous system tumors with uncertain diagnosis or treatment	NGS panel	Known pathogenic mutation, altered diagnosis, targetable with an approved/investigational drug	81	61	19

TRICEPS	Canada	2019	62	Relapsed/refractory, primary high-risk	WES, RNAseq	Targetable, biomarker useful for MRD detection, prognostic risk stratification, change diagnosis	87	87	22
PNOC003	Transnational	2019	15	Primary diffuse intrinsic pontine glioma (DIPG)	WES, WGS, RNAseq	Targetable with an approved/investigational drug	100	100	NR
SMC	South Korea	2019	53	Relapsed/refractory	NGS panel	Targetable with an approved/investigational drug	36	36	NR
SMPAEDS	United Kingdom	2019	209	Relapsed/refractory	Hybrid capture-based NGS panel	Targetable with an approved/investigational drug	51	51	NR
ProfiLER	France	2020	43	Relapsed/refractory, Rare	NSG panel, aCGH	Targetable with an approved/investigational drug	23	23	NR
ZERO Childhood Cancer	Australia	2020	252	Relapsed/refractory, primary high risk	WGS, RNAseq, DNA methylation analysis	Targetable with an approved/investigational drug	71	71	5
PROFYLE	Canada	2020	100	Relapsed/refractory, rare	NGS panel, WGS, RNAseq	Potential to alter diagnosis, risk stratification, prognosis, or treatment plan	82	71	NR

(continued on next page)

Table 1
(continued)

Study Name	Country	Year Published	Successful Samples Analyzed (No)	Tumor Types	Method of Genomic Analysis	Study Definition of Actionable Mutation	Actionable Mutations (%)	Actionable Mutation with Available Targeted Drug (%)	Genomic Analysis Altered Diagnosis (%)
DCOG-iTHER	The Netherlands	2020	80	Relapsed/refractory	WES, lcWGS, RNAseq, DNA methylation analysis	Targetable with an approved/investigational drug	59	34	NR
INFORM	Germany	2021	926	Relapsed/refractory, primary high risk	WES, lcWGS, DNA methylation analysis, RNAseq	Targetable with an approved/investigational drug	85	48	7
MAPPYACTS	France	2022	787	Relapsed/refractory	WES, RNAseq, NGS panel	Targetable with an approved/investigational drug	69	30	NR
MATCH	USA	2022	1000	Relapsed/refractory	NGS panel, IHC	Targetable with an approved/investigational drug	34	31	NR
KiCS	Canada	2023	264	Relapsed/refractory, rare, suspected genetic cancer predisposition	NGS panel, RNAseq, WGS	Targetable with an approved/investigational drug	54	54	NR

Abbreviations: aCGH, array comparative genomic hybridization; IHC, immunohistochemistry; lcWGS, low coverage whole genome sequencing; NGS, next-generation sequencing; NR, not reported; RNAseq, ribonucleic acid sequencing; SNP, single-nucleotide polymorphism; WES, whole exome sequencing; WGS, whole genome sequencing.

performed on recurrent or refractory cancers and use multiple methods of genomic analysis. Although a limitation of these studies is their varied definition of a "clinically actionable mutation," the majority agrees that it is defined by the detection of a known mutation that can be directly or indirectly targeted with an approved or investigational drug; rates vary from 31% to 100% (see **Table 1**).

These studies continue to accrue data worldwide and range from single-center studies to transnational multicenter collaborations (see **Table 1**). Publicly available data repositories also have allowed for data sharing across multiple centers and data pooling to strengthen analytical power (**Box 1**).

ESTABLISHED THERAPEUTIC TARGETS IN PEDIATRIC ONCOLOGY
Cell Surface Targets

Ideal therapeutic targets are diffusely expressed by cancer cells with little-to-no expression on noncancerous cells. Targets can be found on the cell surface (eg, GD2, PD-1) or within the cell (eg, phosphoinositide 3-kinase [PI3K]/mammalian target of rapamycin [mTOR] pathway) but ideally are targetable with available FDA-approved drugs or agents that are under investigation in the clinical or preclinical settings (**Table 2**). As recurrent molecular alterations are discovered across difficult-to-treat pediatric tumors, the overlap in molecular targets between adult and pediatric tumors has allowed for the repurposing of established targeted therapies for off-label use in pediatric oncology (see **Table 2**). Prominent examples include the use of immune checkpoint inhibitors (ICIs) targeting PD-1 and CTLA-4 for Hodgkin lymphoma,[23] melanoma,[24] and microsatellite instability (MSI) high tumors,[25] anti-CD20 monoclonal antibody (rituximab) for non-Hodgkin lymphoma, and ALK inhibitors (crizotinib, ceritinib) for ALK-positive tumors including lymphoma and NB.[26–28] This has not only increased the therapeutic options for refractory disease but has also improved response rates and overall survival (OS) when combined with cytotoxic therapy.[29]

In addition to discovering new indications for existing drugs, ongoing research aims to discover novel therapeutic targets. The discovery of the cell surface marker, tumor-associated disialoganglioside GD2, expressed uniformly by NB tumor cells is a pivotal example of targeted therapy development in pediatric oncology (**Fig. 2**).[30] This led to the development of dinutuximab, an anti-GD2 monoclonal antibody, which demonstrated significant improvement in event-free survival (EFS) (66 ± 5% vs 46 ± 5%, $P = .01$) and OS (86 ± 4% vs 75 ± 5%, $P = .02$) at 2 years in patients with HR-NB.[29] Dinutuximab is currently FDA-approved for use in children with HR-NB and is used as salvage immunotherapy in children with refractory disease.[31] Thus, the discovery of recurrent mutations in difficult-to-treat pediatric cancers has increased therapeutic options and subsequently improved survival through the utilization of existing drugs or the development of novel therapies.

Box 1
List of sequencing data repositories in pediatric oncology

St Jude Cloud (https://pecan.stjude.cloud/)

Gabriella Miller Kids First Data Resource Portal (https://kidsfirstdrc.org/)

R2 Genomics Analysis and Visualization Platform (http://r2.amc.nl/)

Table 2
Molecular targets in pediatric oncology

Molecular Target	Available Drug/Agent(s)	Tumor Types
Cell Surface Targets		
GD2	Dinutuximab	Neuroblastoma
CD20	Rituximab	NHL
ALK	Crizotinib, ceritinib	Anaplastic large cell lymphoma, inflammatory myofibroblastic tumor, neuroblastoma
CD33	Gemtuzumab ozogamicin	AML
PD-1	Pembrolizumab, nivolumab	Hodgkin lymphoma, MSI-H colorectal cancer
CTLA-4	Ipilimumab	Melanoma
SMO	Vismodegib	Medulloblastoma
FGFR	Ponatinib, dovitinib	Rhabdomyosarcoma
Intracellular Targets		
ABL1 kinase	Imatinib, ruxolitinib, dasatinib	ALL, CML
VEGFR/PDGFR kinases	Pazopanib	Rhabdomyosarcoma (PAX3-FOX01 fusion) (Singh 2022)
PARP1	Olaparib, talazoparib	Ewing sarcoma (EWSR1-FLI fusion), medulloblastoma, Wilms tumor
PI3K/mTOR	Everolimus, temsirolimus, rapamycin	Osteosarcoma, subependymal giant cell astrocytoma
MEK	Trametinib, selumetinib	Glioma, neurofibroma, juvenile myelomonocytic leukemia
BRAF	Vemurafenib, dabrafenib	Melanoma, glioma, astrocytoma
NTRK 1/2/3	Larotrectinib	Infantile fibrosarcoma, soft tissue sarcoma, congenital mesoblastic nephroma, thyroid cancer, melanoma, breast cancer
CDK 4/6	Palbociclib, ribociclib	Neuroblastoma
BET	JQ1, IBET726, OTX015	Neuroblastoma, medulloblastoma
AURKA	Alisertib	Neuroblastoma
KDM4B	QC6352	Rhabdomyosarcoma (PAX3-FOX01 fusion)

Abbreviations: AML, acute myeloid leukemia; CML, chronic myeloid leukemia; MSI-H, microsatellite instability-high; NHL, non-hodgkin lymphoma.

APPLICATIONS OF PRECISION ONCOLOGY IN THE DIAGNOSIS AND TREATMENT OF PEDIATRIC CANCERS
Precision Trials in Pediatric Oncology

Early pediatric precision oncology studies highlighted the value of evaluating multiple refractory tumor types to identify clinically actionable mutations among the most difficult-to-treat cancers (see **Table 1**). However, in these early studies, the number

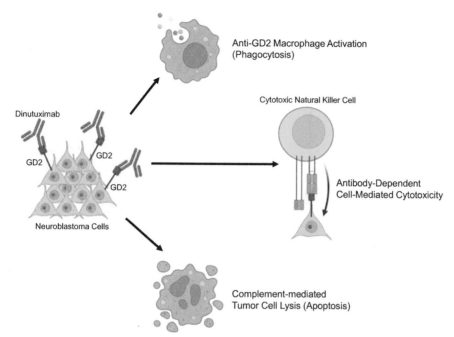

Fig. 2. Targeting of the cell surface marker, GD2, on neuroblastoma cells leads to tumor cell death via multiple mechanisms including antibody-dependent cell-mediated cytotoxicity, complement-mediated cell lysis/apoptosis, and macrophage activation/phagocytosis. (Created with Biorender.com.)

of participants that actually received matched targeted therapy or reported clinical follow-up was low.[32–34] Although conventional tumor-specific clinical trials provided a framework for evaluating the efficacy of novel therapeutic agents, the low (or often unknown) frequency of genomic variants in rare pediatric cancers[6] and our limited understanding of their therapeutic response created unique challenges in applying this framework to pediatric precision oncology.[35]

"Basket trials" provide a solution by recruiting multiple cancer types and allocating participants to treatment arms based on their targetable genomic alteration. Thus, creating a framework to increase access to molecular screening and molecular targeted therapies for cancers with low numbers (ie, refractory or rare tumors) while also evaluating treatment safety and efficacy. At present, the largest ongoing pediatric precision oncology "basket trials" are the National Cancer Institute–Children's Oncology Group Pediatric Molecular Analysis for Therapy Choice (MATCH) trial (NCT03155620, APEC1621) and the Secured Access–European Proof-of-Concept Therapeutic Stratification Trial of Molecular Anomalies in Relapsed or Refractory Tumors (AcSe'-ESMART) trial (NCT02813135, EUDRACT:2016–000133–40) **(Table 3)**.

The Pediatric MATCH trial began recruitment in 2017 and is actively recruiting patients aged 1 to 21 years from Children's Oncology Group institutions with treatment-refractory or recurrent solid tumors, non-Hodgkin lymphoma, or histiocytic disorders.[36] This basket trial uses a centralized system which obtains tumor samples after recurrence or disease progression (except in high-grade glioma), performs targeted NGS amplicon sequencing, RNAseq, and immunohistochemistry, and automatically assigns patients to one of 13 treatment arms previously agreed on by the trial's Target and Agent

Table 3
Comparison of ongoing basket trials in pediatric oncology

Trial Name	Clinical Trial ID	Sponsor	Sequencing Method(s)	Method of Treatment Matching	Treatment Arms
Pediatric-MATCH	NCT03155620	National Cancer Institute–Children's Oncology Group	Uniform gene panel (amplicon DNA sequencing, RNAseq, IHC)	Automated	Monotherapy
AcSe-ESMART	NCT02813135	Gustave Roussy Cancer Campus, Grand Paris	Decentralized advanced molecular testing (WES/WGS ± RNAseq)	Multidisciplinary tumor board	Agent combined with chemotherapy

Table 4
National Cancer Institute–Children's Oncology Group pediatric MATCH trial treatment arms

Arm	Actionable Mutation	Drug	Drug Mechanism of Action
A	NTRK 1/2/3 fusion	Larotrectinib	TRK inhibitor
B	FGFR 1/2/3 mutation/fusion; FGFR4 mutation	Erdafitinib	FGFR kinase inhibitor
C	SMARCB 1/4 mutation/loss	Tazemetostat	EZH2 inhibitor
D	TSC 1/2, mTOR, or PIK3CA mutation; PTEN mutation/loss	Samotolisib	Dual PI3K/mTOR inhibitor
E[a]	BRAF mutation/fusion; NRAS, KRAS, HRAS, NF1, ARAF, GNAQ, GNA11 mutation	Selumetinib	Selective MEK inhibitor
F	ALK mutation/fusion; ROS1 fusion	Ensartinib	ALK inhibitor
G[a]	BRAF V600 mutation	Vemurafenib	BRAF V600 E inhibitor
H	BRCA 1/2, ATM, RAD51 C/D mutation	Olaparib	PARP inhibitor
I	CDK 4/6, CCND 1/2/3 amplification	Palbociclib	Selective CDK inhibitor
J[a]	BRAF mutation/fusion; NRAS, KRAS, HRAS, NF1, ARAF, GNAQ, GNA11, MAP2K1 mutation	Ulixertinib	ERK inhibitor
K	IDH1 R132 mutation	Ivosidenib	IDH1 inhibitor
M[a]	HRAS mutation	Tipifarnib	Farnesyl transferase inhibitor (blocks Ras activation)
N	RET mutation/fusion	Selpercatinib	RET inhibitor

Abbreviations: ALK, anaplastic lymphoma kinase; BRAF, V-raf murine sarcoma viral oncogene homolog B1; CDK, cyclin-dependent kinase; ERK, extracellular signal-regulated kinase; EZH2, enhancer of zeste homolog 2; FGFR, fibroblast growth factor receptor; IDH1, isocitrate dehydrogenase 1; mTOR, mammalian target of rapamycin; PARP, Poly(ADP-ribose)-polymerase; PI3K, phosphoinositide 3-kinase; RET, rearranged during transfection; TRK, tropomyosin receptor kinase.
[a] Arms involved in targeting of mitogen-activated protein kinase (MAPK, MEK signaling pathway).

Prioritization committee (**Table 4**).[37] Of the first 1000 patients enrolled, the majority had non-central nervous system (CNS) solid tumors (72.3%)—primarily sarcomas (50.5%)—and 31.5% were identified to have actionable mutations. Out of those with actionable mutations, 90.2% were matched to a treatment arm, but only 41.6% were ultimately enrolled in a Phase II sub-trial.[36] This study highlights several ongoing challenges in treatment allocation (eg, genomic alterations not yet targetable such as TP53, MYCN, and CTNNB1) as well as patient enrollment (eg, inability for younger patients to take pills, competing non-precision oncology trials).[36] However, this ongoing trial is the first "basket trial" in the United States to demonstrate the feasibility of a centralized nationwide screening and treatment allocation framework.

The AcSe'-ESMART trial began in 2016 led by the Gustave Roussy Cancer Campus, Grand Paris and the Innovative Therapies for Children with Cancer Precision Cancer Medicine Program. This trial is also continuing active enrollment of patients less than 18 years of age with life expectancy $\geq$3 months and hematologic or solid tumors with progression despite standard therapy or no known effective standard therapy.[38]

In contrast to the Pediatric MATCH trial, this uses a decentralized sequencing framework and obtains sequencing results (WES or WGS ± RNAseq), as opposed to tumor samples, and determines treatment allocation based on centralized multidisciplinary tumor board (MTB) consensus (see **Table 3**).[38] This study also differs from its US counterpart by combining targeted therapy with chemotherapy in its treatment arms, in contrast to targeted monotherapy (see **Table 3**). Although both "basket trials" are ongoing, they demonstrate the potential variation in trial design and the feasibility of expanding pediatric precision oncology into clinical practice.

TARGETED THERAPIES IN PEDIATRIC SOLID TUMORS

As surgical resection is a key component in the management of high-risk and difficult-to-treat pediatric solid tumors, the development of targeted therapies for pediatric solid tumors is of particular interest.[39,40] Molecular testing of recurrent or refractory solid tumors has allowed for molecular risk stratification and treatment allocation,[41] whereas extensive preclinical research has also identified recurrent tumor-specific molecular alterations which has provided the rationale for Phase I/II clinical trials (**Table 5**).[42] Targeted therapies can be classified into serving one of two primary functions (1) inhibition of a key tumorigenic pathway (eg, tyrosine kinase inhibitors [TKIs], histone deacetylase [HDAC] inhibitors): or (2) tumor-directed immune system activation (eg, monoclonal antibodies, chimeric antigen receptor T-cell [CAR-T] therapy, DNA vaccines) (see **Table 5**). The following sections review the targeted therapies currently in-use or under investigation among the most common extracranial pediatric solid tumors.

Neuroblastoma

NB originates from neural crest cells and is the most common extracranial pediatric solid tumor—accounting for 7% of childhood cancers and 15% of all childhood cancer deaths.[43] NB is stratified from very low risk to high risk based on the presence or absence of various prognostic factors such as disseminated disease, histologic differentiation, and molecular alterations (eg, *MYCN* oncogene amplification, chromosomal copy number variation).[44] Tumor behavior is also heterogeneous ranging from spontaneous regression in low-risk disease to refractory metastatic disease in HR-NB. Although survival in low-risk disease reaches 90%, 5-year survival remains dismal in HR-NB despite multimodal therapy—with 50% of children ultimately succumbing to this disease.[45] In addition, approximately 50% of HR-NB patients do not respond to first-line therapy, or they relapse within the first 2 years of treatment initiation.[46] The poor prognosis in HR-NB is attributed to posttreatment minimal residual disease or microscopic treatment-refractory disease that proliferates and metastasizes without an effective treatment. Thus, significant work is focused on identifying recurrent molecular alterations that can be targeted in HR-NB.

The discovery of the cell surface marker, disialoganglioside GD2, and the development of the anti-GD2 monoclonal antibody, dinutuximab, is a leading example of targeted therapy development in pediatric precision oncology. GD2 is present in the majority of human NB cell lines, retaining its expression in recurrent disease, and is rarely expressed in normal human tissues—thus making it an ideal target.[47] After extensive preclinical testing and safety evaluation, Phase III investigation of dinutuximab (with granulocyte-macrophage colony-stimulating factor and interleukin-2) in 226 patients with HR-NB demonstrated a clear long-term improvement in 5-year EFS (56.6 ± 4.7% vs isotretinoin alone 46.1 ± 5.1%; $P = .042$) and 5-year OS (73.2 ± 4.2% vs isotretinoin alone 56.5 ± 5.1%; $P = .045$).[48] Since FDA approval in

Table 5
Precision oncology clinical trials for pediatric solid tumors

Trial ID	Sponsor	Phase	Ages Included	Tumor Type	Disease State	Target	Treatment	Targeted Treatment Type	Targeted Treatment Mechanism of Action	Trial Status
NCT04308330	New York Medical College	1	1–30 y	Solid tumors (including CNS)	Recurrent, refractory	Histone deacetylase (HDAC)	Vorinostat + chemotherapy	Small molecular inhibitor	HDAC inhibitor	Recruiting
NCT02644460	Emory University	1	2–25 y	Solid tumors (including CNS)	Recurrent, refractory	CDK 4/6	Abemaciclib	Small molecular inhibitor	Selective CDK 4/6 inhibitor	Recruiting
NCT04928677	Memorial Sloan Kettering Cancer Center	1	1–21 y	GPC3-expressing extra-cranial solid tumors	Recurrent, refractory	GPC3	Codrituzumab	Monoclonal antibody	Anti-GPC3 monoclonal antibody	Recruiting
NCT04851119	COG	1/2	1–30 y	Non-CNS solid tumors (including desmoid tumors) with Wnt pathway aberrations	Recurrent, refractory	Wnt pathway	Tegavivint	Small molecular inhibitor	Inhibits transducin b-like protein 1 (TBL1) binding b-catenin (Wnt pathway)	Recruiting
NCT04897321	St Jude Children's Research Hospital	1	<21 y	Non-CNS solid tumors	Recurrent, refractory	B7-H3	B7-H3 CAR-T cells	CAR-T cell	B7-H3 CAR-T cell therapy	Recruiting
NCT04634357	Eureka Therapeutics Inc	1/2	1–21 y	HLA-A2 positive, liver tumor	Recurrent, refractory	AFP, HLA-A2	ET140203 CAR-T Cells	CAR-T cell	AFP-HLA-A2-CAR T-cell therapy	Recruiting
NCT03107988	New Approaches to Neuroblastoma Therapy Consortium	1/2	1–99 y	ALK-mutated high-risk neuroblastoma	Recurrent, refractory	ALK	Lorlatinib ± chemotherapy	Small molecular inhibitor	ALK inhibitor	Recruiting
NCT02559778	Wake Forest University Health Services	1	<22 y	High-risk neuroblastoma	Primary or recurrent	ALK, receptor tyrosine kinases, HDAC	Ceritinib, dasatinib, sorafenib, or vorinostat ± DFMO	Small molecular inhibitor	Tyrosine kinase inhibitor, HDAC inhibitor	Recruiting
NCT05272371	Jagiellonian University	1/2	1–18 y	High-risk neuroblastoma	Recurrent, refractory	GD2	Dinutuximab + chemotherapy	Monoclonal antibody	Anti-GD2 monoclonal antibody	Recruiting
NCT02914405	University Hospital Southampton NHS Foundation Trust	1	1–18 y	High-risk neuroblastoma	Recurrent, refractory	GD2, PD-1R	Dinutuximab + nivolumab	Monoclonal antibody	Anti-GD2 and anti-PD-1R monoclonal antibody	Recruiting

(continued on next page)

Table 5
(continued)

Trial ID	Sponsor	Phase	Ages Included	Tumor Type	Disease State	Target	Treatment	Targeted Treatment Type	Targeted Treatment Mechanism of Action	Trial Status
NCT03363373	Y-mAbs Therapeutics	2	>1 y	High-risk neuroblastoma	Refractory	GD2	Naxitamab (hu3F8)	Monoclonal antibody	Anti-GD2 monoclonal antibody	Recruiting
NCT03373097	Bambino Gesu Hospital and Research Institute	1/2	1–25 y	GD2-positive tumors	Recurrent, refractory	GD2	GD2-CART01	CAR-T cell	GD2-CAR T-cell therapy	Recruiting
NCT04049864	Belarusian Research Center for Pediatric Oncology	1	1–20 y	Neuroblastoma	Recurrent	NB-associated antigens (TH, Phox2B, survivin, MAGEA 1/3, PRAME)	DNA vaccine	DNA vaccine	Anti-NB DNA vaccine	Recruiting
NCT04936529	Memorial Sloan Kettering Cancer Center	2	All ages	High-risk neuroblastoma	Complete remission	NB-associated antigens	Bivalent DNA vaccine	DNA vaccine	Anti-NB DNA vaccine	Recruiting
NCT05429502	Novartis Pharmaceuticals	1/2	1–21 y	Neuroblastoma, medulloblastoma, high-grade glioma, malignant rhabdoid tumor, rhabdomyosarcoma	Recurrent, refractory	Cyclin-dependent kinase 4/6 (CDK 4/6)	Ribociclib + chemotherapy	Small molecular inhibitor	Selective CDK 4/6 inhibitor	Recruiting
NCT01858168	Massachusetts General Hospital	1	≥16 y	Ewing sarcoma, rhabdomyosarcoma	Refractory	Poly(ADP-ribose) polymerase (PARP)	Olaparib + chemotherapy	Small molecular inhibitor	PARP inhibitor	Recruiting
NCT04299113	Jonsson Comprehensive Cancer Center	1	≥13 y	rhabdomyosarcoma	Recurrent, refractory	HDAC	Mocetinostat + chemotherapy	Small molecular inhibitor	HDAC inhibitor	Recruiting
NCT04417062	Dana-Farber Cancer Institute	2	12–40 y	Osteosarcoma	Recurrent, refractory	PARP, ATR	Olaparib + ceralasertib	Small molecular inhibitor	PARP inhibitor, ATR inhibitor	Recruiting
NCT04833582	K-Group, Beta, Inc.	1/2	≥12 y	Osteosarcoma	Recurrent, refractory	Wee-1	ZN-c3 + chemotherapy	Small molecular inhibitor	Wee-1 inhibitor	Recruiting
NCT02502786	Memorial Sloan Kettering Cancer Center	2	13 months–30 years	Osteosarcoma	Recurrent, refractory	GD2	Humanized 3F8	Monoclonal antibody	Anti-GD2 monoclonal antibody	Recruiting

NCT Number	Sponsor	Phase	Age	Tumor	Target	Condition	Intervention	Type	Mechanism	Status
NCT04294511	Sun Yat-sen University	2	14–65 y	Osteosarcoma	PD1	Primary or recurrent	Camrelizumab + chemotherapy	Monoclonal antibody	Anti-PD1 monoclonal antibody	Recruiting
NCT03628209	H Lee Moffitt Cancer Center	1/2	<39 y	Osteosarcoma	PD1	Recurrent, refractory	Nivolumab ± chemotherapy	Monoclonal antibody	Anti-PD1 monoclonal antibody	Recruiting
NCT03811886	Case Comprehensive Cancer Center	1/2	5–30 y	Pulmonary metastatic osteosarcoma	a4b1-integrin	Refractory	Natalizumab	Monoclonal antibody	Anti-a4b1-integrin monoclonal antibody	Recruiting
NCT03277924	Grupo Espanol de Investigacion en Sarcomas	1/2	12–80 y	Sarcoma (bone, soft tissue)	Receptor tyrosine kinases (VEGFR, PDGFR, c-KIT, RET, CD114, CD135), PD1	Refractory	Sunitinib ± nivolumab + chemotherapy	Small molecular inhibitor, monoclonal antibody	Tyrosine kinase inhibitor, anti-PD1 monoclonal antibody	Recruiting
NCT03462316	Sun Yat-sen University	1	14–70 y	Sarcoma (bone, soft tissue)	NY-ESO-1	Refractory	NY-ESO-1-specific T-cell receptor T-cell therapy	TCR-T therapy	Anti-NY-ESO-1 TCR transduced T-cell therapy	Recruiting
NCT01121588	Pfizer	1	≥15 y	ALK-mutated tumors (excluding NSCLC)	ALK	Primary or recurrent	Crizotinib	Small molecular inhibitor	ALK inhibitor	Active, not recruiting
NCT02909777	Dana-Farber Cancer Institute	1	1–21 y	Solid tumors (including CNS), lymphoma	PI3K, HDAC	Recurrent, refractory	Fimepinostat (CUDC-907)	Small molecular inhibitor	PI3K class 1 inhibitor, HDAC inhibitor	Active, not recruiting
NCT02867592	NCI	2	2–30 y	Solid tumors (including CNS)	Receptor tyrosine kinases	Recurrent, refractory	Cabozantinib-S-Malate	Small molecular inhibitor	Tyrosine kinase inhibitor	Active, not recruiting
NCT05093322	HUTCHMED	1/2	2–21 y	Non-CNS solid tumors, lymphoma	VEGFR, FGFR1, CSFR1	Recurrent, refractory	Surufatinib + chemotherapy	Small molecular inhibitor	VEGF, FGF, CSF inhibitor	Active, not recruiting
NCT05071209	NCI	1/2	1–30 y	Non-CNS solid tumors, lymphoma	Ataxia telangiectasia receptor (ATR)	Recurrent, refractory	Elimusertib	Small molecular inhibitor	Selective ATR inhibitor	Active, not recruiting
NCT02308527	University of Birmingham	2	1–21 y	High-risk neuroblastoma	VEGF	Recurrent, refractory	Bevacizumab + chemotherapy	Monoclonal antibody	Anti-VEGF monoclonal antibody	Active, not recruiting
NCT03294954	Baylor College of Medicine	1	1–21 y	High-risk neuroblastoma	GD2	Recurrent, refractory	GD2-CAR expressing natural killer T cells	CAR-T cell	GD2-CAR NK T-cell therapy	Active, not recruiting

(continued on next page)

Table 5
(continued)

Trial ID	Sponsor	Phase	Ages Included	Tumor Type	Disease State	Target	Treatment	Targeted Treatment Type	Targeted Treatment Mechanism of Action	Trial Status
NCT02998983	Laboratorio Elea Phoenix SA	2	1–12 y	High-risk neuroblastoma	Recurrent, partial remission	N-glycolyl GM3	Racotumomab	Monoclonal antibody	Anti-N-glycolyl GM3 monoclonal antibody	Active, not recruiting
NCT04095221	Memorial Sloan Kettering Cancer Center	1/2	≥1 y	Rhabdomyosarcoma, desmoplastic small round cell tumor	Recurrent, refractory	Checkpoint kinase CHEK 1/2	Prexasertib + chemotherapy	Small molecular inhibitor	CHEK 1/2 inhibitor	Active, not recruiting
NCT04154189	Eisai Inc.	2	2–25 y	Osteosarcoma	Recurrent, refractory	Receptor tyrosine kinases (CEGFR, FGFR, CSFR1, RAF-1, RET, KIT)	Chemotherapy ± lenvatinib	Small molecular inhibitor	Tyrosine kinase inhibitor	Active, not recruiting
NCT04803877	Sarcoma Alliance for Research through Collaboration	2	≥5 y	Osteosarcoma	Recurrent, refractory	Receptor tyrosine kinases (CEGFR, FGFR, CSFR1, RAF-1, RET, KIT), PD1	Regorafenib + nivolumab	Small molecular inhibitor, monoclonal antibody	Tyrosine kinase inhibitor, anti-PD1 monoclonal antibody	Active, not recruiting
NCT01459484	Italian Sarcoma Group	2	<40 y	ABCB1/P-glycoprotein overexpressing high-grade Osteosarcoma	Non-metastatic, primary or recurrent	n/a	Mifamurtide	Muramyl dipeptide (immunostimulant)	Immunostimulant via NOD2 activation	Active, not recruiting
NCT03006848	St Jude Children's Research Hospital	2	12–49 y	Osteosarcoma	Recurrent, refractory	PDL1	Avelumab	Monoclonal antibody	Anti-PDL1 monoclonal antibody	Active, not recruiting
NCT02484443	NCI	2	<29 y	Osteosarcoma	Recurrent, refractory	GD2	Dinutuximab	Monoclonal antibody	Anti-GD2 monoclonal antibody	Active, not recruiting
NCT01953900	Baylor College of Medicine	1	All ages	Osteosarcoma, neuroblastoma	Recurrent, refractory	GD2, varicella zoster	iC9-GD2-CAR-VZV-CTL	CAR-T cell	Anti-GD2-VZV-CAR T-cell therapy	Active, not recruiting

NCT / Sponsor	Phase	Age	Tumor type	Disease status	Target	Drug	Type	Description	Status
NCT01502410 NCI	2	2–30 y	RMS, liver tumors, renal tumors (including Wilms tumor), thyroid tumors	Recurrent, refractory	Raf kinase	Sorafenib tosylate	Small molecular inhibitor	Multi-kinase inhibitor (Raf/BRAF, ERK, MEK), Anti-angiogenic (VEGF, PDGF)	Completed
NCT01598454 Laboratorio Elea Phoenix SA	1/2	1–10 y	Solid tumors (including CNS)	Recurrent, refractory	N-glycolyl GM3	Racotumomab	Monoclonal antibody	Anti-N-glycolyl GM3 monoclonal antibody	Completed
NCT00831844 NCI	2	7 months–30 years	Non-CNS solid tumors	Recurrent, refractory	IGF-1R	Cixutumumab	Monoclonal antibody	Anti-insulin-like growth factor-1 receptor (IGF-1R) monoclonal antibody	Completed
NCT02982941 MacroGenics	1	1–35 y	Non-CNS solid tumors	Recurrent, refractory	B7-H3	Enoblituzumab	Monoclonal antibody	Anti-B7-H3 monoclonal antibody	Completed
NCT02452554 COG	2	1–30 y	Non-CNS solid tumors	Recurrent, refractory	CD56	Lorvotuzumab mertansine (IMGN901)	Monoclonal antibody	Anti-CD56 monoclonal antibody	Completed
NCT04385277 COG	2	<31 y	High-risk neuroblastoma	Post-consolidation therapy, non-progressive	GD2	Dinutuximab + chemotherapy	Monoclonal antibody	Anti-GD2 monoclonal antibody	Suspended (met accrual goal)
NCT04751383 NCI	1	2–35 y	Osteosarcoma, neuroblastoma	Recurrent, refractory	CD47, GD2	Magrolimab + dinutuximab	Monoclonal antibody	Anti-CD47 and anti-GD2 monoclonal antibodies	Suspended (unacceptable toxicity)
NCT01236586 NCI	2	1–21 y	Solid tumors (including CNS), lymphoma	Recurrent, refractory	Gamma secretase (notch signaling)	RO4929097	Small molecular inhibitor	Gamma secretase inhibitor (notch pathway)	Withdrawn

2015, dinutuximab has become the first FDA-approved targeted immunotherapy for HR-NB as part of a first-line multi-agent regimen. Current studies aim to use dinutuximab to augment standard-of-care salvage chemotherapy regimens in refractory disease[49] and mitigate the toxicity profile with the development of a humanized anti-GD2 monoclonal antibody, naxitamab.[50] In addition, bivalent vaccines and CAR-T therapy are also being explored to target HR-NB via the GD2 cell surface marker (NCT03294954, NCT03373097).[51]

In contrast to GD2, MYCN is another potential target in NB that has proved challenging thus far. MYCN is a disordered protein hidden within the cell nucleus which is involved in normal cell proliferation by binding with MAX to act as a transcription factor. However, *MYCN* amplification can lead to uncontrolled cancer cell proliferation, survival, immune evasion, and metastasis.[52] Although *MYCN* amplification occurs in 20% to 30% of NB cases, it is highly correlated with aggressive disease, poor survival, and its presence is a defining factor of high-risk disease.[53] Since the 1990s, MYCN has been identified as a potential target in HR-NB. Approaches to MYCN targeting include blocking MYCN-MAX dimerization or subsequent DNA binding,[54] inhibition of MYCN stabilizer proteins[55] or chaperone molecules,[56] and targeting epigenetic modifications to downregulate MYCN expression.[57] However, the crossover from preclinical to clinical studies has been limited, with the first-in-human Phase I trial of an MYCN inhibitor, PeptoMYC, currently underway (NCT04808362). PeptoMYC preferentially binds MAX to form PeptoMYC-MAX heterodimers, subsequently blocking MYCN oncogene activation.[58,59] Preliminary results seem to demonstrate safety with mild infusion-related reactions reported and eight patients with stable disease (SD, 47.1%) in the first 17 patients enrolled.[60]

Early Phase I/II clinical trials are also investigating the efficacy of targeting key tumorigenic pathways in NB (**Table 6**). Targeting of the ALK signaling pathway with receptor TKIs (eg, crizotinib, lorlatinib)[61] and the PI3k/Akt/mTOR pathway with Akt inhibitors (eg, perifosine)[62] has demonstrated safety with ongoing evaluation of efficacy (see **Table 5**). Preclinical research has also identified additional targets with potential for clinical translation in the Wnt signaling pathway,[63,64] Ras-mitogen-activated protein kinase (MAPK) signal transduction pathway,[65] and *P53*-MDM2 pathway.[66,67] For example, with more than 98% of NB expressing wild-type *P53*,[68] targeted inhibition of the *P53* inhibitor (MDM2) with nutlin-3a has led to *P53* accumulation and downstream reactivation of *P53*-dependent apoptotic pathways decreasing tumor cell proliferation in vitro and tumor growth in preclinical murine models.[69–72] These preclinical findings elucidate the mechanistic understanding of these targetable pathways and provide the rationale for further clinical translation.

Targeting of epigenetic modifications, such as (HDACs and bromodomain and extraterminal (BET) proteins, has also shown promise in the targeted treatment of NB. In a Phase I trial aiming to identify the maximum tolerated dose of the HDAC inhibitor, vorinostat, in refractory pediatric solid tumors, one patient with NB experienced a complete response (CR).[73] Thus, the recognition of recurrent epigenetic modifications in NB has expanded the therapeutic potential of small molecule inhibitors that can alter tumor cell DNA transcription and ultimately tumor cell survival.[74] Future directions in molecular therapy development include targeting of cancer exosomes containing oncogenic microRNAs (miRNA)[75] and DNA vaccines to prevent NB recurrence (NCT04049864).

Wilms Tumor

Wilms tumor (WT), or nephroblastoma, is the most common renal malignancy and the second most common abdominal solid tumor in childhood. Although 5-year survival is favorable at greater than 90% with surgery, chemotherapy, and radiotherapy, survival

Table 6	
Current challenges in pediatric precision oncology	
Limitations in immunotherapy	Immature or depleted immune system
	Lack of biomarkers to predict response of immunotherapy
	Potential for acute and/or late toxicity
	Potential for immune system overactivation
Potential resistance to targeted therapies	Tumor and tumor microenvironment heterogeneity
	Mutations of the target itself
	Activation of alternate pathways (eg, upstream, downstream, parallel)
	Tumor microenvironment cross talk
Lack of access to targeted therapies	Limited overlap with adult tumor molecular targets
	Small number of patients with rare or difficult-to-treat tumors
	Safety concerns in pediatric use
Prohibitive cost	Sequencing
	Data analysis
	Targeted therapy
Lack of logistical infrastructure	Lengthy turnaround time (biopsy to matched therapy initiation)
	Lack of unified framework for pediatric precision oncology
Ethical impact of identifying incidental germline mutations	Unknown implications of incidental germline mutations
	Potential for unnecessary further invasive and/or noninvasive diagnostic testing in healthy individuals

rates decline with advanced disease (metastatic, recurrent).[76,77] The need for alternative therapies in this difficult-to-treat subpopulation, as well as the known toxicity of standard therapeutic regimens (eg, cardiotoxicity from anthracyclines), has driven targeted therapy development for WT.[78]

WTs with an unfavorable prognosis are characterized by an increased ratio of anti-inflammatory (M2) macrophages and low levels of tumor-infiltrating lymphocytes (TILs), which creates an immunologically "cold" environment—protecting the tumor from the immune system.[79,80] This also creates a challenge in the development of targeted immunotherapies against WT. Unlike lymphoma, pediatric solid tumors—especially WTs—express the lowest level of traditional immunotherapy targets, such as immune checkpoint ligands (eg, PD-1, PD-L1)[81–83] and a suboptimal response to ICIs. This was demonstrated by the KEYNOTE-051 study where response to pembrolizumab occurred in only 5.9% of solid tumors as compared with 60% in the lymphoma group.[84] Thus, alternative novel targets are currently being explored.

B7 homolog 3 protein (B7-H3) is an immunoregulatory molecule in the PD-1 pathway that has been linked to cancer cell immune evasion and metastasis. Unlike PD-1, B7-H3 is highly expressed in pediatric solid tumors—with one study observing positive expression in 100% of WT tumor samples.[85] This seems to be a promising target with ongoing studies targeting B7-H3 with CAR-T therapy (NCT04897321) and monoclonal antibody therapy (enoblituzumab; NCT02982941).

Other promising targets include N-glycolyl GM3 and WT 1 (WT1), which demonstrate overexpression in WT. N-glycolyl GM3 is a ganglioside on the outer cell membrane and found in up to 88% of WT tumor samples with low-to-absent expression in normal kidney tissue—making it an ideal therapeutic target.[86] Early investigation of an anti-N-glycolyl GM3 monoclonal antibody, racotumomab, was shown to be safe, but it did not alter disease progression with 12 of 14 patients experiencing disease progression and the other two patients with SD.[87] Similarly, targeting of WT1 with tumor-associated antigen cytotoxic T-cells demonstrated safety and led to disease stability in two of seven patients while increasing 6-month progression-free survival (PFS) from 38% to 73% compared with prior therapy. Additional WT1-targeted therapies are also being explored in adult tumors such as CUE-102 (NCT05360680), an immunogenic fusion protein to mobilize the immune system against WT1, and ASP7517 (NCT04837196), an artificial WT1-loaded artificial immunogenic vector cell. In sum, targeted therapies for WT remain under early investigation but have shown to be safe with early promise with regard to efficacy.

Additional studies also aim to induce cellular apoptosis of tumor cells with the use of recombinant tumor necrosis factor-alpha in combination with actinomycin D.[88,89] Phase II study of combination therapy in 19 patients with recurrent or refractory WT led to 3 patients (15.6%) with a CR, 5 (26.3%) with SD, and 11 (57.9%) with progressive disease (PD). However, widespread adoption remains limited by notable toxicities including thrombocytopenia (40.7%), liver transaminitis (23.7%), neutropenia (20.3%), and leukopenia (13.6%).[88]

Hepatoblastoma

Hepatoblastoma (HB) is the most common primary liver malignancy of childhood with the fastest rising incidence among childhood malignancies in children less than 5 years of age.[90] Advances in cisplatin-based chemotherapy and surgery (resection, liver transplantation) have increased 5-year OS to 82% but similar to NB and WT; recurrent metastatic disease is often refractory to available therapies with poor outcomes.[91] The association of HB with genetic syndromes, such as familial adenomatous polyposis or Beckwith–Wiedemann, suggests potential targetable molecular alterations and pathways.[92,93] However, relative to other pediatric solid tumors, HB retains one of the lowest exon mutational burdens—averaging 2.0 to 3.9 coding mutations per tumor.[94] Despite this, progress in molecular and epigenetic profiling has allowed for disease risk stratification[95,96] and identification of potential therapeutic targets.

One of the major aberrant pathways in HB is the Wnt/β-catenin signaling pathway which is often accompanied by YAP activation leading to cancer cell proliferation and differentiation into cancer stem cells.[97] Targeting of CTNNB1 (gene encoding for β-catenin) and β-catenin itself have demonstrated therapeutic efficacy in preclinical models of hepatocellular cancers which led to the development of small molecule inhibitors of this pathway.[98] Tegavivint is a small molecule inhibitor of β-catenin which was initially developed for desmoid tumors. By selectively disrupting of β-catenin and transducing β-like protein 1 binding, β-catenin nuclear translocation is inhibited leading to β-catenin degradation. This has shown promise in other tumors with Wnt/β-catenin signaling overactivation and is a promising therapy under investigation for refractory HB (NCT04851119). Other promising preclinical targets include TERT promoter regions[94] and receptor tyrosine kinases involved in this pathway.[99] Sorafenib is a multi-kinase inhibitor which has been shown to decrease tumor cell viability and inhibit tumor progression in combination with cisplatin in preclinical studies[100] and has been adopted as adjunct therapy in unresectable disease in the ongoing Phase III Pediatric Hepatic International Tumor Trial (NCT03017326). Additional targeted therapies being evaluated in-human are anti-glypican-3 immunotherapy (monoclonal antibody, CAR-T; NCT04928677) and ICIs (NCT05322187).

The PI3K/Akt/mTOR pathway is also dysregulated in HB and a potential targetable pathway.[101] Preclinical research has demonstrated decreased tumor growth, increased tumor cell apoptosis, and reduced serum alpha fetoprotein (AFP) levels with the inhibition of PI3K,[102] mTOR,[103] and PIM kinases.[104] Additional pathways under preclinical investigation include the TGF-β/SMAD[105] and JAK/STAT signaling pathways.[106]

Epigenetic modifications leading to genetic alterations have also been identified in HB, such as DNA methylation, histone modification, and long non-coding RNAs, with particular interest in HDAC inhibitors for recurrent/refractory HB (NCT04308330). In addition, ongoing preclinical research has identified additional novel therapies (eg, PLK1 inhibitors, PARP1 inhibitors, MDM4 inhibitors, anti-CD326 monoclonal antibodies) which halt tumor growth in combination with cytotoxic therapy.[107–110] Thus, although HB contains a relatively low mutational burden, advances in genomic profiling have identified promising preclinical targets and targetable pathways providing rationale for inclusion in ongoing clinical trials.

Rhabdomyosarcoma

Rhabdomyosarcoma (RMS) originates from immature mesodermal cells and is the most common soft tissue sarcoma in childhood.[111] Although 70% of patients with localized disease are able to achieve complete remission with multimodal therapy (chemotherapy, radiation, surgery), the 5-year EFS for metastatic disease is poor (<20%).[112] RMS is classified by histologic subtype (embryonal, alveolar, pleomorphic, spindle cell/sclerosing) but molecular classification based on the presence or absence of the *PAX-FOXO1* gene fusion may provide more prognostic value with fusion-positive RMS correlating with decreased EFS and OS.[113] Sixty percent of alveolar RMS is fusion-positive and the resultant *PAX-FOXO1* fusion protein acts as an oncogenic transcription factor inducing abnormal gene expression leading to tumorigenesis.[114] Preclinical studies targeting *PAX-FOXO1* either directly with silencing RNA or indirectly with HDAC inhibitors have demonstrated inhibition of tumor growth,[115,116]–and HDAC inhibitors are currently being evaluated for in-human use as an adjunct to chemotherapy (NCT04299113).

Molecular testing has also identified additional targetable pathways—similarly dysregulated in other types of sarcomas—which are involved in tumorigenesis and cancer cell proliferation. Targeting of the PI3K/Akt/mTOR pathway with the mTOR inhibitor, temsirolimus, is promising with disease stabilization in 41% of patients with refractory RMS.[117] Phase II investigation of temsirolimus and bevacizumab (anti- vascular endothelial growth factor [VEGF]) in recurrent RMS was halted early due to superior outcomes with temsirolimus in 6-month EFS (69.1% vs 54.6%) and disease progression (11% vs 28%).[118] Results are currently pending from a Phase III trial examining the efficacy of temsirolimus with or without standard chemotherapy in patients with intermediate-risk RMS (NCT02567435).

However, inhibition of other identified pathways has led to variable outcomes. Phase II investigation of crizotinib (ALK inhibitor) in patients with metastatic RMS led to an objective response rate (ORR) in 14.3% of patients with median OS of 5.6 months, but all participants ultimately succumbed to PD.[119] Similarly, antibody targeting the insulin-like growth factor 1 receptor (IGF-1R) with cixutumumab in 20 patients with refractory RMS led to one partial response (PR) and disease stabilization in three patients,[120] but further studies did not reveal any improvement in survival outcomes.[121,122] Preclinical evaluation of the multi-kinase inhibitor, sorafenib, led to inhibition of xenograft tumor growth, but did not result in an objective response in a Phase II study of refractory RMS.[123] Thus, although prior studies have demonstrated limited success with targeted monotherapy in refractory RMS, ongoing trials indicate that future targeted therapies will likely be used as an adjunct to standard chemotherapy regimens.

Osteosarcoma

Osteosarcoma (OST) is the most common primary malignant bone tumor in children, adolescents, and young adults occurring most frequently in the metaphysis of long bones.[124] Approximately 15% to 20% of patients present with metastatic disease, most commonly to the lung, and have poor survival outcomes (5-year OS 20%).[124] Current treatment involves neoadjuvant chemotherapy, limb-sparing surgical resection of all primary and metastatic disease, and adjuvant chemotherapy, but those with a poor tumor response to neoadjuvant chemotherapy (<90% necrosis) also have poor outcomes (5-year EFS 50%–60%).[125]

Genomic profiling of OST tumor samples has identified regions of localized hypermutations (ie, kataegis) in known tumorigenic genes (TP53, RB1, ATRX, DLG2), as well as differential expression of miRNAs (miR-21/221/106a) that may alter gene expression and contribute to cancer cell proliferation.[126,127] However, structural and immunologic aspects of OST have created challenges in targeted therapy development. The dense calcified matrix intrinsic to OST limits not only the penetration of applied therapies but also contributes to immune system evasion which limits the efficacy of immunotherapy approaches.[128,129] OST is also associated with a high density of immunosuppressive M2 macrophages and low levels of TILs which further limits the ability of targeted molecular therapies to mobilize the immune system against the tumor.[130] Despite these limitations, ongoing research aims to combine forms of targeted therapy to improve survival outcomes in recurrent/refractory OST (see **Table 5**).

Targeting of cell surface markers is an emerging therapeutic avenue in OST. In addition to NB, OST also highly expresses the cell surface marker, GD2, in up to 95% of OST tumor samples.[131] Thus, the use of existing anti-GD2 therapies (monoclonal antibodies, CAR-T cell therapy) to treat OST is currently under investigation (NCT02502786, NCT02484443, NCT03373097). Glycoprotein NMB is also expressed by 92.5% of OST tumor samples and antibody targeting with glembatumumab has demonstrated cytotoxic effects on OST tumor cells with improvements in survival in the preclinical setting.[132,133] Phase II investigation of glembatumumab in 22 patients with refractory OST demonstrated safety, but poor overall response with only one PR and two with disease stabilization.[134] Ongoing research aims to evaluate the utility in targeting alternative cell surface markers, such as a4-integrin, CD47, and RANKL (NCT03811886, NCT04751383).[135]

ICIs are of particular interest given their clinical success in adult solid tumors and preclinical efficacy in OST xenograft models. However, clinical Phase I/II trials have demonstrated safety with limited improvement in PFS and OS.[136] As monoclonal antibody therapy relies on immune system recruitment, this poor response may be due to rapid depletion of cytotoxic T-cells and the immunosuppressive tumor microenvironment (TME) in OST. The combination of TILs and anti-PD1 antibody therapy in patients with metastatic OST led to an ORR of 33.3% and improved median PFS (5.4 months) and OS (15.2 months) compared with ICIs alone, which illustrates the potential value of combining immunotherapy with immune stimulation.[137] Ongoing clinical trials aim to evaluate the efficacy of ICIs as adjunct therapy in difficult-to-treat OST (NCT04294511, NCT03628209).

TME modulation is also being explored to alter the immunosuppressive environment and potentially facilitate improved efficacy of immunotherapies. Agents that decrease M2 macrophage activation and increase pro-inflammatory cytokines, such as mifamurtide and all-trans retinoic acid, have been shown to disrupt cancer stem cell formation and improve survival in localized OST.[138,139] However, the use of these agents in metastatic or refractory OST has not yet been investigated. Thus, although the immunosuppressive TME and structural obstacles of OS have proven challenging in the development of effective targeted therapies for metastatic and refractory OST, the current focus on multifaceted therapeutic regimens that include tumor cell targeting, TME modulation, and immune-stimulation shows great promise.

CHALLENGES TO PRECISION ONCOLOGY IN THE PEDIATRIC POPULATION

Although pediatric precision oncology has the potential to improve survival and mitigate toxicity from current cytotoxic therapies, there are several challenges that must be overcome to make this a clinical reality (see **Table 6**). Here, we discuss the issues with novel targeted therapies (eg, efficacy, toxicity, access) and barriers to clinical implementation of a nationwide pediatric precision oncology program (eg, cost, logistics, ethical impact).

Challenges in Immunotherapy

During the development of novel immunotherapy approaches, it is important to consider the immune milieu of pediatric oncology patients. In addition to immune system depletion after cytotoxic induction chemotherapy, the relatively immature immune system of pediatric patients and the immunologically "cold" TME found in the majority of pediatric solid tumors may affect the efficacy of targeted monotherapy. It should also be emphasized that most of Phase I/II trials include patients who suffer from recurrent and/or treatment refractory disease. Thus, due to known aggressive and resistant tumor biology, combining targeted immunotherapy with cytotoxic chemotherapy or immune stimulation should be considered in trial design. However, this must be weighed carefully with the risk for acute and/or late toxicities from on-target/off-tumor effects from immune system modulation. For example, although rare, the anti-GD2 monoclonal antibody carries the risk of binding to GD2 present on nerve cells leading to severe neuropathic pain. This stresses the importance of careful study design and monitoring for adverse effects during Phase I/II clinical trials evaluating novel immunotherapies.

Challenges with Targeted Therapies

In addition to balancing maximizing efficacy and mitigating toxicity, the potential for resistance to targeted therapies must also be considered. Various mechanisms within known heterogeneous malignancies could lead to future resistance such as mutations in the target itself (eg, GD2 downregulation), reactivation of upstream or downstream pathways (eg, BRAF upregulation with MEK inhibition), or activation of alternate parallel pathways (eg, MAPK signaling activation with mTOR inhibition).[140] This may be mitigated by optimizing therapy administration (ie, combination therapy) or adopting biopsy strategies to ensure all tumors contain the target of interest (eg, recurrent biopsies, biopsies of primary and metastatic disease, "liquid biopsy").

Lack of Access to Novel Targeted Therapies

Relatively small numbers of patients with rare or difficult-to-treat pediatric malignancies, limited overlap with adult molecular targets, and safety concerns with off-label use of adult targeted therapies create challenges in obtaining novel targeted therapies for pediatric patients with cancer. In the United States, the Best Pharmaceuticals for Children Act attempts to address this by allowing off-patent use of drugs for pediatric conditions to assess safety and efficacy, which has improved access to developing agents in pediatric oncology.[141] In addition, due to the Pediatric Research Equity Act, the FDA also has the authority to require testing of relevant drugs in the pediatric population during the drug development process and to accelerate approval of break-through drugs for first-in-human pediatric trials to evaluate potential utility.[141] Increasing collaboration with industry and the development of "basket trials" may further increase access to molecular testing and investigational treatments.

Cost

Prior sequencing studies in pediatric oncology illustrated the high cost associated with precision oncology, which ranges from $6000 to $8000 per sample for whole exome and transcriptome sequencing.[142,143] In addition to the cost of targeted therapy itself, the cost of tumor sample preparation, sequencing, and computational analysis all contribute to a potentially prohibitive cost. A comprehensive economic impact analysis of precision oncology in the pediatric population will be necessary to demonstrate an economic incentive for insurance company approval of molecular testing and targeted therapies.

Logistics

Although the framework for an optimal nationwide pediatric precision oncology program is still under development, current examples such as the US Pediatric MATCH trial and the European AcSe-ESMART trial demonstrate promising frameworks for clinical application. Although prior discovery sequencing studies observed lengthy turnaround times (ie, biopsy to matched therapy initiation), with data analysis alone taking up to 4 weeks, infrastructure development at participating centers, use of uniform genomic panels, and integrating data analysis with treatment matching has the potential to streamline this process further.

Ethical Impact of Incidental Germline Mutations

The ethical impact of identifying incidental germline mutations is also a key consideration to any form of genetic testing. Challenges may arise such as the interpretation of variants of unknown significance and genetic mutations that are potentially attributed to another genetic condition (ie, non-oncogenic). In addition, up to 80% of parents have expressed not wanting to receive the results of incidental germline mutations.[142] Thus, genetic counselor involvement before tissue biopsy should be strongly considered, as well as an opt-in disclosure system for any identified incidental germline mutations.

SURGICAL CONSIDERATIONS
Potential Complications with Targeted Therapies

With the expanding use of novel targeted therapies in pediatric oncology, surgeons should also become familiar with the potential perioperative complications and adverse events requiring surgical intervention that are associated with targeted therapies. These include impaired healing, spontaneous gastrointestinal (GI) perforation, and increased bleeding risk.

Impaired wound healing has been previously reported with the use of anti-angiogenic agents (bevacizumab), TKIs (cabozantinib, pazopanib), and mTOR inhibitors (sirolimus). Bevacizumab was found to be associated with a major wound complication rate of 20% after soft tissue sarcoma resection. Thus, it is recommended to discontinue use for greater than 28 days pre- and post-elective surgery to allow for wound healing.[144] Owing to similar concerns regarding impaired wound healing, TKIs also have recommendations which vary depending on the drug itself (eg, discontinue pazopanib 1 week pre- and 2 weeks post-surgery).[145] Although rates of wound complications with mTOR inhibition have been reported in up to 53% of transplant cases, perioperative dose reduction (ie, omit loading dose) has been shown to reduce rates down to 7% to 8%.[146] Thus, knowledge of these agents and mitigating measures are important during the perioperative management of both elective and emergency cases.

In addition to impaired wound healing, increased risk for major bleeding events and spontaneous GI perforation have been associated with anti-angiogenic agents and TKIs. Systematic review of anti-angiogenic agents (bevacizumab, ramucirumab) demonstrated a significantly increased relative risk for all-grade bleeding events (RR 2.38) and high-grade bleeding events (RR 1.71) which is hypothesized to be secondary to the disruption of tumor vasculature and decreased renewal capacity of vascular endothelium.[147] These agents can also lead to GI perforation anywhere along the GI tract—with the stomach and colon occurring most frequently—at rates of 2% to 3% with bevacizumab.[145] TKIs have also been associated with GI fistula formation with tracheoesophageal fistula occurrence in 4% of patients on cabozantinib and an increased risk in patients on concomitant anti-angiogenic agents, steroids, nonsteroidal anti-inflammatory drugs, or with prior history of peptic ulcer disease.[145,148] Therefore, although relatively uncommon, these serious adverse events are significant in a patient population with existing low physiologic reserve and require emergent surgical care to decrease subsequent morbidity and mortality.

Impact of Precision Oncology on Perioperative Management

Despite the risks of novel targeted therapies, pediatric precision oncology is a promising field with the potential to decrease surgical morbidity by shrinking tumors, as well as improving survival in difficult-to-treat and rare pediatric cancers. As precision oncology programs are implemented, the decisions surrounding when and how to obtain tumor samples for sequencing are important surgical considerations. Although most precision oncology programs agree that tumor samples should be obtained for recurrent or refractory disease, additional tissue may also be required for routine sequencing at the time of diagnosis or due to potential spatial heterogeneity of the tumor itself. Thus, the timeline and approach to surgical biopsy are key considerations in the implementation of precision oncology programs.

The timing of surgery, with regard to targeted therapy use, is also an evolving subject as few drugs have defined recommendations for discontinuation in the perioperative period. Thus, close collaboration with oncologists is paramount during surgical planning, case scheduling, and preoperative counseling in order to safely minimize the time spent off of systemic therapy. As pediatric precision oncology rapidly develops into a clinical reality, surgeons will continue to be significant stakeholders in the care of these patients.

FUTURE DIRECTIONS
Detection of Circulating Tumor DNA ("Liquid Biopsy")

When cancer cells undergo apoptosis or necrosis, the fragmented tumor DNA released into the bloodstream may be used as a biomarker to identify tumor recurrence, monitor treatment response, and evaluate the mutational burden.[149] Detection of this circulating tumor DNA (ctDNA) via peripheral blood sampling has been aptly termed "liquid biopsy." As evolving biopsy strategies in precision oncology rely on recurrent tumor biopsies for molecular profiling and identification of actionable targets, "liquid biopsy" technology provides a promising alternative to the disadvantages associated with conventional biopsy methods (eg, procedural complications, anesthesia ± radiation exposure, pain, inpatient admission). Although its use remains limited, the FDA-approved Foundation One Liquid CDx has been used to evaluate molecular alterations in children with recurrent or refractory cancers. In 45 children, the median time to results was 13 days with targets identified in 56% of samples (eg, *TP53*, *EWS-FLI1*, *ALK*, and *MYC*) and six patients receiving targeted therapy based on these results.[150] Ongoing studies aim to use ctDNA to evaluate treatment response and monitor for disease recurrence or early metastasis.[151,152]

Combining Targeted Therapies

Owing to the complex resistance mechanisms of treatment-refractory pediatric cancers, prior targeted therapy trials have demonstrated poor efficacy with use of monotherapy. Thus, current trials aim to combine targeted therapy with cytotoxic chemotherapy. Combining targeted therapies based on identified targets or aberrant tumorigenic pathways is an approach that has been successful in adult precision oncology[153,154] but is currently being explored in the pediatric population. The INFORM2 study (NCT03838042) is evaluating nivolumab (anti-PD1) and entinostat (HDAC inhibitor) to treat refractory pediatric tumors with high PD-L1 expression and focal MYCN amplification. Dual ICI use is also being actively explored in the Pediatric MATCH "basket trial." Given its success in adult oncology, the future of pediatric precision oncology will likely use multiple targeted therapies, in addition to cytotoxic chemotherapy, in the fight against deadly treatment-refractory disease.

SUMMARY

Pediatric precision oncology is a rapidly developing approach to personalized cancer care with the overarching goals of improving survival and minimizing the morbidity associated with existing therapies. Although ongoing large-scale Phase II clinical trials provide the framework for future clinical implementation, innovative biopsy strategies, advances in sequencing and bioinformatics technology, and increased understanding of targetable mutations/pathways will contribute to its realization. As this develops, pediatric surgical oncologists will be vital stakeholders with key considerations regarding biopsy strategies, timing and extent of surgical resection, and management of immunotherapy-related surgical complications. Multidisciplinary collaboration with oncology, radiology, medical genetics, and pharmacy will be essential in the establishment of pediatric precision oncology programs, which will ultimately provide an avenue of hope for patients with difficult-to-treat or rare pediatric malignancies.

CLINICS CARE POINTS

- Pediatric malignancies harbor low rates of somatic mutations compared with the adult population.
- The use of multiple genetic profiling methods (NGS, RNAseq, proteomics) has allowed for molecular tumor risk stratification and identification of clinically actionable targets.
- Ongoing large-scale "basket trials" (eg, National Cancer Institute–Children's Oncology Group Pediatric MATCH) allocate treatment based on molecular alteration and provide a framework for clinical implementation of pediatric precision oncology.

- Current targeted therapies target cell surface markers (eg, anti-GD2 immunotherapy, immune checkpoint inhibitors) or dysregulated tumorigenic pathways (eg, multi-kinase inhibitors, mammalian target of rapamycin inhibitors).

Targeted therapies (anti-angiogenic agents, tyrosine kinase inhibitors) associated with impaired wound healing, increased bleeding, and spontaneous gastrointestinal perforation.

- Future research focuses on improving biopsy strategies (eg, "liquid biopsy") and combining targeted therapies to improve efficacy in treatment-refractory tumors.

DISCLOSURE

The authors have nothing to disclose.

REFERENCES

1. Ramsey BW, Davies J, McElvaney NG, et al. A CFTR potentiator in patients with cystic fibrosis and the G551D mutation. N Engl J Med 2011;365(18):1663–72.
2. Society AC. Cancer Facts & Figures 2023. American Cancer Society. Accessed March 21, 2023, https://www.cancer.org/content/dam/cancer-org/research/can-cer-facts-and-statistics/annual-cancer-facts-and-figures/2023/2023-cancer-facts-and-figures.pdfhttps://www.cancer.org/content/dam/cancer-org/research/cancer-facts-and-statistics/annual-cancer-facts-and-figures/2023/2023-cancer-facts-and-figures.pdf.
3. Goldstick JE, Cunningham RM, Carter PM. Current causes of death in children and adolescents in the United States. N Engl J Med 2022;386(20):1955–6.
4. Armenian SH, Landier W, Hudson MM, et al, COG Survivorship and Outcomes Committee. Children's Oncology Group's 2013 blueprint for research: survivorship and outcomes. Pediatr Blood Cancer 2013;60(6):1063–8.
5. Matthay KK, Reynolds CP, Seeger RC, et al. Long-term results for children with high-risk neuroblastoma treated on a randomized trial of myeloablative therapy followed by 13-cis-retinoic acid: a children's oncology group study. J Clin Oncol 2009;27(7):1007–13.
6. Ma X, Liu Y, Liu Y, et al. Pan-cancer genome and transcriptome analyses of 1,699 paediatric leukaemias and solid tumours. Nature 2018;555(7696):371–6.
7. Sweet-Cordero EA, Biegel JA. The genomic landscape of pediatric cancers: Implications for diagnosis and treatment. Science 2019;363(6432):1170–5.
8. Lawrence MS, Stojanov P, Polak P, et al. Mutational heterogeneity in cancer and the search for new cancer-associated genes. Nature 2013;499(7457):214–8.
9. Eleveld TF, Oldridge DA, Bernard V, et al. Relapsed neuroblastomas show frequent RAS-MAPK pathway mutations. Nat Genet 2015;47(8):864–71.
10. Schramm A, Köster J, Assenov Y, et al. Mutational dynamics between primary and relapse neuroblastomas. Nat Genet 2015;47(8):872–7.
11. Gröbner SN, Worst BC, Weischenfeldt J, et al. The landscape of genomic alterations across childhood cancers. Nature 2018;555(7696):321–7.
12. Dharia NV, Kugener G, Guenther LM, et al. A first-generation pediatric cancer dependency map. Nat Genet 2021;53(4):529–38.
13. Lawlor ER, Thiele CJ. Epigenetic changes in pediatric solid tumors: promising new targets. Clin Cancer Res 2012;18(10):2768–79.
14. Bolouri H, Farrar JE, Triche T Jr, et al. The molecular landscape of pediatric acute myeloid leukemia reveals recurrent structural alterations and age-specific mutational interactions. Nat Med 2018;24(1):103–12.

15. Morrissy AS, Garzia L, Shih DJ, et al. Divergent clonal selection dominates medulloblastoma at recurrence. Nature 2016;529(7586):351–7.

16. Rosswog C, Fassunke J, Ernst A, et al. Genomic ALK alterations in primary and relapsed neuroblastoma. Br J Cancer 2023;128(8):1559–71.

17. Valentijn LJ, Koster J, Zwijnenburg DA, et al. TERT rearrangements are frequent in neuroblastoma and identify aggressive tumors. Nat Genet 2015;47(12):1411–4.

18. Maraka S, Janku F. BRAF alterations in primary brain tumors. Discov Med 2018;26(141):51–60.

19. Versteege I, Sévenet N, Lange J, et al. Truncating mutations of hSNF5/INI1 in aggressive paediatric cancer. Nature 1998;394(6689):203–6.

20. Lee RS, Stewart C, Carter SL, et al. A remarkably simple genome underlies highly malignant pediatric rhabdoid cancers. J Clin Invest 2012;122(8):2983–8.

21. Schwartzentruber J, Korshunov A, Liu XY, et al. Driver mutations in histone H3.3 and chromatin remodelling genes in paediatric glioblastoma. Nature 2012;482(7384):226–31.

22. Capper D, Jones DTW, Sill M, et al. DNA methylation-based classification of central nervous system tumours. Nature 2018;555(7697):469–74.

23. Ansell SM, Lesokhin AM, Borrello I, et al. PD-1 blockade with nivolumab in relapsed or refractory Hodgkin's lymphoma. N Engl J Med 2015;372(4):311–9.

24. Geoerger B, Bergeron C, Gore L, et al. Phase II study of ipilimumab in adolescents with unresectable stage III or IV malignant melanoma. Eur J Cancer 2017;86:358–63.

25. Subbiah V, Solit DB, Chan TA, et al. The FDA approval of pembrolizumab for adult and pediatric patients with tumor mutational burden (TMB) ≥10: a decision centered on empowering patients and their physicians. Ann Oncol 2020;31(9):1115–8.

26. Mossé YP, Voss SD, Lim MS, et al. Targeting ALK With Crizotinib in Pediatric Anaplastic Large Cell Lymphoma and Inflammatory Myofibroblastic Tumor: A Children's Oncology Group Study. J Clin Oncol 2017;35(28):3215–21.

27. Pacenta HL, Macy ME. Entrectinib and other ALK/TRK inhibitors for the treatment of neuroblastoma. Drug Des Devel Ther 2018;12:3549–61.

28. Foster JH, Voss SD, Hall DC, et al. Activity of Crizotinib in Patients with ALK-Aberrant Relapsed/Refractory Neuroblastoma: A Children's Oncology Group Study (ADVL0912). Clin Cancer Res 2021;27(13):3543–8.

29. Yu AL, Gilman AL, Ozkaynak MF, et al. Anti-GD2 antibody with GM-CSF, interleukin-2, and isotretinoin for neuroblastoma. N Engl J Med 2010;363(14):1324–34.

30. Schulz G, Cheresh DA, Varki NM, et al. Detection of ganglioside GD2 in tumor tissues and sera of neuroblastoma patients. Cancer Res 1984;44(12 Pt 1):5914–20.

31. Ladenstein R, Pötschger U, Valteau-Couanet D, et al. Interleukin 2 with anti-GD2 antibody ch14.18/CHO (dinutuximab beta) in patients with high-risk neuroblastoma (HR-NBL1/SIOPEN): a multicentre, randomised, phase 3 trial. Lancet Oncol 2018;19(12):1617–29.

32. Harris MH, DuBois SG, Glade Bender JL, et al. Multicenter Feasibility Study of Tumor Molecular Profiling to Inform Therapeutic Decisions in Advanced Pediatric Solid Tumors: The Individualized Cancer Therapy (iCat) Study. JAMA Oncol 2016;2(5):608–15.

33. Harttrampf AC, Lacroix L, Deloger M, et al. Molecular Screening for Cancer Treatment Optimization (MOSCATO-01) in Pediatric Patients: A Single-

Institutional Prospective Molecular Stratification Trial. Clin Cancer Res 2017; 23(20):6101–12.

34. Wong M, Mayoh C, Lau LMS, et al. Whole genome, transcriptome and methylome profiling enhances actionable target discovery in high-risk pediatric cancer. Nat Med 2020;26(11):1742–53.

35. Forrest SJ, Geoerger B, Janeway KA. Precision medicine in pediatric oncology. Curr Opin Pediatr 2018;30(1):17–24.

36. Parsons DW, Janeway KA, Patton DR, et al. Actionable Tumor Alterations and Treatment Protocol Enrollment of Pediatric and Young Adult Patients With Refractory Cancers in the National Cancer Institute-Children's Oncology Group Pediatric MATCH Trial. J Clin Oncol 2022;40(20):2224–34.

37. Allen CE, Laetsch TW, Mody R, et al. Target and Agent Prioritization for the Children's Oncology Group-National Cancer Institute Pediatric MATCH Trial. J Natl Cancer Inst 2017;109(5). https://doi.org/10.1093/jnci/djw274.

38. Pasqualini C, Rubino J, Brard C, et al. Phase II and biomarker study of programmed cell death protein 1 inhibitor nivolumab and metronomic cyclophosphamide in paediatric relapsed/refractory solid tumours: Arm G of AcSé-ESMART, a trial of the European Innovative Therapies for Children With Cancer Consortium. Eur J Cancer 2021;150:53–62.

39. Mullassery D, Farrelly P, Losty PD. Does aggressive surgical resection improve survival in advanced stage 3 and 4 neuroblastoma? A systematic review and meta-analysis. Pediatr Hematol Oncol 2014;31(8):703–16.

40. Zwaveling S, Tytgat GA, van der Zee DC, et al. Is complete surgical resection of stage 4 neuroblastoma a prerequisite for optimal survival or may >95 % tumour resection suffice? Pediatr Surg Int 2012;28(10):953–9.

41. Pfister SM, Reyes-Múgica M, Chan JKC, et al. A Summary of the Inaugural WHO Classification of Pediatric Tumors: Transitioning from the Optical into the Molecular Era. Cancer Discov 2022;12(2):331–55.

42. Casey DL, Cheung NV. Immunotherapy of Pediatric Solid Tumors: Treatments at a Crossroads, with an Emphasis on Antibodies. Cancer Immunol Res 2020;8(2):161–6.

43. Matthay KK, Maris JM, Schleiermacher G, et al. Neuroblastoma. Nat Rev Dis Primers 2016;2:16078. https://doi.org/10.1038/nrdp.2016.78.

44. Cohn SL, Pearson AD, London WB, et al. The International Neuroblastoma Risk Group (INRG) classification system: an INRG Task Force report. J Clin Oncol 2009;27(2):289–97.

45. Berlanga P, Cañete A, Castel V. Advances in emerging drugs for the treatment of neuroblastoma. Expert Opin Emerg Drugs 2017;22(1):63–75.

46. London WB, Castel V, Monclair T, et al. Clinical and biologic features predictive of survival after relapse of neuroblastoma: a report from the International Neuroblastoma Risk Group project. J Clin Oncol 2011;29(24):3286–92.

47. Nazha B, Inal C, Owonikoko TK. Disialoganglioside GD2 Expression in Solid Tumors and Role as a Target for Cancer Therapy. Front Oncol 2020;10:1000.

48. Yu AL, Gilman AL, Ozkaynak MF, et al. Long-Term Follow-up of a Phase III Study of ch14.18 (Dinutuximab) + Cytokine Immunotherapy in Children with High-Risk Neuroblastoma: COG Study ANBL0032. Clin Cancer Res 2021;27(8):2179–89.

49. Mody R, Yu AL, Naranjo A, et al. Irinotecan, Temozolomide, and Dinutuximab With GM-CSF in Children With Refractory or Relapsed Neuroblastoma: A Report From the Children's Oncology Group. J Clin Oncol 2020;38(19):2160–9.

50. Cheung NK, Guo H, Hu J, et al. Humanizing murine IgG3 anti-GD2 antibody m3F8 substantially improves antibody-dependent cell-mediated cytotoxicity while retaining targeting in vivo. OncoImmunology 2012;1(4):477–86.

51. Kushner BH, Cheung IY, Modak S, et al. Phase I trial of a bivalent gangliosides vaccine in combination with β-glucan for high-risk neuroblastoma in second or later remission. Clin Cancer Res 2014;20(5):1375–82.

52. Villanueva MT. Long path to MYC inhibition approaches clinical trials. Nat Rev Cancer 2019;19(5):252.

53. Katzenstein HM, Bowman LC, Brodeur GM, et al. Prognostic significance of age, MYCN oncogene amplification, tumor cell ploidy, and histology in 110 infants with stage D(S) neuroblastoma: the pediatric oncology group experience–a pediatric oncology group study. J Clin Oncol 1998;16(6):2007–17.

54. Müller I, Larsson K, Frenzel A, et al. Targeting of the MYCN protein with small molecule c-MYC inhibitors. PLoS One 2014;9(5):e97285.

55. Yang Y, Ding L, Zhou Q, et al. Silencing of AURKA augments the antitumor efficacy of the AURKA inhibitor MLN8237 on neuroblastoma cells. Cancer Cell Int 2020;20:9.

56. Hogarty MD, Norris MD, Davis K, et al. ODC1 is a critical determinant of MYCN oncogenesis and a therapeutic target in neuroblastoma. Cancer Res 2008; 68(23):9735–45.

57. Puissant A, Frumm SM, Alexe G, et al. Targeting MYCN in neuroblastoma by BET bromodomain inhibition. Cancer Discov 2013;3(3):308–23.

58. Soucek L, Whitfield J, Martins CP, et al. Modelling Myc inhibition as a cancer therapy. Nature 2008;455(7213):679–83.

59. Demma MJ, Mapelli C, Sun A, et al. Omomyc Reveals New Mechanisms To Inhibit the MYC Oncogene. Mol Cell Biol 2019;39(22). https://doi.org/10.1128/mcb.00248-19.

60. Direct MYC Inhibitor Passes First Clinical Test. Cancer Discov 2023;13(1):4. https://doi.org/10.1158/2159-8290.Cd-nb2022-0067.

61. Mossé YP, Lim MS, Voss SD, et al. Safety and activity of crizotinib for paediatric patients with refractory solid tumours or anaplastic large-cell lymphoma: a Children's Oncology Group phase 1 consortium study. Lancet Oncol 2013;14(6): 472–80.

62. Kushner BH, Cheung NV, Modak S, et al. A phase I/Ib trial targeting the Pi3k/Akt pathway using perifosine: Long-term progression-free survival of patients with resistant neuroblastoma. Int J Cancer 2017;140(2):480–4.

63. Zins K, Schäfer R, Paulus P, et al. Frizzled2 signaling regulates growth of high-risk neuroblastomas by interfering with β-catenin-dependent and β-catenin-independent signaling pathways. Oncotarget 2016;7(29):46187–202.

64. Flahaut M, Meier R, Coulon A, et al. The Wnt receptor FZD1 mediates chemoresistance in neuroblastoma through activation of the Wnt/beta-catenin pathway. Oncogene 2009;28(23):2245–56.

65. Eleveld TF, Schild L, Koster J, et al. RAS-MAPK Pathway-Driven Tumor Progression Is Associated with Loss of CIC and Other Genomic Aberrations in Neuroblastoma. Cancer Res 2018;78(21):6297–307.

66. Van Maerken T, Ferdinande L, Taildeman J, et al. Antitumor activity of the selective MDM2 antagonist nutlin-3 against chemoresistant neuroblastoma with wild-type p53. J Natl Cancer Inst 2009;101(22):1562–74.

67. Ramaiah MJ, Pushpavalli SN, Lavanya A, et al. Novel anthranilamide-pyrazolo[1,5-a]pyrimidine conjugates modulate the expression of p53-MYCN associated

micro RNAs in neuroblastoma cells and cause cell cycle arrest and apoptosis. Bioorg Med Chem Lett 2013;23(20):5699–706.

68. Vogan K, Bernstein M, Leclerc JM, et al. Absence of p53 gene mutations in primary neuroblastomas. Cancer Res 1993;53(21):5269–73.

69. Kim ES, Shohet JM. Reactivation of p53 via MDM2 inhibition. Cell Death Dis 2015;6(10):e1936.

70. Kim E, Shohet J. Targeted molecular therapy for neuroblastoma: the ARF/MDM2/p53 axis. J Natl Cancer Inst 2009;101(22):1527–9.

71. Lakoma A, Barbieri E, Agarwal S, et al. The MDM2 small-molecule inhibitor RG7388 leads to potent tumor inhibition in p53 wild-type neuroblastoma. Cell Death Discov 2015;1:15026.

72. Patterson DM, Gao D, Trahan DN, et al. Effect of MDM2 and vascular endothelial growth factor inhibition on tumor angiogenesis and metastasis in neuroblastoma. Angiogenesis 2011;14(3):255–66.

73. Fouladi M, Park JR, Stewart CF, et al. Pediatric phase I trial and pharmacokinetic study of vorinostat: a Children's Oncology Group phase I consortium report. J Clin Oncol 2010;28(22):3623–9.

74. Henssen A, Althoff K, Odersky A, et al. Targeting MYCN-Driven Transcription By BET-Bromodomain Inhibition. Clin Cancer Res 2016;22(10):2470–81.

75. Haug BH, Hald Ø H, Utnes P, et al. Exosome-like Extracellular Vesicles from MYCN-amplified Neuroblastoma Cells Contain Oncogenic miRNAs. Anticancer Res 2015;35(5):2521–30.

76. Irtan S, Ehrlich PF, Pritchard-Jones K. Wilms tumor: "State-of-the-art" update, 2016. Semin Pediatr Surg 2016;25(5):250–6.

77. Dome JS, Graf N, Geller JI, et al. Advances in Wilms Tumor Treatment and Biology: Progress Through International Collaboration. J Clin Oncol 2015;33(27):2999–3007.

78. Palmisani F, Kovar H, Kager L, et al. Systematic review of the immunological landscape of Wilms tumors. Mol Ther Oncolytics 2021;22:454–67.

79. Tian K, Wang X, Wu Y, et al. Relationship of tumour-associated macrophages with poor prognosis in Wilms' tumour. J Pediatr Urol 2020;16(3):376, e1-e8.

80. Maturu P, Overwijk WW, Hicks J, et al. Characterization of the inflammatory microenvironment and identification of potential therapeutic targets in Wilms tumors. Transl Oncol 2014;7(4):484–92.

81. Pinto N, Park JR, Murphy E, et al. Patterns of PD-1, PD-L1, and PD-L2 expression in pediatric solid tumors. Pediatr Blood Cancer 2017;64(11). https://doi.org/10.1002/pbc.26613.

82. Mochizuki K, Kawana S, Yamada S, et al. Various checkpoint molecules, and tumor-infiltrating lymphocytes in common pediatric solid tumors: Possibilities for novel immunotherapy. Pediatr Hematol Oncol 2019;36(1):17–27.

83. Silva MA, Triltsch N, Leis S, et al. Biomarker recommendation for PD-1/PD-L1 immunotherapy development in pediatric cancer based on digital image analysis of PD-L1 and immune cells. J Pathol Clin Res 2020;6(2):124–37.

84. Geoerger B, Kang HJ, Yalon-Oren M, et al. Pembrolizumab in paediatric patients with advanced melanoma or a PD-L1-positive, advanced, relapsed, or refractory solid tumour or lymphoma (KEYNOTE-051): interim analysis of an open-label, single-arm, phase 1-2 trial. Lancet Oncol 2020;21(1):121–33.

85. Majzner RG, Theruvath JL, Nellan A, et al. CAR T Cells Targeting B7-H3, a Pan-Cancer Antigen, Demonstrate Potent Preclinical Activity Against Pediatric Solid Tumors and Brain Tumors. Clin Cancer Res 2019;25(8):2560–74.

86. Scursoni AM, Galluzzo L, Camarero S, et al. Detection and characterization of N-glycolyated gangliosides in Wilms tumor by immunohistochemistry. Pediatr Dev Pathol 2010;13(1):18–23.

87. Cacciavillano W, Sampor C, Venier C, et al. A Phase I Study of the Anti-Idiotype Vaccine Racotumomab in Neuroblastoma and Other Pediatric Refractory Malignancies. Pediatr Blood Cancer 2015;62(12):2120–4.

88. Meany HJ, Seibel NL, Sun J, et al. Phase 2 trial of recombinant tumor necrosis factor-alpha in combination with dactinomycin in children with recurrent Wilms tumor. J Immunother 2008;31(7):679–83.

89. Seibel NL, Dinndorf PA, Bauer M, et al. Phase I study of tumor necrosis factor-alpha and actinomycin D in pediatric patients with cancer: a Children's Cancer Group study. J Immunother Emphas Tumor Immunol 1994;16(2):125–31.

90. Hubbard AK, Spector LG, Fortuna G, et al. Trends in International Incidence of Pediatric Cancers in Children Under 5 Years of Age: 1988-2012. JNCI Cancer Spectr 2019;3(1):pkz007.

91. Siegel RL, Miller KD, Fuchs HE, et al. Cancer Statistics, 2021. CA Cancer J Clin 2021;71(1):7–33.

92. Giardiello FM, Offerhaus GJ, Krush AJ, et al. Risk of hepatoblastoma in familial adenomatous polyposis. J Pediatr 1991;119(5):766–8.

93. DeBaun MR, Tucker MA. Risk of cancer during the first four years of life in children from The Beckwith-Wiedemann Syndrome Registry. J Pediatr 1998;132(3 Pt 1):398–400.

94. Sumazin P, Chen Y, Treviño LR, et al. Genomic analysis of hepatoblastoma identifies distinct molecular and prognostic subgroups. Hepatology 2017;65(1):104–21.

95. Hooks KB, Audoux J, Fazli H, et al. New insights into diagnosis and therapeutic options for proliferative hepatoblastoma. Hepatology 2018;68(1):89–102.

96. Carrillo-Reixach J, Torrens L, Simon-Coma M, et al. Epigenetic footprint enables molecular risk stratification of hepatoblastoma with clinical implications. J Hepatol 2020;73(2):328–41.

97. Wang W, Smits R, Hao H, et al. Wnt/β-Catenin Signaling in Liver Cancers. Cancers 2019;11(7). https://doi.org/10.3390/cancers11070926.

98. Tao J, Zhang R, Singh S, et al. Targeting β-catenin in hepatocellular cancers induced by coexpression of mutant β-catenin and K-Ras in mice. Hepatology 2017;65(5):1581–99.

99. Hishiki T. Current therapeutic strategies for childhood hepatic tumors: surgical and interventional treatments for hepatoblastoma. Int J Clin Oncol 2013;18(6):962–8.

100. Eicher C, Dewerth A, Thomale J, et al. Effect of sorafenib combined with cytostatic agents on hepatoblastoma cell lines and xenografts. Br J Cancer 2013;108(2):334–41.

101. Wu PV, Rangaswami A. Current Approaches in Hepatoblastoma-New Biological Insights to Inform Therapy. Curr Oncol Rep 2022;24(9):1209–18.

102. Hartmann W, Küchler J, Koch A, et al. Activation of phosphatidylinositol-3'-kinase/AKT signaling is essential in hepatoblastoma survival. Clin Cancer Res 2009;15(14):4538–45.

103. Wagner F, Henningsen B, Lederer C, et al. Rapamycin blocks hepatoblastoma growth in vitro and in vivo implicating new treatment options in high-risk patients. Eur J Cancer 2012;48(15):2442–50.

104. Stafman LL, Mruthyunjayappa S, Waters AM, et al. Targeting PIM kinase as a therapeutic strategy in human hepatoblastoma. Oncotarget 2018;9(32): 22665–79.

105. Buenemann CL, Willy C, Buchmann A, et al. Transforming growth factor-beta1-induced Smad signaling, cell-cycle arrest and apoptosis in hepatoma cells. Carcinogenesi 2001;22(3):447–52.

106. Nagai H, Naka T, Terada Y, et al. Hypermethylation associated with inactivation of the SOCS-1 gene, a JAK/STAT inhibitor, in human hepatoblastomas. J Hum Genet 2003;48(2):65–9.

107. Kats D, Ricker CA, Berlow NE, et al. Volasertib preclinical activity in high-risk hepatoblastoma. Oncotarget 2019;10(60):6403–17.

108. Johnston ME 2nd, Rivas MP, Nicolle D, et al. Olaparib Inhibits Tumor Growth of Hepatoblastoma in Patient-Derived Xenograft Models. Hepatology 2021;74(4): 2201–15.

109. Woodfield SE, Shi Y, Patel RH, et al. MDM4 inhibition: a novel therapeutic strategy to reactivate p53 in hepatoblastoma. Sci Rep 2021;11(1):2967.

110. Armeanu-Ebinger S, Hoh A, Wenz J, et al. Targeting EpCAM (CD326) for immunotherapy in hepatoblastoma. OncoImmunology 2013;2(1):e22620.

111. Ognjanovic S, Linabery AM, Charbonneau B, et al. Trends in childhood rhabdomyosarcoma incidence and survival in the United States, 1975-2005. Cancer 2009;115(18):4218–26.

112. Breneman JC, Lyden E, Pappo AS, et al. Prognostic factors and clinical outcomes in children and adolescents with metastatic rhabdomyosarcoma–a report from the Intergroup Rhabdomyosarcoma Study IV. J Clin Oncol 2003; 21(1):78–84.

113. Skapek SX, Anderson J, Barr FG, et al. PAX-FOXO1 fusion status drives unfavorable outcome for children with rhabdomyosarcoma: a children's oncology group report. Pediatr Blood Cancer 2013;60(9):1411–7.

114. Barr FG. Gene fusions involving PAX and FOX family members in alveolar rhabdomyosarcoma. Oncogene 2001;20(40):5736–46.

115. Rengaswamy V, Zimmer D, Süss R, et al. RGD liposome-protamine-siRNA (LPR) nanoparticles targeting PAX3-FOXO1 for alveolar rhabdomyosarcoma therapy. J Control Release 2016;235:319–27.

116. Bharathy N, Berlow NE, Wang E, et al. The HDAC3-SMARCA4-miR-27a axis promotes expression of the PAX3:FOXO1 fusion oncogene in rhabdomyosarcoma. Sci Signal 2018;11(557). https://doi.org/10.1126/scisignal.aau7632.

117. Geoerger B, Kieran MW, Grupp S, et al. Phase II trial of temsirolimus in children with high-grade glioma, neuroblastoma and rhabdomyosarcoma. Eur J Cancer 2012;48(2):253–62.

118. Mascarenhas L, Chi YY, Hingorani P, et al. Randomized Phase II Trial of Bevacizumab or Temsirolimus in Combination With Chemotherapy for First Relapse Rhabdomyosarcoma: A Report From the Children's Oncology Group. J Clin Oncol 2019;37(31):2866–74.

119. Schöffski P, Wozniak A, Leahy MG, et al. The tyrosine kinase inhibitor crizotinib does not have clinically meaningful activity in heavily pre-treated patients with advanced alveolar rhabdomyosarcoma with FOXO rearrangement: European Organisation for Research and Treatment of Cancer phase 2 trial 90101 'CREATE'. Eur J Cancer 2018;94:156–67.

120. Weigel B, Malempati S, Reid JM, et al. Phase 2 trial of cixutumumab in children, adolescents, and young adults with refractory solid tumors: a report from the Children's Oncology Group. Pediatr Blood Cancer 2014;61(3):452–6.

121. Malempati S, Weigel BJ, Chi YY, et al. The addition of cixutumumab or temozolomide to intensive multiagent chemotherapy is feasible but does not improve outcome for patients with metastatic rhabdomyosarcoma: A report from the Children's Oncology Group. Cancer 2019;125(2):290–7.

122. Wagner LM, Fouladi M, Ahmed A, et al. Phase II study of cixutumumab in combination with temsirolimus in pediatric patients and young adults with recurrent or refractory sarcoma: a report from the Children's Oncology Group. Pediatr Blood Cancer 2015;62(3):440–4.

123. Kim A, Widemann BC, Krailo M, et al. Phase 2 trial of sorafenib in children and young adults with refractory solid tumors: A report from the Children's Oncology Group. Pediatr Blood Cancer 2015;62(9):1562–6.

124. Bielack SS, Kempf-Bielack B, Delling G, et al. Prognostic factors in high-grade osteosarcoma of the extremities or trunk: an analysis of 1,702 patients treated on neoadjuvant cooperative osteosarcoma study group protocols. J Clin Oncol 2002;20(3):776–90.

125. Bacci G, Avella M, Capanna R, et al. Neoadjuvant chemotherapy in the treatment of osteosarcoma of the extremities: preliminary results in 131 cases treated preoperatively with methotrexate and cisdiamminoplatinum. Ital J Orthop Traumatol 1988;14(1):23–39.

126. Chen X, Bahrami A, Pappo A, et al. Recurrent somatic structural variations contribute to tumorigenesis in pediatric osteosarcoma. Cell Rep 2014;7(1):104–12.

127. Nakka M, Allen-Rhoades W, Li Y, et al. Biomarker significance of plasma and tumor miR-21, miR-221, and miR-106a in osteosarcoma. Oncotarget 2017;8(57):96738–52.

128. Isakoff MS, Bielack SS, Meltzer P, et al. Osteosarcoma: Current Treatment and a Collaborative Pathway to Success. J Clin Oncol 2015;33(27):3029–35.

129. Lu Y, Zhang J, Chen Y, et al. Novel Immunotherapies for Osteosarcoma. Front Oncol 2022;12:830546.

130. Wolf-Dennen K, Gordon N, Kleinerman ES. Exosomal communication by metastatic osteosarcoma cells modulates alveolar macrophages to an M2 tumor-promoting phenotype and inhibits tumoricidal functions. OncoImmunology 2020;9(1):1747677.

131. Roth M, Linkowski M, Tarim J, et al. Ganglioside GD2 as a therapeutic target for antibody-mediated therapy in patients with osteosarcoma. Cancer 2014;120(4):548–54.

132. Roth M, Barris DM, Piperdi S, et al. Targeting Glycoprotein NMB With Antibody-Drug Conjugate, Glembatumumab Vedotin, for the Treatment of Osteosarcoma. Pediatr Blood Cancer 2016;63(1):32–8.

133. Kolb EA, Gorlick R, Billups CA, et al. Initial testing (stage 1) of glembatumumab vedotin (CDX-011) by the pediatric preclinical testing program. Pediatr Blood Cancer 2014;61(10):1816–21.

134. Kopp LM, Malempati S, Krailo M, et al. Phase II trial of the glycoprotein non-metastatic B-targeted antibody-drug conjugate, glembatumumab vedotin (CDX-011), in recurrent osteosarcoma AOST1521: A report from the Children's Oncology Group. Eur J Cancer 2019;121:177–83.

135. Beristain AG, Narala SR, Di Grappa MA, et al. Homotypic RANK signaling differentially regulates proliferation, motility and cell survival in osteosarcoma and mammary epithelial cells. J Cell Sci 2012;125(Pt 4):943–55.

136. Xie L, Xu J, Sun X, et al. Apatinib plus camrelizumab (anti-PD1 therapy, SHR-1210) for advanced osteosarcoma (APFAO) progressing after chemotherapy:

a single-arm, open-label, phase 2 trial. J Immunother Cancer 2020;8(1). https://doi.org/10.1136/jitc-2020-000798.

137. Wang C, Li M, Wei R, et al. Adoptive transfer of TILs plus anti-PD1 therapy: An alternative combination therapy for treating metastatic osteosarcoma. J Bone Oncol 2020;25:100332.

138. Múdry P, Kýr M, Rohleder O, et al. Improved osteosarcoma survival with addition of mifamurtide to conventional chemotherapy - Observational prospective single institution analysis. J Bone Oncol 2021;28:100362.

139. Shao XJ, Xiang SF, Chen YQ, et al. Inhibition of M2-like macrophages by all-trans retinoic acid prevents cancer initiation and stemness in osteosarcoma cells. Acta Pharmacol Sin 2019;40(10):1343–50.

140. Ramos P, Bentires-Alj M. Mechanism-based cancer therapy: resistance to therapy, therapy for resistance. Oncogene 2015;34(28):3617–26.

141. Institute of Medicine Forum on Drug Discovery D, Translation. The national academies collection: reports funded by national institutes of health. Addressing the barriers to pediatric drug development: workshop summary. Washington, DC: National Academy of Sciences; 2008. National Academies Press (US) Copyright © 2008.

142. Mody RJ, Wu YM, Lonigro RJ, et al. Integrative Clinical Sequencing in the Management of Refractory or Relapsed Cancer in Youth. JAMA 2015;314(9):913–25.

143. Worst BC, van Tilburg CM, Balasubramanian GP, et al. Next-generation personalised medicine for high-risk paediatric cancer patients - The INFORM pilot study. Eur J Cancer 2016;65:91–101.

144. Yoon SS, Duda DG, Karl DL, et al. Phase II study of neoadjuvant bevacizumab and radiotherapy for resectable soft tissue sarcomas. Int J Radiat Oncol Biol Phys 2011;81(4):1081–90.

145. Shah DR, Dholakia S, Shah RR. Effect of tyrosine kinase inhibitors on wound healing and tissue repair: implications for surgery in cancer patients. Drug Saf 2014;37(3):135–49.

146. Tiong HY, Flechner SM, Zhou L, et al. A systematic approach to minimizing wound problems for de novo sirolimus-treated kidney transplant recipients. Transplantation 2009;87(2):296–302.

147. Xiao B, Wang W, Zhang D. Risk of bleeding associated with antiangiogenic monoclonal antibodies bevacizumab and ramucirumab: a meta-analysis of 85 randomized controlled trials. OncoTargets Ther 2018;11:5059–74.

148. Davis LE, Bolejack V, Ryan CW, et al. Randomized Double-Blind Phase II Study of Regorafenib in Patients With Metastatic Osteosarcoma. J Clin Oncol 2019; 37(16):1424–31.

149. Deveson IW, Gong B, Lai K, et al. Evaluating the analytical validity of circulating tumor DNA sequencing assays for precision oncology. Nat Biotechnol 2021; 39(9):1115–28.

150. Cahn F, Revon-Riviere G, Min V, et al. Blood-Derived Liquid Biopsies Using Foundation One(®) Liquid CDx for Children and Adolescents with High-Risk Malignancies: A Monocentric Experience. Cancers 2022;14(11). https://doi.org/10.3390/cancers14112774.

151. Bratman SV, Yang SYC, Iafolla MAJ, et al. Personalized circulating tumor DNA analysis as a predictive biomarker in solid tumor patients treated with pembrolizumab. Nat Cancer 2020;1(9):873–81.

152. Dawson SJ, Tsui DW, Murtaza M, et al. Analysis of circulating tumor DNA to monitor metastatic breast cancer. N Engl J Med 2013;368(13):1199–209.

153. Sicklick JK, Kato S, Okamura R, et al. Molecular profiling of cancer patients enables personalized combination therapy: the I-PREDICT study. Nat Med 2019; 25(5):744–50.
154. Sicklick JK, Kato S, Okamura R, et al. Molecular profiling of advanced malignancies guides first-line N-of-1 treatments in the I-PREDICT treatment-naïve study. Genome Med 2021;13(1):155.

Current Multidisciplinary Lymphoma and Myeloma Management for Surgeons

William B. Pearse, MD, Erin G. Reid, MD, MS*

KEYWORDS

- Lymphomas • Non-Hodgkin lymphoma • Hodgkin lymphoma
- Plasma cell disorders • Multiple myeloma

KEY POINTS

- Lymphoid neoplasms are composed of more than 100 clinically relevant subtypes, which have in common relatively high sensitivity to glucocorticoids, cytotoxic chemotherapy, and radiation.
- Many lymphoid malignancies have high rates of long-term disease control or are curable even when presenting in advanced stages.
- The large clinical diversity of lymphomas translates to importance of high-quality excisional lymph node biopsies for accurate pathologic classification. Core needle biopsies are preferred only when excisional biopsy would be associated with significant risk of morbidity or prolonged surgical recovery, which may delay definitive systemic chemoimmunotherapy.
- The relative merits and risks of surgical, medical, and radiotherapeutic approaches to managing an oncologic emergency arising from lymphoma or myeloma should be weighed through multidisciplinary case discussion among surgical, hematology/ oncology, and radiation oncology specialists.

INTRODUCTION

Tumors of lymphoid tissue comprise a heterogeneous group of neoplasms originating from clonally expanded B-lymphocytes and T-lymphocytes, generally as a consequence of environmental, infectious, or genetic factors allowing for dysregulated cellular proliferation, growth, and evasion of host immunity. Lymphomas represent approximately 5% of all malignancies and generally enjoy a favorable treatment response profile, even in patients who present with advanced stage or high burden

Division of Hematology/Oncology, University of California, San Diego Moores Cancer Center, 3855 Health Sciences Drive, La Jolla, CA 92093, USA
* Corresponding author.
E-mail address: egreid@health.ucsd.edu
Twitter: @ErinReidMD (E.G.R.)

Surg Oncol Clin N Am 33 (2024) 447–466
https://doi.org/10.1016/j.soc.2023.12.009
1055-3207/24/© 2023 Elsevier Inc. All rights reserved.
surgonc.theclinics.com

of disease.[1] As such, a thorough understanding of the diversity of lymphoproliferative diseases is essential when considering the optimal diagnostic, treatment, and inter-professional care coordination approaches for such patients, particularly from the perspective of the surgical oncologist.

As patients with hematologic malignancies will typically present with multifocal or widespread involvement, the role of surgery is typically diagnostic as opposed to ther-apeutic. In this regard, the biological diversity of lymphomas can have significant im-plications on surgical goals when considering an approach to tissue sampling. The high chemotherapy and radiation sensitivity of lymphomas typically translates to effective nonsurgical treatment strategies that can rapidly reduce the size of lymphoid tumors impairing or threatening organ function in the acute setting. Despite this, there are discrete clinical circumstances where more extensive surgical intervention is warranted.

The emerging landscape of precision oncology within lymphoma care is particularly relevant from a diagnostic and therapeutic perspective. Most recently, 126 discrete diagnoses have been identified as subtypes of mature lymphoid, histiocytic, and den-dritic cell tumors as published by the joint Clinical Advisory Committee of the Society for Hematopathology and the European Association for Haematopathology.[2] Many of these classifications were described from recent advances in immunohistochemistry, flow cytometry, cytogenetic, and gene sequencing studies, which are now widely available in clinical practice and are a component of contemporary diagnostic strate-gies for treatment optimization. Such studies ordered at the time of tissue sampling can ensure timeliness of accurate diagnosis and risk stratification for tumor-directed therapies.

Given the extensive diversity of lymphoma subtypes, understanding common prin-ciples distinguishing categories of lymphomas is of practical significance. The first ma-jor line of distinction is classic Hodgkin lymphoma (cHL) versus non-Hodgkin lymphomas (NHLs). Classic Hodgkin lymphoma is distinct from NHLs in being charac-terized by a contiguous pattern of lymphadenopathy, attributed to the clonal Reed-Sternberg cells spreading from one nodal or lymphoid structure through lymphatic channels to an adjacent anatomic lymphoid structure. By contrast, NHLs are often characterized by noncontiguous patterns of involvement, attributed to hematogenous spread. Within the NHLs, 2 broad independent categories with clinical relevance are recognized: (1) B-cell versus T/NK-cell NHL, with B-cell NHLs comprising approxi-mately 85% of all NHLs, and (2) clinically indolent versus aggressive NHLs. Many forms of aggressive NHLs, characterized by more rapid rates of proliferation and pro-gression, are often curable. By contrast, indolent NHLs, characterized by slow rates of progression, are not currently curable outside of infrequent cases presenting with very early stage disease where involved site radiation can be curative in more than 50%.[3] Due to the typically slow rate of progression, even advanced cases of indolent NHLs may not require therapy at the time of diagnosis and sometimes remain stable for months or years before requiring therapy.

NON-HODGKIN LYMPHOMAS

NHLs are neoplasms of the lymphoid tissues originating from B cell precursors, mature B cells, T cell precursors, and mature T cells. NHLs comprise approximately 82% of lymphoid, histiocytic, and dendritic cell tumor diagnoses.[4] There are currently 92 discrete B-cell and T-cell neoplasms that comprise NHLs, each with different etiologies, immunophenotypes, genetic and clinical features, as well as prognoses and responses to therapy.[2] As such, it is clinically relevant to categorize such tumors as "B-cell" versus

"NK/T-cell" based on cell of origin, and "aggressive" versus "indolent" lymphomas, based on clinical course and prognosis, given tumor biology strongly influences treatment goals, therapeutic approaches, and anticipated outcomes of therapy.

Clinical Features

Common aggressive NHLs include discrete histologies such as Burkitt lymphoma, diffuse large B-cell lymphomas (DLBCLs), mantle cell lymphoma (MCL), primary central nervous system (CNS) lymphoma, and mature T-cell lymphomas (**Table 1**). Patients are often symptomatic at diagnosis and may present with complaints of painless lymphadenopathy, lethargy, loss of appetite, and infection, as well as characteristic "B symptoms," which comprise fevers, weight loss, and/or drenching night sweats. Such symptoms typically develop during the course of weeks to months and are often progressive. Tumor biology will drive clinical presentation, with high-grade tumors such as Burkitt lymphoma and high-grade DLBCL often presenting with rapidly increasing lymphadenopathy, spontaneous tumor lysis syndrome, and sometimes neurologic complications of CNS involvement. Seventy percent of patients with an aggressive NHL will present with advance-stage (stage III/IV) disease.[5] Approximately 50% of patients may develop secondary extranodal disease, whereas between 10% and 35% will have primary extranodal lymphoma at the time of diagnosis.[6] Typical sites of extranodal disease include the bowel, stomach, liver, lungs, pleura, anterior mediastinum, bones, spleen, testes, breast tissue, orbits, sinuses, and brain/spine. The presence of multiple sites of extranodal involvement typically portends an aggressive clinical course with higher risk of CNS involvement and poorer prognosis but are nonetheless potentially curable. Patients with either primary (isolated to the CNS) or secondary CNS involvement may present with headache, lethargy, altered mental status, focal neurologic deficits, seizures, paralysis, spinal cord compression, or lymphomatous meningitis.

Table 1 Aggressive non-Hodgkin lymphoma	
	Proportion of Lymphoma Diagnoses (US SEER Data, 2020)
Mature B-Cell Lymphomas	
DLBCL	32.5%
MCL	4.1%
PMBL lymphoma	2%–3%
Lymphoblastic lymphoma	2%
Lymphoblastic lymphoma	<1%
Primary CNS lymphoma	<1%
HIV-associated diffuse large B-cell lymphoma	<1%
Mature T-cell and NK cell lymphomas	
Peripheral T-cell lymphoma, NOS	6%
Systemic anaplastic large cell lymphoma	2%
Angioimmunoblastic T-cell lymphoma	1%
Extranodal NK/T-cell lymphoma	0.2%
Enteropathy-associated intestinal T-cell lymphoma	<0.1%
Hepatosplenic T-cell lymphoma	<0.1%
Adult T-cell leukemia/lymphoma	0.03%

Common indolent NHLs include follicular lymphoma (FL), marginal zone lymphomas (MZLs—also known as mucosal associated lymphoid tissue [MALT] lymphomas), small lymphocytic lymphoma (SLL), and mycosis fungoides (MF; **Table 2**). Some mantle cell lymphomas will also follow an indolent clinical course. Patients are often asymptomatic at the time of diagnosis and diagnosed incidentally when pursuing medical evaluations for unrelated clinical concerns. Waxing and waning painless lymphadenopathy is a hallmark of indolent lymphomas. Symptoms, if they develop, often take months to years to manifest. Laboratory abnormalities are often absent and only 20% of patients will present with B symptoms.[7]

Clinical Evaluations and Diagnostic Considerations

Routine clinical and laboratory evaluations for patients with NHL include history and physical examination, assessment of performance status, complete blood count (CBC) with differential, complete metabolic profile (CMP), phosphorus, uric acid, and lactate dehydrogenase (LDH). Baseline staging involves imaging with 18-fluoro-deoxyglucose positron emission tomography/computed tomography (^{18}F-FDG PET/CT) with or without diagnostic-quality CT studies of the neck, chest, abdomen, and pelvis, using iodinated contrast when renal function permits.[8] Several conventional staging criteria exist although the 2014 Lugano classification for NHL is widely used as the conventional clinical standard[9] (**Table 3**). Infection screening for human immunodeficiency virus (HIV), hepatitis C virus, and hepatitis B virus is also essential as the presence of these viruses warrants concurrent antiviral therapy, and HIV-associated malignancies typically present with aggressive clinical phenotypes often warranting dedicated treatment protocols.[9] Bone marrow biopsies are standard for staging of most indolent NHL. PET-CT scans are sensitive to bone marrow involvement in aggressive NHL where bone marrow biopsy is reserved for cases where cytopenias are present without clear marrow involvement on PET-CT. Sampling of cerebrospinal fluid for flow cytometry and cytology review and MRI assessments of the complete spine and brain should be pursued for neurologic deficits, or if extranodal disease presentation is appreciated in breast tissue, testes, kidneys, or adrenal glands, as well as in very high grade forms of NHL (ie, Burkitt, lymphoblastic).

Table 2
Indolent non-Hodgkin lymphoma

	Proportion of Lymphoma Diagnoses (US SEER Data, 2020)
Mature B-Cell Lymphomas	
Chronic lymphocytic leukemia/SLL	18.6%
FL	17.1%
MZLs (splenic, nodal, and extranodal MALTs)	10.0%
MCL	4.1%
LPL	1%
Waldenstrom macroglobulinemia	<1%
Mature T-Cell and NK Cell Lymphomas	
Primary cutaneous T-cell lymphoma (MF and Sezary syndrome)	4.0%
Primary cutaneous anaplastic large cell lymphoma	<1%
Subcutaneous panniculitis-like T-cell lymphoma	<1%

Table 3
Lugano staging criteria

Stage	Involvement	Extranodal (E) Status
Limited		
Stage I	One node or a group of adjacent nodes	Single extranodal lesion without nodal involvement
Stage II: nonbulky	Two or more nodal groups on the same side of the diaphragm; all nodes/masses are <7.5 cm at the widest diameter	Stage I or II by nodal extent with limited contiguous extranodal involvement
Stage II: bulky	Two or more nodal groups on the same side of the diaphragm; at least one node or mass is > 7.5 cm	N/A
Extensive (Advanced)		
Stage III	Nodes on both sides of the diaphragm or nodes above the diaphragm with spleen involvement	N/A
Stage IV	Nodes on both sides of the diaphragm with noncontiguous extralymphatic involvement	N/A

Abbreviation: NA, not applicable.

Surgical excisional biopsy (SEB) of a lymph node is the gold standard for lymphoma diagnosis and is essential for accurate tumor classification.[9] Although core needle biopsy (CNB) typically offers a more clinically practicable approach to tissue sampling, CNBs fail to completely capture nodal architecture and significantly contribute to diagnostic uncertainty and sometimes inaccurate lymphoma classification. These limitations result in clinically meaningful delays in delivery of lymphoma-directed care and also increase the need for subsequent biopsies. Thus, it is our clinical practice to request SEB without antecedent CNB sampling, wherever possible when suspicion of lymphoma is high. Nevertheless, clinical circumstances may heavily influence tissue sampling practicability, and CNB may be appropriate as initial sampling of masses or lymph nodes where excisional biopsy would be exceedingly invasive—for example, nodes localized in mediastinal, abdominal, retroperitoneal, or intrathoracic regions. Exposure to steroids before biopsy may result in initial necrosis preventing accurate diagnosis. High-grade lymphomas may also have high degrees of necrosis even before the initiation of steroids or lymphoma therapy, necessitating repeat biopsies or more invasive sampling. In certain cases, such as primary mediastinal B-cell lymphoma or primary effusion lymphoma, mediastinoscopy with tissue sampling or thoracentesis with flow cytometry, respectively, may be necessary for diagnosis. Patient age and performance status influence the clinical decision to pursue excisional lymph node biopsy, with retrospective data showing those of advanced age and worse performance status/medical comorbidity pursing CNB significantly more often than SEB in patients with suspected lymphoma.[10] Despite these practicability concerns, multicenter international registry data have consistently documented the superiority of SEB relative to CNB in providing accurate diagnosis and distinction among the many distinct type of lymphomas.[10–12]

The largest multicenter inventory of lymph nodes sampled either by CNB or by SEB in patients with suspected lymphoma was recently published by the French Lymphopath Network. They assessed 32,285 cases by evaluating the percentage accurate diagnoses using CNB and surgical excision approaches, according to the 2018 World Health Organization (WHO) classification.[11] Although CNB provided a definitive diagnosis in 92.3% of cases and seemed to be a reliable method of investigation for most patients with suspected lymphoma, it remained less conclusive than SEB, which provided a definitive diagnosis in 98.1% of cases. Discordance rates between referral and expert diagnoses were higher on CNB (23.1%) than on SEB (21.2%; $P = .004$), and referral pathologists provided more cases with unclassified lymphoma or equivocal lesion through CNB. In such cases, expert review improved the diagnostic workup by classifying ~90% of cases, with higher efficacy on SEB (93.3%) than CNB (81.4%; $P < .000001$). Moreover, diagnostic concordance for reactive lesions was higher on SEB than CNB ($P = .009$). Overall, although CNB accurately diagnoses lymphoma in most instances, it increases the risk of erroneous or nondefinitive conclusions and can significantly delay the initiation of therapy. This large-scale survey also emphasizes the need for systematic expert review in cases of lymphoma suspicion, especially in those sampled by CNB. If institutional resources are absent for consensus hematopathology review, SEB is greatly favored over CNB.

Molecular Characteristics and Precision Oncology

Pathologic evaluations of B-cell and T-cell neoplasms require a variety of immunohistochemical, cytogenetic, and in some cases gene sequencing methods for accurate diagnosis within the modern classification systems for NHL diagnoses, particularly when considering the heterogeneity of tumor types and therapies. Morphologic features remain the cornerstone of evaluation for both aggressive and indolent NHL; however, ancillary studies are important in virtually all cases.

Immunophenotyping is helpful in both the diagnosis and classification of lymphoproliferative disorders, with common B-cell markers including immunoglobulin light and heavy chains, CD5, CD10, CD19, CD20, CD22, CD79, PAX5, and FMC7, and common T-cell markers including CD2, CD3, CD4, CD7, CD8, CD25, and CD30. Polymerase chain reaction (PCR) assays directed against rearrangement of the light chain genes, the kappa-deleting segment, or immunoglobulin heavy chain genes are also useful in the detection of B-cell clonality in mature B cell proliferations and are reported to detect clonality in up to 50% of B-cell lymphomas.[13] PCR assays for T cell clonality are usually directed against either T-cell receptor beta (TCRβ) or TCRγ. Specific cytogenetic translocations are also associated with specific NHL subtypes, including t(8;14) in Burkitt Lymphoma, t(11;14) in MCL, and t(14;18) in FL. Fluorescence in situ hybridization (FISH) is also an essential component for assessment of lymphomas, and in particular large cell lymphomas where concurrent *MYC*, *BCL2*, and/or *BCL6* gene rearrangements typically portend higher risk disease warranting consideration of more aggressive induction chemoimmunotherapy.[14]

The molecular heterogeneity of DLBCL was initially appreciated from gene expression profiling studies where subtypes were identified by cell-of-origin: germinal center B-cell (GCB), activated B-cell (ABC), and primary mediastinal B-cell (PMBL) were described.[15,16] The 2016 revision of the WHO classification recognized ABC DLBCL and GCB DLBCL as distinct molecular subtypes of DLBCL. FISH-based assays have similarly distinguished germinal center (GC) from nongerminal center (non-GC), which approximate the molecular GCB and ABC subtypes.[1] Prospective studies have not clearly identified superior treatment approaches relative to conventional standard-of-care chemoimmunotherapy for DLBCL subtypes; however, high-risk subgroups may benefit from specific targeted agents, particularly in the relapsed/refractory setting, therefore subtyping is an important pathologic distinction for the treating hematologist/oncologist and should be component of diagnostic studies when tissue samples are obtained.

Next-generation sequencing studies of the whole genome, whole exome, and transcriptome have further delineated the genetic landscapes within and across cell-of-origin subtypes, as well as can further subclassify DLBCL into discrete genotypic categories specific to common classes of driver mutations that contribute to lymphomagenesis.[15,16] Although potential molecular targets have been identified, further studies are needed to understand the clinical impact of these newly minted subtypes regarding their role of targeted therapy and may inform eligibility for clinical trials or management of highly refractory disease.

Prognosis, Treatment Considerations, and Surgical Interventions

The prognosis of NHL is contingent on specific histopathology, stage at presentation, presence of extranodal disease, discrete laboratory data, and patient-specific factors. The International Prognostic Index (IPI) and its disease-specific variants help to determine overall survival (OS) after delivery of standard-of-care therapy and are used as the main prognostic tools in patients with NHL (**Table 4**). IPI is calculated by the following specific clinical variables: (1) age greater than 60 years, (2) serum LDH greater than upper limit of institutional normal, (3) Eastern Cooperative Oncology Group (ECOG) performance status 2 or greater, (4) clinical stage III/IV disease, and (5) greater than 1 extranodal site of involvement. One point is given for each factor, a total score from which determines the degree of risk. These are classified as low risk (0–1 adverse factor), intermediate risk (2 adverse factors), and poor risk (3 or more adverse factors).[17] The IPI scoring system has been modified for most NHL subtypes for better assessment of prognosis each discrete histopathologies (eg, FLIPI for FL, MIPI for MCL, and so forth).

Treatment of NHL is generally based on stage at presentation, histopathological features, burden of disease (eg, "bulky" vs "nonbulky" disease), and symptoms. Despite the biological heterogeneity of NHLs, these tumors show exquisite sensitivity to chemoimmunotherapy and radiotherapy approaches, which have become the standards of care. The goal of therapy for an aggressive NHL is curative, with 55% to 95% of patients achieving functional cure of their malignancy.[18,19] This wide variability in outcomes further reflects the clinic heterogeneity of aggressive NHL subtypes, although generally speaking the prognosis for aggressive lymphomas is favorable.

The goal of therapy for indolent NHL is disease control as indolent lymphomas are typically not curable with current treatment strategies.[20] Indolent lymphomas with low disease burden can be observed and treatment deferred unless symptomatic.[21] The preferred treatment in early stage disease, if indicated, is radiotherapy, which in rare circumstances may provide cure for some histologies such as FL.[3] *Helicobacter pylori* eradication therapy is often curative for gastric MALT, a specific type of indolent MZL that is driven by chronic antigenic stimulation and inflammation.[22] Treatment of patients with advanced stage III/IV disease or bulky stage II disease (tumors >7 cm) involves combination chemotherapy with monoclonal antibody therapy (rituximab or obinutuzumab).[9] Relapse is common after several years posttreatment in patients with indolent NHL; however, subsequent second-line, third-line, and fourth-line therapies are readily available, which provide durable remissions typically measured on the order of years.

Table 4
International prognostic index

	IPI Scoring	5-y PFS	5-y OS
Prognostic Indices			
Age >60 y	1	—	—
ECOG PS ≥ 2	1	—	—
Extranodal site ≥1	1	—	—
Stage III/IV disease	1	—	—
LDH > ULN	1	—	—
Risk categories			
Low	0–1	70%	73%
Low-intermediate	2	50%	51%
High-intermediate	3	49%	43%
High	4–5	40%	26%

Abbreviations: ECOG, Eastern Cooperative Oncology Group; LDH, lactate dehydrogenase; OS, overall survival; PFS, progression-free survival; PS, performance status; ULN, upper limit normal.

HODGKIN LYMPHOMAS

Hodgkin lymphomas (HL) comprise a group of 5 discrete histopathologic diagnoses that are characterized by the presence of rare Reed-Sternberg (R-S) cells amid a background of reactive inflammatory cells. There are 4 classic HL (cHL) subtypes, which include nodular sclerosis, mixed-cellularity, lymphocyte-depleted, and lymphocyte-rich (**Table 5**). These subtypes are considered aggressive diseases and warrant urgent initiation of curative-intent therapy. A fifth, nonclassic Hodgkin lymphoma (HL) subtype described as nodular lymphocyte-predominant HL is a separate and indolent disease, which rarely requires emergent intervention; treatment is typically provided with the intention of disease control because it is considered noncurable.[23]

Clinical Features

An estimated 83,087 new cases of cHL were diagnosed globally in 2020 with an age-standardized incidence rate of 0.98 per 100,000 people.[24] The incidence is highest in young adult patient populations (ages 20–24 years) with a second peak appreciated in patients aged older than 55 years. Regardless of stage, cHL is considered highly curable.[25]

Clinical Features, Prognosis, and Therapy

Classic Hodgkin lymphoma
Patients with cHL will commonly present with painless supradiaphragmatic lymphadenopathy presenting in a contiguous pattern of spread or symptoms from cervical nodes or a mediastinal mass (cough, dyspnea, or chest pain—particularly after ingestion of alcohol). B-symptoms are reported in approximately 30% of patients and are generally more common in advanced-stage disease, mixed-cellularity, or lymphocyte-depleted cHL subtypes. CNS involvement is exceedingly rare.

The contiguous pattern of lymphatic spread characteristic of cHL accounts for it being one of the first malignancies for which cure was possible before availability of cytotoxic chemotherapy because radiation could be directed at the known sites of disease and the adjacent lymphatic structures with curative intent.[26] This contiguous disease pattern is attributed to dependence of the R-S cells on the microenvironment of the

Table 5				
Classic Hodgkin lymphomas and nodular lymphocyte predominate Hodgkin lymphoma				
Biomarker	**NS**	**MC**	**LD**	**LR**	**NLP**
CD30	Positive	Positive	Positive	Positive	Negative
CD15	Usually positive (~80%)	Usually positive (~80%)	Usually positive (~80%)	Usually positive (~80%)	Negative
IRF4	Positive	Positive	Positive	Positive	Positive
CD20	Occasionally positive (~20%) with variable intensive	Occasionally positive (~20%) with variable intensive	Occasionally positive (~20%) with variable intensive	Occasionally positive (~20%) with variable intensive	Positive
PAX5	Positive	Positive	Positive	Positive	Positive
B-cell transcription factors	Usually negative	Usually negative	Usually negative	Positive or negative	Positive
EBV	Positive (10%–20%)	Positive (~75%)	Positive (~75%)	Positive (~30%)	Negative

Abbreviations: LD, lymphocyte depleted; LR, lymphocyte rich; MC, mixed cellularity; NLP, nodular lymphocyte predominate Hodgkin lymphoma which is now recoined as NLP B-cell lymphoma; NS, nodular sclerosing.

inflammatory infiltrate noted in the nodal architecture. Radiation continues to be an important modality for cHL, although doses and fields have been dramatically reduced with modern radiotherapy techniques, and it is now used as an adjunct to systemic therapy in specific circumstances: following chemotherapy in favorable risk early stage disease or directed to bulky sites of disease as consolidation of systemic therapy in advanced stage disease.

Even in the highest risk category, cHL is curable in more than 50% of patients, with long-term progression-free survival rates (PFS, a surrogate of cure rates) greater than 90% in the most favorable risk groups.[27,28] It should be noted that those presenting with cHL at age greater than 45 years have inferior PFS and OS relative to younger counterparts.[29] Management of cHL is based on 3 major prognostic groups where stage is determined by the Ann Arbor staging classification[30] with the Lugano update (see **Table 3**)[31] incorporating the use of FDG-PET: early stage (stages I–II) favorable disease, early stage unfavorable disease, and advanced stage (stages III–IV) disease.

The distinction between favorable or unfavorable risk early stage disease depends on factors such as bulky disease, erythrocyte sedimentation rate, B symptoms, number of nodal sites, and the ratio of the size of mediastinal mass to the intrathoracic diameter on chest imaging.[27] Durable complete remission rates with favorable risk early stage cHL are greater than 90% with 2 cycles of ABVD (doxorubicin, bleomycin, vinblastine, dacarbazine) chemotherapy followed by 20 Gy of involved field radiotherapy.[32] The use of chemotherapy alone is also an option particularly when complete metabolic remission is present on postchemotherapy FDG-PET/CT.[33] This strategy may be preferable in some circumstances based on location of cHL involvement when considering long-term complications of radiation, including secondary malignancies; the trade-off is a slightly increased risk of relapse, which would necessitate additional therapy to achieve cure. Management of unfavorable early stage disease involves additional cycles of chemotherapy with or without involved site radiation, incorporating risk-adapted strategies escalating or deescalating therapy based on results of interim FDG-PET/CT.[34] ABVD has been the standard frontline therapy for advanced stage disease,[35] with recent trials demonstrating feasibility of substituting the anti-CD30 antibody–drug conjugate, brentuximab vedotin,[36] or the checkpoint inhibitor, nivolumab, for bleomycin.

NODULAR LYMPHOCYTE PREDOMINATE HODGKIN LYMPHOMA: "NODULAR LYMPHOCYTE PREDOMINATE B-CELL LYMPHOMA"

Highlighting major biologic and clinical differences between nodular lymphocyte predominate HL and classic HL, the International Consensus Classification Clinical Advisory Committee proposed a new name removing reference to HL altogether: nodular lymphocyte predominant B-cell lymphoma.[2] Most cases present with early stage disease and pursue an indolent clinical course. Management principles are similar to indolent NHLs, including the options of observation versus involved site radiotherapy for early stage cases. Observation versus chemotherapy including rituximab with or without radiation may be appropriate for advanced stage disease depending on whether patients are symptomatic or have high-risk features.[37]

TARGETED THERAPIES IN LYMPHOMAS

Monoclonal antibodies directed at lymphoma antigens such as CD20 were the first targeted therapies to become standard in the management of lymphomas, effecting antibody-dependent cellular cytotoxicity.[38] Antibody–drug conjugates (ADCs) have further developed this strategy, delivering a cytotoxic payload into cells with the target antigen (ie, CD19, CD30, and CD79b). Additional categories of lymphoma therapy have recently exapnded the lymphoma therapeutic toolbox, such as immunomodulatory drugs (IMiDs), and kinase inhibitors, which have activity in specific NHL subtypes. Autologous and allogeneic hematopoietic stem cell transplant have been important in the management of relapsed and refractory lymphomas in patients who are medically fit.[37,39] Immune checkpoint inhibitors are an active component of therapy for HL but have disappointing activity in NHL.[37] Recent immunotherapeutic approaches also include strategies using chimeric antigen receptor T-cells (CAR-T) directed against lymphoma antigens, as well as bispecific antibodies adding direct T-cell engagement to the antigen targeting mechanism[9] (**Table 6**).

PLASMA CELL NEOPLASMS

Plasma cell neoplasms (PCNs) are a group of mature B-cell lymphoid malignancies typically manifesting excessive production of monoclonal heavy-chain immunoglobulins referred to as "paraproteins." This class of diseases includes entities such as monoclonal gammopathy of undetermined significance (MGUS), plasmacytomas, monoclonal immunoglobulin deposition diseases, Waldenstrom Macroglobulinemia/lymphoplasmacytic lymphoma (LPL), and multiple myeloma (MM). These abnormal plasma cell clones can cause lytic bone lesions due to aberrant osteoclast stimulation by serum free light chains, inhibit normal hematopoiesis due to rapid expansion within the bone marrow, and can cause deterioration of renal function through the deposition of abnormal immunoglobulin in the renal glomeruli and renal tubules. Light-chain amyloidosis (AL) is a distinct clinical entity, which may complicate clonal plasma cell disorders manifesting as amyloid fibril deposition in nonlymphoid tissues interfering with native organ function. Given the clinical heterogeneity of this class of malignancies, a multimodality approach to therapy is generally considered with surgical interventions warranted in select circumstances.

Table 6
Examples of targeted therapies active in lymphomas

Category	Target	Examples	Type of Lymphoma
Monoclonal antibody	CD20	Rituximab Ofatumumab	B-cell lymphomas, both indolent and aggressive
ADCs	CD19 CD30	Loncastuximab teserine Brentuximab vedotin	DLBCL cHL, selected T cell lymphomas
	CD79b	Polatuzumab vedotin	DLBCL
Bispecific T cell engager	CD20 + CD3	Mosunetuzumab	FL
CAR-T immunotherapy	CD19	Axicabtagene ciloleucel Brexucabtagene Tisagenlecleucel	Acute lymphoblastic leukemia/lymphoma, DLBCL, FL
Kinase inhibitors	Bruton's tyrosine kinase	Ibrutinib Acalabrutinib Zanubrutinib Pirtubrutinib	CLL/SLL, MCL, Waldenstrom macroglobulinemia
	Phosphoinositide 3′-kinase	Idelalisib Duvelisib	CLL/SLL
Immune checkpoint inhibitor monoclonal antibody	PD-1	Nivolumab Pembrolizumab	cHL

Abbreviations: CLL, chronic lymphocytic leukemia; DLBCL, diffuse large B-cell lymphoma; SLL, small lymphocytic lymphoma.

Clinical Features

PCNs comprise approximately 1% of all newly diagnosed malignant tumors in the United States annually and account for 15% of new hematologic malignancy diagnoses.[40] PCNs are generally a disease of older age with the median age of diagnosis at 66 years; there is increased risk in men and African Americans.[41]

Clinical manifestations of these diseases are not uniform and can vary widely, with many patients lacking symptoms (**Table 7**). Diseases such as MGUS or smoldering MM are unlikely to be referred for surgical interventions specifically associated to their monoclonal gammopathy because, by definition, these patients have no identifiable end-organ damage caused by their malignancy. Those with focal diseases such as extramedullary/osseous plasmacytomas may only note symptoms at the location of their tumor, whereas patients with systemic diseases such as MM may report fatigue and exertional dyspnea from anemia or renal insufficiency, symptoms of hypercalcemia, and possible focal symptoms at areas of immunoglobulin deposition such as bone or nerve pain.

Clinical Evaluations and Diagnostic Considerations

Routine clinical and laboratory evaluations for patients with PMNs include history and physical examination, assessment of performance status, CBC with differential, CMP with creatinine clearance assessment, serum uric acid, serum phosphorus, serum LDH, serum beta-2 microglobulin, serum protein electrophoresis (SPEP) with immunofixation, serum kappa and lambda free light chain assessment, bone marrow aspirate and biopsy with plasma cell-enriched interphase fluorescence in situ hybridization

Table 7
Clinical characteristics of plasma cell neoplasms

Plasma Cell Neoplasm	M Protein Type	Pathology	Clinical Presentation
MGUS	IgG kappa or lambda; or IgA kappa or lambda	<10% plasma cells in bone marrow	Asymptomatic, without evidence of disease (aside from the presence of an M protein)
Isolated plasmacytoma of bone	IgG kappa or lambda; or IgA kappa or gamma	Solitary lesion of bone; <10% plasma cells in marrow of uninvolved site	Asymptomatic or symptomatic at the location of the affected bone
Extramedullary plasmacytoma	IgG kappa or lambda; or IgA kappa or gamma	Solitary lesion of soft tissue; most commonly occurs in the nasopharynx, tonsils, or paranasal sinuses	Asymptomatic or symptomatic at the location of tumor involvement
MM	IgG kappa or lambda; or IgA kappa or gamma	Typically presents with CRAB criteria and >10% clonal plasma cells in bone marrow; >60% clonal plasma cells in bone marrow and/or involved:uninvolved light chain ratio >100 is also diagnostic; often with multiple lesions of bone	Typically symptomatic, with systemic manifestations of disease (eg, fatigue, bone pain, infections, and so forth)
Waldenstrom macroglobulinemia	IgM kappa or lambda	>10% clonal plasma cells in bone marrow, monoclonal IgM paraprotein on SPEP/IFE	—

(iFISH), NT-proBNP, and whole-body low-dose CT or ^{18}F-FDG PET/CT to assess for lytic lesions. X-ray films are not sufficiently sensitive to assess for lytic lesions and are not considered acceptable as screening tools for patients with symptomatic PCNs.

MM is the main disease entity in PCNs and presents variably, with symptoms ranging from asymptomatic to aggressive. The diagnosis is based on the assessment of discrete pathologic, radiological, and clinical features.[42] Diagnosis requires bone marrow biopsy showing at least greater than 10% clonal plasma cell involvement and requires any combination of the following: evidence of end-organ damage attributable to the underlying plasma cell clone ("CRAB" criteria) as manifest by hyperCalcemia, Renal failure, Anemia, or lytic Bone lesions. Alternate biomarker criteria for patients who do not meet CRAB-criteria were added to the IMWG diagnostic guidelines in 2016 and include involved-to-uninvolved serum free light chain ratio of 100 or greater and/or clonal plasma cell bone marrow involvement of 60% or greater.[43] Symptoms of MM include B-symptoms related to bone marrow infiltration, specifically fatigue and pallor, bleeding, and infection, as well as symptoms related to CRAB complications. Secondary extramedullary involvement with plasmacytomas is present in a minority of cases, with the most common sites including lymph nodes, liver, spleen, and bones. Advanced disease often manifests with poor performance status, unintentional weight loss, oliguric renal failure, or pathologic fracture requiring surgical fixation.[43]

Plasmacytomas present with 2 distinct clinical phenotypes: solitary plasmacytoma of bone (SPB) and extramedullary plasmacytoma (EMP). Surgical sampling of affected tissue is required for diagnosis because there are no pathognomonic radiographic features to definitively diagnose these entities. SPB refers to the involvement of cortical bone with monoclonal plasma cells; the most common bone sites include the vertebrae, ribs, and skull. EMP refers to localized PCNs that originate in tissues other than bone, with approximately 80% of patients presenting with pathology in the upper respiratory tract (eg, sinuses, nasopharynx, oropharynx, and so forth). Other tissues of origin for EMPs include gastrointestinal (GI) tract, CNS, breast tissue, lungs, parotid glands, and skin.[44] CNB of an associated mass is acceptable for diagnosis, although crush artifact in osseous lesions may require a more extensive surgical bone biopsy. These neoplasms are primary tumors without measurable systemic involvement of a monoclonal PCN. As such, a thorough assessment must be pursued at diagnosis to exclude PCM with secondary extramedullary involvement, including tests to assess serum monoclonal protein, bone marrow aspirate and biopsy, and advance imaging studies such whole-body CT, PET, or MRI. Patients will typically present with localized pain; those with osseous disease can show evidence for soft tissue extension and those with soft tissue disease can show associated osseous erosions. SPB shows progression to MM or multifocal plasmacytoma in up to 70% of cases; therefore, referral to a hematologist/oncologist for serial longitudinal follow-up is essential for these patients. Although EMP is considered curative with either involved-field radiation and/or complete surgical resection, observation for systemic disease progression is prudent.

Monoclonal immunoglobulin deposition diseases include amyloid light-chain (AL) disease and heavy chain diseases. Both disorders are characterized by clonal plasma cells that secrete either intact or fragmented immunoglobulins, which thereafter deposit nonspecifically in soft and visceral tissues, leading to organ dysfunction.[45] The major difference between these 2 disease entities is that AL amyloidosis stains positive with Congo red stain, whereas heavy chain deposition diseases require immunofluorescence assays. Approximately 20% of patients with evidence of amyloidosis will have primary MM; therefore, thorough systemic assessments as outlined above remain crucial. Sites of clinical significance in patients with amyloidosis include subcutaneous fat, kidney, heart, liver, gastrointestional tract, peripheral nerves, and bone marrow. Clinical symptoms are extremely variable and depend on the organs involved. For example, cardiac involvement can present as congestive heart failure, kidney involvement can present as nephrotic syndrome, gastrointestinal involvement may present as a protein-losing enteropathy and profuse diarrhea, and liver involvement may present as hepatomegaly with or without synthetic liver dysfunction. Tissue sampling of the affected organ is essential for this diagnosis and can be made sufficiently with core needle samples. If the affected organ is not clinically amenable to biopsy, fat pad biopsy may be pursued as a surrogate diagnostic tool.

Molecular Characteristics and Precision Oncology

Conventional immunohistochemical and cytogenetic assessments for PCNs show some general similarities when considering histopathologic diagnoses. The combination of antibodies to CD138 or 38, Bcl-2, CD79a, and CD20 enables classification of malignant plasmacytosis in the bone marrow, considering occasional heterogeneity in tumor antigen expression.[46] Immunoglobulin heavy and light chain staining is useful for identifying plasma cells and for demonstrating the presence of clonal restriction. Activating mutations in MYD88 are present in 93% to 97% of patients with Waldenstrom macroglobulinemia and 50% to 70% of patients with IgM MGUS.[47] Cyclin D1 is a cell cycle regulator that is overexpressed in 24% to 40% of patients with MM, and positivity is associated with higher tumor grade and stage[48] while being associated with shorter survival.[49]

Conventional cytogenetic analysis in myeloma is difficult because of the low proliferation rate of malignant plasma cells and, together with a variable degree of bone marrow infiltration, this type of analysis grossly underestimates karyotypic changes in MM. When plasma cells are identified in metaphases for chromosomal and cytogenetic assessment, it has been shown that they typically originate from the normal hemopoietic compartment and underrepresent driver mutations important for risk stratification and optimal therapy.[50] As such, interphase fluorescence in situ hybridization (FISH) is vastly preferred for diagnosis and risk stratification because it enriches the assessable cellular pool for malignant plasma cells, rendering it superior in the detection of plasma cell dyscrasia cytogenetic aberrations.

As with NHL tumor subtypes, recent advances in DNA and RNA sequencing techniques have begun to characterize the molecular landscape of PCNs by better delineating the role that somatic mutations play in regulating physiologic B-cell development and resultant clonal evolution through oncogenic pathways and tumor suppressor genes, epigenetic alterations, and tumor-promoting bone marrow microenvironments. Next generation DNA sequencing can be considered at the time of diagnosis, particularly if there are plans for clinical trial enrollment or candidacy, however this degree of precision oncology rarely influences diagnostic interventions or frontline therapeutic decisions as the individual drugs that constitute current standards of care are agnostic to molecular characteristics and biomarkers.

Prognosis, Treatment Considerations, and Surgical Interventions

The prognoses for patients with PCNs are variable and contingent on the discrete disease subtype. MM and light-chain deposition diseases are aggressive and incurable malignancies that typically take a progressive clinical course. Although life expectancy is measured in years, patients will typically require multiple lines of therapy and show diminishing degrees of tumor response with subsequent treatments. Isolated SPBs and EMPs are curative malignancies with involved-field radiotherapy and/or complete surgical excision. Patients with Waldenstrom macroglobulinemia and other LPLs enjoy a very favorable prognosis with a life expectancy measured in years to decades; these are chronic and indolent conditions with multiple treatments options, though they remain incurable diseases.

The 2 most significant drivers of prognosis in MM are stage and disease biology. The Revised Multiple Myeloma International Staging System (R-ISS) is used to characterize patients with newly diagnosed disease and is composed of 4 discrete clinical variables: (1) serum beta 2 microglobulin level, (2) serum albumin, (3) risk class as defined by iFISH [that is, presence or absence of either del(17p), translocation t(4;14), and/or translocation t(14;16)], and (4) serum LDH. Patients with R-ISS Stage I disease showed a 5-year OS of 82% and PFS of 55% compared with 5-year OS of 40% and PFS of 24% in stage III.[51] High-risk cytogenetic abnormalities including t(4:14), t(14:16), gain of 1q, and/or t(14:20) adversely affect survival.

Initial management of patients with MM should involve evaluations for acute concerns that threaten organ function, such as the management of severe anemia, hypercalcemia, and renal dysfunction. Isotonic saline administration for rapid volume expansion is the hallmark of hypercalcemia management, along with the selective use of calcitonin and/or bisphosphonates. Red cell transfusion should be pursued to maintain adequate hemoglobin concentrations. Medical optimization should be undertaken for the management of myeloma-associated kidney injury, including assessment of volume status with appropriate volume expansion where indicated, avoidance of nephrotoxic agents, dose adjustments for medications that may further affect renal function, and discussion of hemodialysis if severe renal impairment is noted. Clinicians should assess patients for signs of serum hyperviscosity (eg, headaches, acute vision changes, hypoxia, abnormal bleeding, acute renal failure, and so forth) and should pursue plasmapheresis, if present.

Spinal cord compression resulting from a pathologic vertebral fracture or the presence of a secondary plasmacytoma is a medical emergency and should be managed aggressively by neurosurgery and/or orthopedic interventions. Dexamethasone is typically used as a means of mitigating vasogenic spinal cord edema in preparation for spinal cord decompression. Surgical intervention and tissue sampling should be pursued within 24 hours of steroid initiation if used for spinal cord compromise because tumor necrosis will rapidly ensue in this context, threatening accurate diagnosis and disease staging.

Frontline induction therapy for MM is driven by risk stratification and transplant eligibility. Autologous hematopoietic stem cell transplantation (autoHSCT) is typically considered to deepen remission and improve on PFS, particularly for those with high-risk disease. Eligibility for autoHSCT is assessed on a case-by-case basis and is often influenced by age, performance status, and medical comorbidities, as well as response to induction therapy. Regardless of the clinical appropriateness of autoHSCT relative to patient-specific factors, long-term maintenance therapy is typically used to improve on PFS and OS in patients with both standard and high-risk MM.

The additions of proteasome inhibitors, immunomodulating agents, and anti-CD38 antibodies to the MM treatment arsenal have greatly improved survival among patients with all stages and risk factors.[52] In recent years, further incremental gains have been made in the relapsed/refractory setting through the use of agents with novel mechanisms, such as panobinostat (histone deacetylase inhibitor), selinexor (selective inhibitor of nuclear export compound), belantamab mafodotin (anti-BCMA ADC), and idecabtagene vicleucel (CAR-T cell therapy). Although treatment approaches can be adjusted to patients' comorbidities, cytogenetic risk, functional status, and response to therapy, the individual drugs that constitute current standards of care are agnostic to molecular characteristics and biomarkers. Despite these remarkable advances in therapy, depth and duration of responses to current agents can vary widely and unpredictably due in large part to extensive intertumor and intratumor genetic variability.[53] Drug-refractory relapse remains an inevitability in most patients and each successive line of therapy generally produces shorter responses.

SPB and EMP are radiosensitive, and radiotherapy is the treatment of choice in these diseases, with cure rates approaching 80%.[54,55] Fractionated radiotherapy with a cumulative dose of 40 to 50 Gy during a duration of 4 weeks is given at the rate of 1.8 to 2.0 Gy per fraction and intensity-modulated radiotherapy or proton therapy can be used to mitigate locoregional toxicity of the ocular, salivary gland, or oropharyngeal mucosa.[44] Upfront radical surgery of head and neck plasmacytomas should be avoided because these tumors are highly radiosensitive relative to the high potential for surgery-associated morbidity. In other areas, surgery can be pursued where feasible because combination surgery with adjuvant radiotherapy contributes to an improved PFS, particularly in SPB.[44] Surgery is also indicated for vertebral instability, fractures, or neurologic involvement. It should be noted that surgical resection without RT shows increased rates of recurrence.[56]

Patients with Waldenstrom macroglobulinemia/LPL are typically treated similarly to patients with other indolent B-cell lymphomas and initially monitored without therapy if asymptomatic. A retrospective analysis of 439 patients with asymptomatic Waldenstrom macroglobulinemia[57] found 4 variables associated with an increased risk of progression warranting therapy: (1) IgM 4500 mg/dL or greater, (2) bone marrow lymphoplasmacytic infiltration 70% or greater, (3) beta 2 microglobulin 4.0 mg/dL or greater, and (4) serum albumin 3.5 g/dL or lesser. Wild-type MYD88 was also an independent risk factor for progression. Treatment of symptomatic patients typically involves the use of anti-CD20 monoclonal antibody therapy ± chemotherapy or a bruton's tyrosine kinase inhibitor.[58] Patients with IgM concentrations greater than 4000 mg/dL may present with symptoms of serum hyperviscosity for which plasmapheresis is a useful temporizing measure while treatment of the underlying lymphoma is pursued.

SURGICAL CONSIDERATIONS FOR LYMPHOMAS AND PLASMA CELL NEOPLASMS BEYOND DIAGNOSTIC BIOPSIES

It is not possible to overstate the importance of multidisciplinary discussion among surgeons, hematology/oncology, and radiation oncology specialists in the decision to pursue surgical interventions beyond diagnostic biopsies for lymphoid malignancies. The decision for surgical intervention in patients with lymphomas and PCNs with oncologic emergencies must be carefully weighed against options for less-invasive treatment modalities such as temporizing glucocorticoid, immunotherapy, radiation, or even definitive systemic therapy. This is of particular concern in that systemic treatments for lymphoma and PCN often involve high-dose glucocorticoids and myelosuppressive therapy. Hence, procedures requiring prolonged recovery may significantly delay initiation of often curative-intent therapy due to the risk of impaired wound healing and infectious complications, and may therefore ultimately contribute to longitudinal harm. Although surgical decompression is occasionally indicated, the high chemotherapy and radiation sensitivity of lymphomas and PCNs translates to effective nonsurgical options to rapidly reduce the size of lymphoid tumors impairing or threatening organ function in many but not all circumstances. Common clinical scenarios likely to require surgical assessment and possible intervention include acute neurologic compression, bowel obstruction or suspected perforation, airway obstruction, and destructive osseous lesions at high risk of presenting as pathologic fractures.[59–61]

SUMMARY

In summary, the lymphoid malignancies comprise an extremely diverse group of diseases. Most are highly sensitive and may respond rapidly to glucocorticoids, cytotoxic chemotherapy, and radiation. Since the turn of the century, many novel immunotherapies and targeted therapies have improved disease control and cure rates for nearly all subtypes of lymphomas and PCNs, with further promising therapeutic candidates in development. Because surgery is not typically a mainstay of therapy, surgical oncologists will primarily be involved in obtaining biopsies of sufficient sample size and quality to allow accurate determination of the diagnosis, distinguishing between the many types of lymphoid malignancies. However, there are scenarios in which surgical intervention may be considered to address an oncologic emergency originating because of acute neurologic, respiratory, or other organ compromise; such cases benefit from early engagement in multidisciplinary review with hematology/oncology and radiation oncology specialists to weigh the relative merits and risks of surgical, medical, and radiotherapeutic approaches to individualize management.

CLINICS CARE POINTS

- Classic HL is characterized by a contiguous pattern of lymphadenopathy, attributed to the clonal B lymphocyte spreading through lymphatic channels, whereas NHLs are often characterized by noncontiguous patterns of involvement, attributed to hematogenous spread.

- Classic HL and aggressive NHLs (ie, Burkitt lymphoma and diffuse large B-cell lymphoma) have high cure rates. By contrast, indolent NHLs (ie, follicular and MZLs) and MM are not typically curable but may be associated with prolonged disease control rates.

- Indolent NHLs and myeloma may not require treatment at the time of initial diagnosis and sometimes remain stable for months or years before requiring therapy.

- During the last 3 decades, the development of targeted therapies, including immunotherapeutic approaches, have contributed to improved disease control and survival rates for those affected by lymphomas and myeloma.

REFERENCES

1. Swerdlow SH, Campo E, Pileri SA, et al. The 2016 revision of the World Health Organization classification of lymphoid neoplasms. Blood 2016;127(20): 2375–90.
2. Campo E, Jaffe ES, Cook JR, et al. The International Consensus Classification of Mature Lymphoid Neoplasms: a report from the Clinical Advisory Committee. Blood 2022;140(11):1229–53.
3. Brady JL, Binkley MS, Hajj C, et al. Definitive radiotherapy for localized follicular lymphoma staged by. Blood 2019;133(3):237–45.
4. SEER Preliminary Cancer Incidence Rate Estimates for 2017, and diagnosis years 2000 to 2017, SEER 18, National Cancer Institute. Bethesda, MD, https:// seer.cancer.gov/statistics/preliminary-estimates/, based on the February 2019 SEER data submission and the November 2018 SEER data submission. Posted to the SEER web site, September 2019.
5. Nair R, Bhurani D, Rajappa S, et al. Diffuse Large B-Cell Lymphoma: Clinical Presentation and Treatment Outcomes From the. Front Oncol 2021;11:796962.

6. Anderson T, Chabner BA, Young RC, et al. Malignant lymphoma. 1. The histology and staging of 473 patients at the National Cancer Institute. Cancer 1982;50(12): 2699–707.

7. Freedman A. Follicular lymphoma: 2018 update on diagnosis and management. Am J Hematol 2018;93(2):296–305.

8. Ricard F, Cheson B, Barrington S, et al. Application of the Lugano Classification for Initial Evaluation, Staging, and Response Assessment of Hodgkin and Non-Hodgkin Lymphoma: The PRoLoG Consensus Initiative (Part 1-Clinical). J Nucl Med 2023;64(1):102–8.

9. Zelenetz AD, Gordon LI, Abramson JS, et al. NCCN Guidelines® Insights: B-Cell Lymphomas, Version 6.2023. J Natl Compr Canc Netw 2023;21(11):1118–31.

10. Johl A, Lengfelder E, Hiddemann W, et al. Core needle biopsies and surgical excision biopsies in the diagnosis of lymphoma-experience at the Lymph Node Registry Kiel. Ann Hematol 2016;95(8):1281–6.

11. Syrykh C, Chaouat C, Poullot E, et al. Lymph node excisions provide more precise lymphoma diagnoses than core biopsies: a French Lymphopath network survey. Blood 2022;140(24):2573–83.

12. Assaf N, Nassif S, Tamim H, et al. Diagnosing Lymphoproliferative Disorders Using Core Needle Biopsy Versus Surgical Excisional Biopsy: Three-Year Experience of a Reference Center in Lebanon. Clin Lymphoma Myeloma Leuk 2020; 20(8):e455–60.

13. Stevenson F, Sahota S, Zhu D, et al. Insight into the origin and clonal history of B-cell tumors as revealed by analysis of immunoglobulin variable region genes. Immunol Rev 1998;162:247–59.

14. Cortese MJ, Wei W, Cerdeña S, et al. A multi-center analysis of the impact of DA-EPOCH-R dose-adjustment on clinical outcomes of patients with double/triple-hit lymphoma. Leuk Lymphoma 2023;64(1):107–18.

15. Rosenwald A, Wright G, Chan WC, et al. The use of molecular profiling to predict survival after chemotherapy for diffuse large-B-cell lymphoma. N Engl J Med 2002;346(25):1937–47.

16. Alizadeh AA, Eisen MB, Davis RE, et al. Distinct types of diffuse large B-cell lymphoma identified by gene expression profiling. Nature 2000;403(6769):503–11.

17. International Non-Hodgkin's Lymphoma Prognostic Factors Project. A predictive model for aggressive non-Hodgkin's lymphoma. N Engl J Med 1993;329(14): 987–94.

18. Sehn LH, Berry B, Chhanabhai M, et al. The revised International Prognostic Index (R-IPI) is a better predictor of outcome than the standard IPI for patients with diffuse large B-cell lymphoma treated with R-CHOP. Blood 2007;109(5):1857–61.

19. Gisselbrecht C, Gaulard P, Lepage E, et al. Prognostic significance of T-cell phenotype in aggressive non-Hodgkin's lymphomas. Groupe d'Etudes des Lymphomes de l'Adulte (GELA). Blood 1998;92(1):76–82.

20. Solal-Céligny P, Roy P, Colombat P, et al. Follicular lymphoma international prognostic index. Blood 2004;104(5):1258–65.

21. Horning SJ, Rosenberg SA. The natural history of initially untreated low-grade non-Hodgkin's lymphomas. N Engl J Med 1984;311(23):1471–5.

22. Stathis A, Chini C, Bertoni F, et al. Long-term outcome following Helicobacter pylori eradication in a retrospective study of 105 patients with localized gastric marginal zone B-cell lymphoma of MALT type. Ann Oncol 2009;20(6):1086–93.

23. Hoppe RT, Advani RH, Ai WZ, et al. Hodgkin lymphoma, version 2.2015. J Natl Compr Canc Netw 2015;13(5):554–86.

24. American Cancer Society. Key statistics for Hodgkin lymphoma 2023. Available at: https://www.cancer.org/cancer/types/hodgkin-lymphoma/about/key-statistics.html.
25. Huang J, Pang WS, Lok V, et al. Incidence, mortality, risk factors, and trends for Hodgkin lymphoma: a global data analysis. J Hematol Oncol 2022;15(1):57.
26. Witkowska M, Majchrzak A, Smolewski P. The role of radiotherapy in Hodgkin's lymphoma: what has been achieved during the last 50 years? BioMed Res Int 2015;2015:485071.
27. Klimm B, Goergen H, Fuchs M, et al. Impact of risk factors on outcomes in early-stage Hodgkin's lymphoma: an analysis of international staging definitions. Ann Oncol 2013;24(12):3070–6.
28. Hasenclever D, Diehl V. A prognostic score for advanced Hodgkin's disease. International Prognostic Factors Project on Advanced Hodgkin's Disease. N Engl J Med 1998;339(21):1506–14.
29. Evens AM, Hong F, Gordon LI, et al. The efficacy and tolerability of adriamycin, bleomycin, vinblastine, dacarbazine and Stanford V in older Hodgkin lymphoma patients: a comprehensive analysis from the North American intergroup trial E2496. Br J Haematol 2013;161(1):76–86.
30. Carbone PP, Kaplan HS, Musshoff K, et al. Report of the Committee on Hodgkin's Disease Staging Classification. Cancer Res 1971;31(11):1860–1.
31. Cheson BD, Pfistner B, Juweid ME, et al. Revised response criteria for malignant lymphoma. J Clin Oncol 2007;25(5):579–86.
32. Engert A, Plütschow A, Eich HT, et al. Reduced treatment intensity in patients with early-stage Hodgkin's lymphoma. N Engl J Med 2010;363(7):640–52.
33. Radford J, Illidge T, Counsell N, et al. Results of a trial of PET-directed therapy for early-stage Hodgkin's lymphoma. N Engl J Med 2015;372(17):1598–607.
34. Johnson P, Federico M, Kirkwood A, et al. Adapted Treatment Guided by Interim PET-CT Scan in Advanced Hodgkin's Lymphoma. N Engl J Med 2016;374(25):2419–29.
35. Duggan DB, Petroni GR, Johnson JL, et al. Randomized comparison of ABVD and MOPP/ABV hybrid for the treatment of advanced Hodgkin's disease: report of an intergroup trial. J Clin Oncol 2003;21(4):607–14.
36. Connors JM, Ansell SM, Fanale M, et al. Five-year follow-up of brentuximab vedotin combined with ABVD or AVD for advanced-stage classical Hodgkin lymphoma. Blood 2017;130(11):1375–7.
37. Hoppe RT, Advani RH, Ai WZ, et al. NCCN Guidelines Insights: Hodgkin Lymphoma, Version 1.2018. J Natl Compr Canc Netw 2018;16(3):245–54.
38. Grillo-López AJ, White CA, Dallaire BK, et al. Rituximab: the first monoclonal antibody approved for the treatment of lymphoma. Curr Pharm Biotechnol 2000;1(1):1–9.
39. Philip T, Guglielmi C, Hagenbeek A, et al. Autologous bone marrow transplantation as compared with salvage chemotherapy in relapses of chemotherapy-sensitive non-Hodgkin's lymphoma. N Engl J Med 1995;333(23):1540–5.
40. Seer Data. Available at: https://seer.cancer.gov/archive/csr/1975_2016/.
41. Bray F, Ferlay J, Soerjomataram I, et al. Global cancer statistics 2018: GLOBOCAN estimates of incidence and mortality worldwide for 36 cancers in 185 countries. CA Cancer J Clin 2018;68(6):394–424.
42. Rajkumar SV. Updated Diagnostic Criteria and Staging System for Multiple Myeloma. Am Soc Clin Oncol Educ Book 2016;35:e418–23.
43. Kyle RA, Rajkumar SV. Multiple myeloma. N Engl J Med 2004;351(18):1860–73.

44. Caers J, Paiva B, Zamagni E, et al. Diagnosis, treatment, and response assessment in solitary plasmacytoma: updated recommendations from a European Expert Panel. J Hematol Oncol 2018;11(1):10.
45. Palladini G, Merlini G. How I treat AL amyloidosis. Blood 2022;139(19):2918–30.
46. Wei A, Juneja S. Bone marrow immunohistology of plasma cell neoplasms. J Clin Pathol 2003;56(6):406–11.
47. Guerrera ML, Tsakmaklis N, Xu L, et al. mutated and wild-type Waldenström's Macroglobulinemia: characterization of chromosome 6q gene losses and their mutual exclusivity with mutations in. Haematologica 2018;103(9):e408–11.
48. Athanasiou E, Kaloutsi V, Kotoula V, et al. Cyclin D1 overexpression in multiple myeloma. A morphologic, immunohistochemical, and in situ hybridization study of 71 paraffin-embedded bone marrow biopsy specimens. Am J Clin Pathol 2001;116(4):535–42.
49. Sonoki T, Hata H, Kuribayashi N, et al. Expression of PRAD1/cyclin D1 in plasma cell malignancy: incidence and prognostic aspects. Br J Haematol 1999;104(3): 614–7.
50. Weh HJ, Gutensohn K, Selbach J, et al. Karyotype in multiple myeloma and plasma cell leukaemia. Eur J Cancer 1993;29A(9):1269–73.
51. Palumbo A, Avet-Loiseau H, Oliva S, et al. Revised International Staging System for Multiple Myeloma: A Report From International Myeloma Working Group. J Clin Oncol 2015;33(26):2863–9.
52. Seer Data. Available at: https://seer.cancer.gov/statfacts/html/mulmy.html.
53. Lohr JG, Stojanov P, Carter SL, et al. Widespread genetic heterogeneity in multiple myeloma: implications for targeted therapy. Cancer Cell 2014;25(1):91–101.
54. Tsang RW, Campbell BA, Goda JS, et al. Radiation Therapy for Solitary Plasmacytoma and Multiple Myeloma: Guidelines From the International Lymphoma Radiation Oncology Group. Int J Radiat Oncol Biol Phys 2018;101(4):794–808.
55. Tanrivermis Sayit A, Elmali M, Gün S. Evaluation of Extramedullary Plasmacytoma of the Larynx with Radiologic and Histopathological Findings. *Radiologia (Engl Ed)*. 2020:S0033-8338(20)30121-1. doi: 10.1016/j.rx.2020.07.006.
56. Kilciksiz S, Karakoyun-Celik O, Agaoglu FY, et al. A review for solitary plasmacytoma of bone and extramedullary plasmacytoma. ScientificWorld J 2012;2012: 895765.
57. Bustoros M, Sklavenitis-Pistofidis R, Kapoor P, et al. Progression Risk Stratification of Asymptomatic Waldenström Macroglobulinemia. J Clin Oncol 2019; 37(16):1403–11.
58. Castillo JJ, Ghobrial IM, Treon SP. Biology, prognosis, and therapy of waldenström macroglobulinemia. Cancer Treat Res 2015;165:177–95.
59. Panneerselvam K, Goyal S, Shirwaikar Thomas A. Ileo-colonic lymphoma: presentation, diagnosis, and management. Curr Opin Gastroenterol 2021; 37(1):52–8.
60. Grommes C, Rubenstein JL, DeAngelis LM, et al. Comprehensive approach to diagnosis and treatment of newly diagnosed primary CNS lymphoma. Neuro Oncol 2019;21(3):296–305.
61. Harrington KD. Orthopedic surgical management of skeletal complications of malignancy. Cancer 1997;80(8 Suppl):1614–27.

Moving?

Make sure your subscription moves with you!

To notify us of your new address, find your **Clinics Account Number** (located on your mailing label above your name), and contact customer service at:

Email: journalscustomerservice-usa@elsevier.com

800-654-2452 (subscribers in the U.S. & Canada)
314-447-8871 (subscribers outside of the U.S. & Canada)

Fax number: 314-447-8029

Elsevier Health Sciences Division
Subscription Customer Service
3251 Riverport Lane
Maryland Heights, MO 63043

*To ensure uninterrupted delivery of your subscription, please notify us at least 4 weeks in advance of move.

Printed and bound by CPI Group (UK) Ltd, Croydon, CR0 4YY

03/10/2024

01040474-0011